S0-CCK-231

WRESTLING WITH RHINOS

The Adventures of a Glasgow Vet in Kenya

DR. JERRY HAIGH

ECW PRESS

Copyright © Jerry Haigh, 2002

All rights reserved. No part of this publication may be reproduced, stored in
a retrieval system, or transmitted in any form by any process — electronic,
mechanical, photocopying, recording, or otherwise — without the prior
written permission of the copyright owners and ECW PRESS.

NATIONAL LIBRARY OF CANADA CATALOGUING IN PUBLICATION DATA

Haigh, J. C. (Jerry C.)
Wrestling with rhinos: the adventures of a Glasgow vet in Kenya

ISBN 1-55022-507-3

1. Haigh, J. C. (Jerry C.) 2. Wildlife veterinarians — Kenya — Biography.
1. Title.

SF613.H29A3 2002   636.089´092   C2001-904134-9

Cover and text design by Tania Craan
Layout by Mary Bowness

Printed by AGMV

Distributed in Canada by
General Distribution Services,
325 Humber College Blvd.,
Toronto, ON M9W 7C3

Distributed in the United States by
Independent Publishers Group,
814 North Franklin St.,
Chicago, IL, USA 60610

Published by ECW PRESS
2120 Queen Street East, Suite 200
Toronto, ON M4E 1E2
ecwpress.com

This book is set in Bembo and Copperplate.

PRINTED AND BOUND IN CANADA

The publication of *Wrestling with Rhinos* has been generously supported by the
Canada Council, the Ontario Arts Council, and the Government of Canada through
the Book Publishing Industry Development Program. Canada

TABLE OF CONTENTS

I speak of Africa and golden days.

— Henry IV, Part 2, Act v, Sc 3

Memory, my dear Cecily, is the diary that
we all carry about with us.

— Oscar Wilde. The Importance of Being Ernest

ACKNOWLEDGEMENTS

For our many friends of Kenya days I hope that this offering provides enjoyment and some happy memories. A special *asante sana* to Paul Sayer, for sharing so many memories over the years and helping to tighten up parts of the story. Thanks to Ian Parker for sharing his Baedekker-like knowledge of wildlife issues and helping to proof important segments. To Tony Parkinson and the late John Seago, so many thanks for giving me the chance to start on a new career path, but of course before that the admissions committee at Glasgow for having the faith to let me fulfill a boyhood dream and the faculty and staff of that institution for guidance and a sound education. Naturally, untold thanks to my parents, who chose to move to Kenya, and then had the foresight to let me do my own thing, while encouraging a sense of adventure, pursuit of intellectual avenues and a love of the outdoors. Also, of course, to Brigid, for ideas, and reminders of a shared childhood.

A special thank you to Elma Sayer and Kipsiele arap Kurgat who are sadly no longer with us. To others who helped me tidy up loose ends, or were part of the mosaic of life in Kenya in the period of which I write, I offer sincere thanks. They include Jonny Baxendale, Jimmy Caldwell, Tony and Velia Carn, John and Lillemore Carnegie, Miles and Liz Coverdale, Frank Douglas, Jimmy and Timmy Duncan, Tony and Rose Dyer, Rodney Elliott, Peter and Judy Gamble, Paddy and Pam Grattan, Peter Holt, Don and Iris Hunt, Wilber James, the late Peter and Sarah Jenkins, Hugh Miller, Karl Morthole, Bilasius Mutua Mugambi, George and Irralie Murray, Lily Mwenda, Erastus and Anna Nkabu, Dick and Jenny Neal, Njeru

Nyaga, Court Parfet, Vagn and Jean Pedersen, John and Ros Poulton, Tim and Judy Roberts, Peter and Pat Scott, Charlie and Anne Stonewigg, Stanley and Dorothy Tirima, Nigel and Muffet Trent, and Anne Wallen. If I have forgotten others, mea culpa, I hope they will forgive me. If some of their stories have not been included, the honeypot beckons.

Several people generously shared their photographs and allowed them to be used. The striking photograph on the cover was taken by Peter Beard whose work as a wildlife photographer and author is as distinctive as it is classy. Many thanks Peter for allowing us to use it. Henk Faberij de Jonge allowed me free access to his wonderful collection of pictures, both in colour and black and white, and Giles Camplin took most of the photographs in Rwanda. Jonny Baxendale and Andrew Botta went to great lengths to find and print the pictures of George and Joy Adamson respectively. Iris Hunt took the picture on the back cover and others at the camp near Maralal and Dick Neal took the photo that heads the epilogue.

To Kay and Peter Mehren, thanks for shared memories of Kenya, and a pile of work with an edit of an early draft.

Thanks to Juliane Deubner, Trudy Janssens and Katherine Sopotyk who played invaluable parts with technical help on photographs and maps.

I owe more than I realized at the time to Joan Givner, whose encouragement, coaching and critical judgment helped turn a dry text into something that I could take forward. It was the folks at the Saskatchewan Writer's Guild who put me on to her, and I thank them for that.

To Penny Dickens and the folks at the Writers Union of Canada for thoughtful input and Jim Russell for useful advice, many thanks.

Without the faith of Jack David at ECW, the dedication of Mary Bowness and the ECW staff and the vision and meticulous work of my editor, Nadia Halim, this book would never have made it past the starting line. To them, a sincere debt of gratitude. They picked up on grammatical and factual mistakes. Any that are left are entirely my own responsibility.

Of course, to Jo, for a shared life. All and everything that matters.

For Jopie, Karen, and Charles

CHAPTER 1

THE NEW GRADUATE

*In which I leave for Kenya after graduating from vet school.
I see my first cases, get involved in local sports, and meet
Tony Parkinson, a wild animal trapper who will have
a major influence upon my career.*

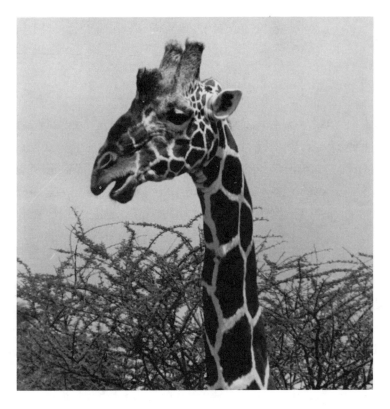

Sixteen feet from top to toe, ten feet above my head.

THE TRANSITION FROM MY cushioned college days to my veterinary career in Kenya began with a bit of a jolt. Less than a month before, I had nervously boarded a plane in Scotland. Now, here I was, staring up at the head of a giraffe some ten feet above me, wondering how I was going to examine his swollen foot, which was about the size of a dinner plate. There was no point in just staring, so with some trepidation I bent down and gingerly felt around the foot. When the animal did not kick out, or try to embed my teeth in the back of my throat, I slipped a finger between the two enormous hooves.

In 1965 there was a shortage of giraffes, lame or otherwise, in Glasgow. This animal brought home, in spades, the realization that despite five years of veterinary education I was still a greenhorn.

Normally, to examine a dairy cow, one would catch her in a headstall and get on with it. This giant patient needed a different approach. The owner, Tony Parkinson, had climbed a ladder set in front of the pen, and the giraffe had at once come limping around the side and entered its own stall. A bar was slipped behind its thighs and it stood there and started to chew on the fodder. Ignoring the ongoing activity far above my head I continued my inspection. The foot was obviously swollen. If the patient were a cow, I would have picked up the foot, taken out a hoof knife, scraped the dirt off the sole, and checked for cracks, sharp objects or other causes of trouble. But there was no way I'd be able to try that with this character.

My finger emerged from between the hooves, bringing with it an unmistakable sickly-sweet smell, known to every large animal vet all over the world. The black muck I'd found more or less clinched the diagnosis of footrot, giraffe or not.

The opportunity to revisit the country of my birth, and work as an intern for a year in the Kabete veterinary college, had arisen several months before my graduation from the veterinary school at Bearsden, near Glasgow, and I had seized it gladly.

I'd been in Glasgow for six years. Prior to that, after living my first few years in Kenya, I'd had a typical "military brat" childhood, constantly moving from one army house to another. From the age of nine I had been educated in British boarding schools, while my father was posted to Germany, English army towns, and trouble spots like Cyprus and Suez; the family either went with him or stayed in the family home on the Isle of Wight, off England's south coast. My mother, perhaps ahead of her time in her view of equal opportunities, had insisted that my sister Brigid also get a boarding school education. What the double dose of school fees had cost the family I only appreciated much later. While most of the other boys at school had been visited by parents in smart cars, some very smart, we didn't get our first car in England until I was about 15. This was a small, second-hand, slab-sided, black Austin 7, promptly christened "The Matchbox" by my unforgiving housemates.

All my life at home, I had been a Jeremy, with its various tones according to mood, or a Dickensian Jem when in good books. In public school tradition, I had, of course, been Haigh, until I reached Scotland. Jeremy was obviously deemed far too English by my vet school classmates, and within about ten minutes of arrival I was Jerry, except of course to the family.

After twenty-some years in the Highland Light Infantry, my father had followed me to live in Scotland, where he had joined Distillers (makers of amber liquid Scottish products such as Johnnie Walker and Black & White). Scotland became home for all of us.

My decision to try and get into veterinary school had followed naturally upon my boyhood ambitions, first, to be a zookeeper, when my classmates had all wanted to be train drivers, and then to be a farmer. From the age of 12, veterinary medicine had been the single option, as far as I was concerned, despite the fact that no medical ancestor of any sort could be found in the family tree. The decision to go to Glasgow was simple. It was the only veterinary school in Britain that offered me a place, which is not very surprising when I recall that during my interview at Bristol I had naïvely told the committee that their school was my third choice. I really had no clear vision of what a veterinary career would be, but I was certain that it would involve a country life. City streets did not appeal.

The chance to go to Kenya came out of the blue. The professor of medicine at Glasgow, Ian McIntyre, was also dean at the school in Kabete, just outside Nairobi. The program in Kenya was new, and when I heard that internship positions were opening, I applied, more or less on spec. The chance to visit my birth country, and have a job as well, seemed too good to miss.

I had, from time to time, wondered about Kenya, a few faint memories surfacing sometimes and getting mixed up with family stories. One pseudo-memory, which surfaced fairly frequently in family discussions, was my mother's account of the time that I was heard screaming fit to burst after eating a bright red pepper in the garden, having mistaken it for a tomato. Definite mind's eye images included standing with my father as he shot birds that flew out of the forest — he told me it was during a posting to Moshi, in Tanganyika (now Tanzania) — and being fascinated by stately giraffes as they peered, seemingly legless, at the car over treetops or loped away in seven-league strides.

The familiar face of my former classmate Jimmy Duncan, part of the group of interns that had preceded me, was a welcome sight across the barrier outside the customs hall at the Nairobi airport. His dark good looks and almost Roman nose suggested some Italian ancestry, despite his most Scottish of names and sonorous brogue.

"Morning Jerry. Had a good flight? How was Glasgow?" Jimmy came from the west of Scotland, and was eager for first-hand news of home, so I tried to oblige.

"I hope you've brought your tennis racquet. You're playing with me in a club tournament tonight." Jimmy had somehow got wind of my love of the game.

As we turned right at the T junction leading from the airport road into town, I was startled to see the swaying forms of three giraffes not more than 400 yards away. Jimmy explained that we were seeing animals right on the boundary of Nairobi National Park.

We passed through the edge of the industrial area, and I began to relax. The incredible array of colours of the bougainvillea in the median strip of Uhuru Highway, and the dark red soil, are my strongest memories of that first morning, as they must have been for millions of visitors over the years. As we drove along, I noticed the sharp contrast between the town site on our right and the hill on our left with its masses of tall trees, many of them Australian eucalyptus. Several buildings were half hidden amongst the greenery.

Jimmy acted as my tour guide as we circumnavigated the round-abouts and took our chances with the traffic.

"That's the Railway Club golf course. . . . There's the old post office. It was built way back in colonial times. The New Stanley Hotel is on the right down that street. . . . The Norfolk, where Lord Delamere is supposed to have ridden his horse into the bar, is behind these university buildings. You must make sure you get to it. . . . Up there is the Coryndon Museum. Fascinating, especially the paintings of the various tribes in traditional costumes done by Joy Adamson."

Soon we were on more open road, heading towards Fort Smith and Kabete, where the veterinary college was located. I recalled an old photo in my parents' album, taken on this very road some 26 years before. It showed them as cheerful, smiling newly marrieds beside an early 1930s Morris, the dickey seat opened up. There were only two narrow strips of tarmac on the road. Anytime a motorist saw something coming towards him, he had to pull over and leave the one strip on the other side available. The left-hand wheel took its chances in the dirt.

After dropping off my luggage at the flat I was to share with an intern who would arrive later, I reported to Dr. McIntyre. First I had to run the gauntlet of his efficient secretary, Elma McGruer. I recognized her red hair, stocky figure, and friendly grin.

"Och, hello Jerry, it's good to see you again," she said in her soft west-of-Scotland brogue. "We met at Bearsden in February, when I was home on leave. I'll just see if he's free. Have a seat while I check."

Dean McIntyre greeted me in his brusque fashion, standing up and limping slightly on his built-up shoe. His high domed forehead and receding hairline gave the appearance of a huge intellect. As final year students we had been petrified of him, hoping that he would not hone in and ask us a question in front of our classmates.

"Good morning Haigh. I trust you had a good flight. Jimmy Duncan was there to meet you?"

"Oh yes sir, we had no trouble, and I've already dropped my stuff off at the flat."

"Take a couple of days to get yourself organized. Find yourself some sort of vehicle. Ask Elma about arrangements for financing. She can also help you with an advance on your salary. You can start work on Monday."

The bombardment of new sights and sounds continued as I was shown around the impressive new facilities, and Jimmy informed me that the official opening would soon take place, although the place had been in use for a few months.

"President Kenyatta himself will do the honours. All the money for these buildings has come from foreign aid. The veterinary college has grown out of a less ambitious set of buildings. I'll take you back to the stock barns and you'll see."

"Where do the other staff and faculty come from?" I asked.

"Faculty have been recruited from Glasgow, Giessen and Colorado. Most of the staff are local, and many of them were here in the days when this place only offered a diploma course. Now the graduates get a proper degree."

On that first day it was impossible to take in all the colours and sensations, so different from the drab dirt and fog of Glasgow in 1965. Pepper trees, bottle-brush trees, canna lilies, Kikuyu grass, all were foreign. Even stranger, to my unfamiliar eye, was the sight of a diminutive woman carrying an enormous bundle of firewood on her back. A leather thong stretched over her head seemed to be the only means of support for what looked like a very heavy load.

The birds too were colourful, quite different than anything one might see in Scotland. A colony of bright yellow weaver birds were busy building nests in a roadside tree. Superb starlings fussed around the car park and trees at the clinic, and I marveled at their gaudy red-and-blue uniforms, with a white crossbar on the breast. Like foot soldiers of some long past war.

Thiongo brought us lunch. A gap-toothed, wizened old Kikuyu, he acted as houseboy-cum-cook for Jimmy and the two other ex-Glasgow interns, Paul Sayer and Hugh Miller, who shared the flat. Today, he would be called a house servant. Twenty-six years earlier, my father's house staff, over and above his batman and shared with one other subaltern, had consisted of a cook, a gardener, an assistant gardener and a kitchen *toto*, or assistant. Quite a contrast.

I opted out of more introductions and sightseeing, went to my own new flat, and hit the sack for a while after unpacking. Jimmy warned me to be ready for tennis by 4:30 and returned to the clinic. He gave me 15 minutes grace, no doubt recalling his own exhaustion upon arrival six months earlier, and I awoke when he pounded on my door at 4:45.

"Right you are. Let's go, Jerry. Are you not ready yet?"

I struggled into my shorts and we were soon off to tennis at the local Vet Lab Sports Club, a handy two minutes' drive away.

Kabete lies at an altitude of just over 6,000 feet. Trying to play sports at this height fresh from a departure point at sea level would be tough enough. Being exhausted after the long flight was no help, and I soon found that my only chance was to go for broke with my left-handed serve and hope that my opponent wouldn't be able to handle it. If he was, I was in no position to run after the return. The lack of oxygen, and my thin, unacclimatized blood, made breathing the first priority.

The racial mix at the club was interesting. There were no Africans present that evening, except the barman, although I later found out that there were a few African members of the golf section of the club, where Jimmy's flatmate Hugh later excelled by playing well below his handicap and winning the *Sungura* (rabbit) cup. Virtually all members seemed to be of European descent. I heard one extremely cultured accent which sounded straight out of the poshest English public school, and turned to see a generously built East Indian man (all people from the Indian sub-continent were generically termed Asian). Jimmy and I found ourselves playing against him and being soundly beaten as he produced an array of elegant shots. His name was Sushil Gurram, and he was an Oxford-educated lawyer who had won a blue at squash, and was obviously a natural athlete, despite his shape.

Another of our opponents that evening was Tony Parkinson. About an inch shorter than me, but a good ten pounds lighter than my 13 and a half stone (189 lbs.), his tennis owed little to coaching, but a great deal to the power of dogged determination and a natural athletic flair. His left-handed strokes were deceptively powerful, and his blond wavy hair, parted on the right, and natural good looks also made him seem younger than me. He had been an amateur boxing champion and had played league soccer in Kenya. Our shared enjoyment of tennis was to play a pivotal role in the future.

"So you're another of these Glasgow vets," he said. "You must come down and meet my family and see our collection some time. We're just on Lower Kabete road."

"What sort of collection?"

"Well, right now we've got some wildebeest and a couple of giraffe. Also half a dozen zebra."

"What are they for?"

"Tony and his partner, John Seago, are animal trappers, otherwise known as zoological collectors," said Jimmy. "They catch animals for zoos, and translocate them out of settlement areas."

■

The morning after my first game of tennis in Kenya, and my first full day in Africa in 18 years, I woke to a view that still acts like a magnet on me. From the front window of the flat, the land dropped sharply across a meadow. Then one's eye was drawn across a huge undulating green carpet of mist-enshrouded treetops, here and there punctuated by a bright red crown of a flame tree or the more subtle purplish-blue of a jacaranda, to the crown of Mount Kenya with its spiked peaks reaching over 17,000 feet up, some 80 miles away. Less imposing was the hump of the Aberdares, 3,000 feet lower, but 25 miles closer.

"The mountain was great this morning" was a common conversational opener.

Although the monthly payments left little spending money for nights out or beer, I bought my first car, a white MG 1100 with red upholstery. I can still remember the registration number: KHQ 597.

I was soon embroiled in my work. My colleagues ensured that I would not lack experience; that first weekend, I was left on duty as they headed for more relaxing activities. I had been assigned to the field service unit, which meant that I would go out on farm calls. Of course I had no clue where to go, but fortunately there were members of staff who could act as guide, driver and technician. Lawrence Gitau and Paul Kinyanjui were relatively new members of staff, while Charlie Kiengo had been around for many years, serving as the essential link between farmer and vet in the days when the college had only offered a diploma course. Lawrence and Paul were both about five foot seven, but where Lawrence was slim, with an oval head, Paul was stockier, and had a head shaped more like a soccer ball. Charlie was taller, and beginning to get the grizzled hair of an older man. All three spoke excellent English, which was a relief to me.

Early on my first Saturday morning, Lawrence arrived at my door just as I was finishing breakfast and told me that we had a call to go and assist a young heifer that was having trouble delivering her calf. The farmer's messenger piled into the back of the Land Rover, on top of the several boxes of drugs and equipment that Lawrence had already packed, and we were on our way. We left Kabete, turned right where a road sign read Limuru and Naivasha and began a steady climb.

At this stage my Swahili (Kiswahili) was rudimentary, but I had undertaken to learn two new words a day. Before I left Scotland, my mother had bought me a 1964 copy of *Up Country Swahili,* the updated version of the book that she had used herself 26 years earlier. My father had dug into his phenomenal memory banks and written out four foolscap pages of useful Swahili phrases with their English translations. He had not been in Kenya for over 18 years, but still remembered the language clearly and spoke it fluently when he visited another five years later. Most of his phrases would prove useful on many occasions, but one had become dated, and highlighted the differences between the Kenya which Dad remembered from his wartime days and the newly independent one to which I was going. The phrase was *"weka nguo maredadi,"* which translates as "Put up smart clothes." This was how my father had instructed his houseboy to put out his full dress uniform, which he had been required to wear each night to dine in the officers' mess. For a 1965 veterinary graduate sharing a flat and relying on a single man to cook, wash clothes and keep the apartment tidy, such a phrase would have produced a justifiably blank stare.

Work-related terms were what I most needed to learn. I asked Lawrence, "What's the Swahili for a rope, and for a cattle crush?"

"Rope is *kamba,* crush, *munanda.*"

"*Kamba,* rope; *munanda,* crush," I repeated to myself, like a mantra, as we drove along.

I had spoken Swahili with my *ayah* (nanny) of the Kipsigis tribe at the same time as I was learning English from my mother, and perhaps this was why I could converse freely in Swahili within about three months. Perhaps it had been stored in a shoulder-top "computer chip" for 18 years but had taken time to emerge as the connections were made. Swahili yes, but not the true Swahili of the coastal peoples. Most up-country people, of whatever stripe, spoke a simplified version. The *safi* (smart) version was used on the local "Voice of Kenya" radio station, and I could only get snatches of it by listening carefully.

After leaving the main road we followed a series of rutted lanes that twisted and turned between tall hedges of pale green plants with large bright yellow flowers. It dawned on me that the greens themselves had a different hue from those of Europe. Somehow harsher, almost metallic. Perhaps it was the strong overhead light, perhaps something more intrinsic.

Suddenly we were on a slope, and a spectacular view over the wall of the Great Rift Valley opened up. I asked Lawrence to stop. Immediately below us a patchwork quilt of small farms continued down the hill and I could see a volcano-shaped mountain in the hazy distance. Lawrence told me it was called Suswa.

We continued on, and soon pulled in through a gap in the hedge. The farm itself was small, no more than three or four acres. In the middle stood two grass thatch-roofed huts, and in a corner was a much smaller one, no more than about three or four feet across. This was the outdoor lavatory. The walls of all three were made of mud caked on a woven patchwork of thin sticks, as was plain from a look at the partially completed hut standing to one side.

The farmer emerged from one of the houses, wiping his hands on a cloth. There was a very specific protocol involved in a greeting.

"Jambo daktari." (Good morning, doctor.)

"Jambo mzee." (Good morning, old man. "Old man" is a term of respect, whatever the age of the man.)

"Habari?" (What news?)

"Mzuri, habari yako?" (Good news, what is your news?)

"Mzuri, lakini . . ." (Good news, but . . .)

The "but" could be anything from a minor inconvenience to a major catastrophe. The essential thing was to observe the niceties of form and start the conversation politely.

A small cross-bred Ayrshire heifer was standing in a homemade crush. It was plain that the *"lakini"* in this case was pretty serious, and the heifer had no chance of delivering a live calf. Lawrence asked a couple of questions in the local Kikuyu language, which was quite beyond me, and found out that she was only 18 months old. Somehow she had come into season at a very early age, and one of the local bulls had picked up the chemical signals and done all too efficient a job.

Things might have been all right if the calf had decided to exit from the birth canal in the normal feet-first position, but there was an ominous lack of feet showing, and the head that had appeared was already swollen. "What a way to start one's solo career," I thought to myself. "No chance of success with a Caesarean section, no chance of getting at the legs, and only one option." Lawrence, too, knew what must happen. I don't suppose that he translated my English exactly, but he hardly needed to.

Twenty minutes later the calf was on the ground in two parts, and the heifer was walking stiffly back to her grazing spot, relieved of the burden and alive, at least.

This was the only consolation we had as we headed back to Kabete. Lawrence was more philosophical about it than I, and to take my mind off the unfortunate animal and her owner, who had lost an important source of potential income, we got back to the language lessons.

"Lawrence, is Gitau your father's name?" I asked.

"No. My father's name is Thaiya. In the Kikuyu tribe we have a strict system for naming children. The first-born boy is called for his father's father. The next for his mother's father. Each child has a father's name, followed by 'son of.' So I am Gitau wa Thaiya. Lawrence is my Christian name."

"What about girls, do they have a similar system?"

"Yes, using their mothers' names."

And then came my encounter with the giraffe. About four weeks and several more games of tennis after my arrival, Tony and I were chatting at the bar, and he said, "We have a lame giraffe down at the animal yards. Would you have time to pop down in the morning and have a look at it?"

Here was an opportunity to get a hands-on experience with the towering animal of my early memories. So pop down I did, and that's how I wound up finding that familiar black muck in a very unfamiliar situation. Next, I had to decide what to do about it. At least there were no stones or sharp objects embedded in the crack between the hooves. I couldn't be certain that the animal had no nail in the sole of its foot; I would just have to hope on that one.

"I can't be 100% sure," I said to Tony, "but it looks just like footrot in cattle. I'm glad you've caught it early, before it gets up into the joint." I offered my hand for him to smell. He sniffed, and curled up his nose. Footrot is also known by the more expressive name "foul-of-foot."

Trusting to luck, and realizing that a giraffe is basically an elongated version of a cow, with its four stomach compartments, its cloven feet and its habit of chewing the cud, I worked out a dose of antibiotic based on Tony's knowledge of its weight. Standing on the bottom rail of the chute and reaching up a couple of feet above my head to give a penicillin injection was a novel experience, but the patient hardly noticed. I later learned that giraffe skin was the favoured material for bucket manufacture among the peoples of Kenya's northeast, because it is both durable and thick. Luckily my needle was razor sharp and long enough to penetrate the tough hide. The other challenge was to persuade this less-than-domestic animal to let us apply some sort of poultice.

"We need to get him to stand in hot water and Epsom salts for at least 20 minutes, twice a day; a double handful dumped in a couple of gallons is about the right mix," I explained.

"Don't worry Jerry. I'll dig a pit below the feed bunk, big enough to take a rubber feed bowl, and we'll get him to stand in it when he comes for hay and pellets," said Tony.

Tony was able to get a full course of penicillin into my tall patient, and when I visited again a few days later, the giraffe showed no sign of lameness and the swelling in his foot had gone right down.

Unwilling to sell anything except a perfect specimen, Tony obtained permission from the game department to exchange this animal for another one, and a month later he took the fully recovered patient back to the Northern Frontier District where it had been captured.

CHAPTER 2

TROPICAL CHALLENGES

I deal with cases in cattle, many of them specific to the tropics and quite new to me, and learn about the problems of communication by radio-phone. My father's recollections of his military days during WWII show how much the country has changed.

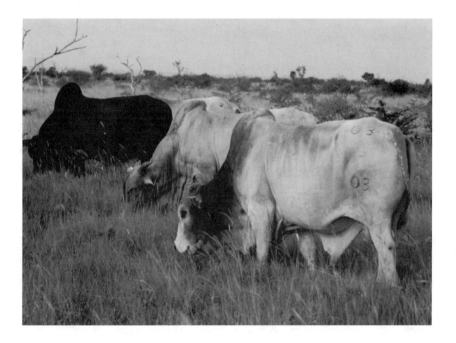

Boran bulls.

T HE DAILY ROUTINE STARTED with a gathering at the clinic office, at which we divided up the day's cases. There were usually two of us on the large animal circuit; the area we had to cover was too large to be adequately serviced by a single person. It included a mix of farms, from the small holdings like the one where I had tried to help the young heifer to large ones where dozens of sleek and gentle Channel Island cows, of Guernsey or Jersey breeds, produced high-quality milk for the Nairobi market. We also had other dairy breeds to deal with, and some beef cattle, as well as the odd riding stable that trained race horses.

Other large properties in the area included coffee or tea estates where a few cows were kept to supply milk for the numerous staff, and a few horses for the owners' recreation. Coffee grew at low altitudes, tea high, and sometimes estates in the middle region between the two would grow both crops in nearly adjacent plots, neither thriving like they would if planted in their ideal environments. The best known of these intermediate estates was gone before my time, but has become the subject of one of the great books of all time, as well as an evocative film. Karen Blixen's *Out of Africa* famously begins, "I had a farm in Africa," and the area covered by our practice included the Nairobi suburb named for her, where she had struggled to make a go of it, although the coffee was gone and when we went there it was usually to treat the horses of the white residents.

One farm to which we paid regular visits was the East African Veterinary Research Organization's research centre at Muguga, some ten miles from Kabete. Here, beef cattle management was studied, among other things, and a large herd of Hereford cattle seemed to need constant attention.

My first visit to Muguga was to see a cow with an eye problem. Our route took us up the main road towards the tea-growing country of Limuru, through an extensive area of small holdings in the so-called Kikuyu reserve. We turned off down a steep scarp to the railway crossing at Sigona and then up to the research station. Instead of small holdings there were extensive paddocks. Most striking was the large number of Australian gum trees — an import that had thrived, although the ground underneath them was devoid of the shrubs that grew freely under other trees.

There were three cows waiting in the corral. One was a Hereford, with the typical reddish-brown coat and white face. The others were large, sleek versions of the rather scruffy native humped cattle that one saw almost everywhere by the side of the roads. One was a pale dun colour, the other a dark cream. Their humps were so big that they wobbled above the shoulders, and seemed to have trouble standing upright.

"What breed are those?" I asked Paul, the animal health technician traveling with me.

"Those are Boran cattle. Here at Muguga they are comparing the success of these with European breeds."

After the usual greetings, the herdsman said, "We have three cows for you this time, doctor. This grade one (grade cattle were those of

European origin) has a bad eye, and I'd like to know if these other two are pregnant."

The herdsman made short work of getting them into the crush, a stoutly built affair made of gum tree logs, and I examined the eyes of the Hereford. Each had a small growth in one corner, at the edge of the third eyelid. In each eye Paul placed a couple of drops of local anesthetic, and we waited for a few minutes for it to take effect. The growths were easily removed with a pair of scissors.

Later, when I discussed these animals with Jimmy and the dean, an interesting story emerged.

"The data are interesting," said Dean McIntyre, or Mac as we definitely did not call him to his face. "There's little doubt that the Herefords grow faster and put on much more weight than the Borans. However, the Herefords also tend to get cancer of the tissues around the eye. It seems that the lack of pigment on the head makes them susceptible to the effects of the sun. The Borans don't seem to be affected. Growing cattle is not just a question of weight gains and food conversion. Hardiness and immunity are part of the equation."

An easily dealt-with case of eyelid cancer was virtually nothing compared to the host of novel challenges which had faced European cattle owners since they first began to arrive, bringing their stock with them. Early accounts of farming and ranching describe many problems — not least of which was the little matter of marauding lions, which could devastate a herd once they got the taste for prey that couldn't run nearly as fast as buffalo, antelope or zebra. The most gruesome of the "lion problems" was the plague of man-eaters that preyed upon railroad crews as the Uganda Railway was being pushed up-country from Mombasa, early in the 20th century. It was only the determined and long-lasting campaign by J.H. Patterson, documented in his book *Man-Eaters of Tsavo*, that put an end to this particular problem. Elsewhere, lions continued to be a nuisance, and later, in the Mount Kenya area, it was not unusual for me to hear of a farmer sitting up in a hide all night waiting for a pride that had already taken some cattle to revisit the site. One rancher described the leopard to me as "the greater spotted sheep-eater."

Predation was not limited to big cats. For some young men of the Masai, Samburu and other tribes, a cattle raid on a European-owned farm was nothing short of an opportunity to prove their manhood and acquire some new wealth at the same time. They could cut fences and get a stolen herd moving at an astonishing rate, covering many miles in a single night, and mixing tracks up with other cattle in order to confuse the tracking team, which would not be able to set out after them until daylight came. Not all such raiders were caught.

Diseases, about which I had only read, included several viral conditions that could be rapidly fatal, and a series of blood-borne parasites that continued to kill cattle in large numbers. Our practice was outside the area in which tsetse flies could thrive, so we did not have to deal with the sleeping sickness that made some areas of the country totally unsuitable for cattle. As I quickly learned, we had four blood parasites that caused trouble enough of their own. Each was transmitted by ticks, and there was no shortage of these little creatures. The most serious condition was East Coast Fever, and grade cattle that developed this disease, with its high fever, swollen glands and fluid-filled lungs, almost always died. The only defence was prevention through rigorous attention to tick control, which for the small-holder meant once- or twice-weekly application with a hand-held spray, and on larger farms meant herding the cattle into corrals from which the only exit was via a plunge bath full of some solution poisonous enough to kill the ticks, but not the cattle. A herder would stand by and ensure that even the heads went under for a brief moment, as the main vector of this scourge was the aptly-named "brown ear tick" which liked to set up shop inside the ears, where it could be sure of a good meal of the blood that it needed to complete its life cycle.

Teams of scientists at Muguga tried for many years to develop a vaccine for this condition, or a treatment, or both. The small hardy native cattle were immune to East Coast Fever and the other three conditions that affected local grade cattle: anaplasmosis, redwater (which caused the cattle to pass dark red urine, as parasites ruptured their red blood cells and the pigment ended up in the bladder) and heartwater, which was also a killer. These three could often be treated if seen early enough, but would severely reduce milk yield and productivity. We seemed to see at least one of these each day, usually in the Kikuyu reserve, where the use of dips and sprays for tick control was not always optimum.

Diseases were not confined to infections, and their causes often took a long time to unravel. For many years the settlers found that imported cattle in the Rift Valley did not thrive, and they could not figure out why. The name that they coined for the condition was "Nakuruitis," which implies some sort of infection (the "itis" finishes up the names of many such diseases), and was based upon the name of the most important town in the region. Eventually it was discovered that Nakuruitis had nothing to do with infection, and was in fact due to a deficiency of cobalt in the diet. As cobalt is an essential building block for the hemoglobin that carries oxygen in red blood cells, it's no wonder that its absence would cause cattle to fade.

We left Muguga and crossed the main road en route to our next call. The dark red colour of the soil remained predominant in the roads, banks, and valleys, but the plant mix changed as we climbed to higher elevations. At first we saw banana trees interspersed with the dark green stands of coffee bushes. Along stream beds there were the arrow-shaped leaves of yams; along the contours, pale yellowish-green clumps of Napier grass stood in rows. Then suddenly there were larger areas of pale-green tea plants, shade trees standing amongst them. The green of the tea reminded me of an Irish rugby jersey.

Life was not all work, work, work. I soon learned that sports, and in particular the sports club, was at the core of social life for most white people — *Wazungu* (*wa-* is the plural prefix, *m-* *is* the singular prefix) or Europeans as they were collectively known, whatever their origins. Besides providing fun and recreation, sporting activities were the main place for informal, non-professional social contact. Aside from tennis at the club, games took place at weekends. During the week there was only a period of about 90 minutes for exercise between the end of the working day and dusk, there being no floodlights.

As was the case in British colonial settlements in many countries, the social importance of the sports club was a tradition that went back many years. Twenty-six years before my arrival as an adult in Nairobi, the Nairobi Club had been the centre of my parents' social lives — along with the tight-knit community of the army. My father had been posted in Kenya in July 1939, and was active in the African theatre of WW II, helping fight the Italians back into Ethiopia. My mother, meanwhile, had flown from England to Kenya in late December of the same year. In fact, she was the last unmarried woman allowed to travel out to Kenya after the declaration of the war.

"I boarded a Solent flying boat in Southampton water," she recalled one evening before I left, "and we flew via Marseilles, Alexandria, Khartoum, Entebbe and Kisumu, stopping overnight at each place. The heat and noise were frightful, but I was engaged and going out to get married, so what did it matter. At Entebbe I was bumped by some general and had to wait an extra 24 hours."

Dad had taken up the tale. "Of course I had driven out to Naivasha, which was the landing site for the seaplanes, to meet her. That's about 50 miles from Nairobi, and the road was pretty frightful. Lo and behold, no Margery. Luckily I was able to wait for a day, and so we drove back to

Olive Collyer's coffee farm at Kabete, near Kikuyu, where your mother stayed until the wedding. I wonder if it's still there?"

They had met at a series of parties in the Isle of Wight, where they belonged to the same social set, and they became engaged before Dad left for Kenya. Dad had joined the Nairobi Club within a month of his arrival, and so mother had a ready-made social group to join right after their honeymoon.

Kenya around the start of the war was an interesting place. Those were the declining days of the infamous Happy Valley set, which had begun its activities in the 1920s and is so well described in James Fox's literary reconstruction of the murder of Lord Errol, *White Mischief*. As Fox writes, the "legend grew up of a set of socialites in the Aberdares whose existence was a permanent feast of dissipation and sensuous pleasure." The murder happened in 1941, so Dad was well aware of the stories of sexual shenanigans, and of hostesses assigning partners by random draws. As a military man, he observed these goings-on from a safe distance, but the social environment did lead to some interesting moments in his military career.

Dad had been stationed for a time at the depot battalion in Nairobi, where soldiers were allowed to billet in individual houses with their wives (only one wife at a time if they had more). One day, he was the junior officer at an Orderly Room session, where soldiers who had been accused of discipline infractions, or had queries, were brought before officers. The company sergeant major, a Nandi called C.S.M. Limo, marched in a very tall Acholi (Ugandan) soldier followed by his newlywed wife. Through a translator — who had a hard time keeping control of his giggles while working from the tribal language into Swahili — the wife complained about the treatment meted out by her husband. The substance of the complaint was that while she had no objections to an after-parade liaison, and others after the evening meal and before they went to sleep or if he happened to wake in the middle of the night, or indeed again before early morning parade at 6:00 a.m. or even at breakfast time, she simply wasn't going to put up with a run-through at half past eleven during morning break, and could the *bwana* Captain kindly tell this man not to do it then. As the flummoxed officers tried to make appropriate, noises and keep straight faces, the wife even admitted that a 2:00 p.m. session was OK, but the 11:30 one was a definite no-no.

While this tortured conversation was going on, Dad looked into an open drawer and saw a letter from a well-known white woman. He later admitted he should not have read it, but temptation had got the better of him. The exploits described in this letter made the soldier's activities seem rather mundane. To put it briefly, it appeared the letter-writer would have no qualms about the kind of schedule the soldier's wife was complaining about. My father showed the letter to his superior in the Orderly Room, and by mutual agreement they promptly took it outside and burned it, to prevent a scandal from spreading. I never heard any details or names of those involved, but one could easily conclude that the lady in question might have been a member of the Happy Valley set.

Perhaps it was this letter, among other things, that prompted Dad's advice to me, as I was about to set off for Kenya, to watch out for women who lived at altitudes above 8,000 feet. He was convinced that this was some sort of magic number that removed all inhibitions and induced in women (but not, somehow, in the men) an unbridled show of libido!

On Sundays off we could explore as much as we wished or could afford. I soon got to Nairobi National Park. It was easy to reach, cheap to enter, and full of fascinating species. Giraffes browsing high up on flat-topped acacias. Wildebeest staring, moving nothing except their tails, until they suddenly snorted, swiveled, and started to move away *en masse* with a rocking motion. A waterbuck looking strangely unbalanced with one horn broken off close to his skull.

In the middle of the hockey season, some of the other interns and I headed to Kericho for a weekend of games and socializing. We drove past the Muguga turn-off and on up past the country town of Limuru, with its heavily advertised Bata shoe factory. Roadside vendors offered sheepskins and fruit. Suddenly the road began to drop, and down we went into the rift valley. The road twisted and turned as we passed a tiny church and came to the valley floor, still at 7,000 feet. The dormant volcanic cone of Longonot rose in front of us. Huge multi-branched euphorbia were dotted around the plain and yellow fever trees were everywhere. We passed through Naivasha and Gil Gil. As we drove by Lake Nakuru, we had a stunning view of the shoreline, which appeared pink because it was edged by up to a million flamingos. Our route led us up to the Timboroa summit, a spectacular climb during which we passed a yellow-and-black sign claiming to be exactly on the equator. Finally we arrived at Kericho, tea-growing capital of Kenya. Here the tea estates were huge; the rolling carpets of bushes seemed to go on forever. In some fields women stood waist-deep among the plants, throwing leaves over their shoulders into large wicker baskets on their backs.

After a weekend of true rural hospitality we headed home and back to reality, and work. Apart from their duties in the field service unit, all the interns had responsibilities with the in-clinic animals, cattle and horses that had been admitted for a variety of reasons. One such animal was a pedigree Aberdeen Angus bull who had been trucked all the way from a farm high on the northern slopes of Mount Kenya. The local veterinarian had been unable to help him with his continued difficulty in breathing, and he had not responded to antibiotics. We too were foxed. Even the dean, whose particular expertise was in medical, as opposed to surgical, problems, came down and examined him.

"He sounds as if he's got pneumonia, but it's certainly not typical," he said in his typical brusque manner. "There are fluid sounds throughout his chest. The swelling on his brisket is full of fluid. I've not seen anything like this before. Try him on Penbritin. I know it's expensive, but as it's a new product, it may kill any resistant bacteria."

Try him we did. The course was set to last ten days, but suddenly, on a Sunday morning when I had the misfortune to be on duty, the bull dropped dead. I had completed my rounds of the stables about three hours earlier, and when the barn man came to feed him at 11:00 a.m., there he was, stretched out on his side.

There was nothing to do. I arranged for him to be shipped for a post-mortem, and on the following morning I reported to the dean, who just about had a fit.

"What do you mean, dead?" he said. "You were on duty, why didn't you check him to see how he was?"

"Oh I did sir, about 8:00 a.m. He was no worse than usual." I had the medical file showing the recorded visit and treatment in my hand. Mac had a reputation as a fire eater, and woe betide anyone who was not prepared.

"Well, you should have checked him more often," he said. Silence was the best option.

The results of the post-mortem let me off the hook, although the dean made no apology. Hugh and his colleagues determined that the bull had been suffering from a condition known as high mountain disease, or altitude sickness.

Altitude sickness is well recognised in the Rocky Mountain regions of Colorado, and also in the Andes. Some animals, cattle and sheep especially, are unable to manage the thin air at high elevations, and their lungs react by filling up with fluid. There is usually severe permanent damage if they are not brought down to lower levels quickly, and this bull had gone well past the point of no return by the time he was admitted to the college. He had come from Marania, a farm that lies at an altitude of about 8,000 feet. The college, at 6,000 feet, was still over a mile high, and in retrospect I wonder if a trip to a truly low altitude would have helped him.

I had the unenviable task of informing the clients of the sudden demise of this expensive imported animal, which meant I had to face the business of using the radio-phone. My first try at noon was a failure. The operator said, "You can only make contact at a fixed time. Mr. Murray will be up on his radio at six o'clock. Call then."

Six o'clock came around.

"Hello, is that Mr. Murray?" This question was followed by a longish pause. Then up he came, over a line that was as much extraneous noise as words.

"Good *crackle zzzzt* Haigh. *Bzzzz zzzzt* say 'over' each time you finish. *Bzzzz*, this is George Murray. Over."

"Mr. Murray. I have some bad news. The Angus bull you sent here last week has died of high mountain disease, otherwise known as altitude sickness. Over."

"I only got half of that *zzzzzzzzt zzzzzzt* understand you to say that the bull has died. Over."

"Yes, that is correct. I will send you a report as soon as it is ready. Over."

Mr. Murray's end of the conversation continued to sound like a disjointed mixture of bubble and squeak, with the odd word thrown in. I had no way of knowing how much of my own message was getting through in an intelligible form, but we proceeded as best we could. It was only much later that I learned that a substantial number of his neighbours would have been able to listen in, as we broadcast over a wavelength used by at least a couple of dozen farmers in the area around Mount Kenya. Finally the call came to a muddled conclusion.

"Right you are. *Zzzzt* you for telling me. I look forward to seeing the full report. Over and out."

Now I understood the origin of another Swahili word. The language is full of onomatopoeic words, many borrowed from other tongues, all based upon the African trait of using characteristics of things that the people have observed. A diesel engine is a *tinka-tinka*, a motor scooter (and a motor bike) is a *piki-piki*. Both of these, repeated aloud several times, demonstrate their appropriateness. Virtually all Swahili words end in a vowel, and the word for a two-way radio or radio-phone is *ova-ova*.

Quite soon afterwards I was able to get back into the dean's better books. Charlie Kiengo and I were called up to Limuru to see a cow that was supposed to have pneumonia.

After the ritual greetings the owner, a farmer with only three cows and half a dozen sheep on his rather ill-kept plot, said, "She has been sick for five days. She is not eating, and her milk has gone. She started with a cold, with water coming from her nostrils, but yesterday her eyes became cloudy, and she cannot see."

"What's her temperature?" I asked Charlie, who had already put a thermometer where it would do its job.

"Mia moja na tano," he said, testing my Swahili comprehension, just for the devilment.

"A hundred and five. Wow, that's up there," I thought to myself. To show Charlie that I was with him I said the last phrase out loud in Swahili: *"Kumbe! moto sana."*

The "cold" that the farmer had described had turned into a really nasty runny nose, with crusts over the bare skin on the muzzle, and pus streaked through the mucus. There were several ugly ulcers inside her mouth. No wonder she was not eating.

"This cow is very sick indeed, Charlie. I don't think that it will live, whatever we do, but if the farmer is willing I may be able to persuade the dean to buy it as a teaching case. By the way, how long has the farmer had this animal here?"

Charlie turned to the farmer, explained my proposal in Kikuyu, and translated my question.

"The cow was born here, and has never left the farm, except to go to the neighbours for servicing when she wants the bull," was the reply.

The farmer agreed to our suggestion, and when I got back I went looking for the head of the field service section, Dr. Bill Luke. I found him walking the large animal wards, dapper as usual in blue shorts, with white knee stockings and a white shirt. He was leaning over a stable door and stroking his equally white beard.

"*Jambo* Jerry. What's up?" he asked.

"I think that there might be an interesting teaching case. It may be malignant catarrh, but there is no history of wildebeest contact. I don't imagine there are any wildebeest within 70 miles. The fellow does have a few sheep."

"Let's go and see Mac about it, and see whether he has any funds for teaching cases," he said, straightening up.

The dean seemed interested, but was cautious.

"Hmph. Call me as soon as she arrives. I'd like to take a look."

The animal arrived the next day, even sicker than when I had seen her. Mac was delighted and congratulated me generously on spotting the possibilities. By the time the cow died three days later all the students and faculty had had a chance to examine it, at the dean's insistence.

At that time the way in which this usually fatal disease was transmitted to cattle was not completely understood, although it was well-known to be associated with wildebeest and sometimes cropped up in association with sheep. The Masai, who had lived among wild animals of the plains for centuries, knew better than to let their cattle anywhere near wildebeest at their calving time. They believed that the fluids associated with birthing carried something that the cattle could catch. If that happened, their precious cattle almost always died. The wildebeest never showed any signs of sickness from the condition. It was yet another in the host of plagues to which cattle were susceptible as they arrived from

Europe. For those settlers who knew nothing of the Masai experiences, it must have been a nasty shock.

Scientists at the veterinary laboratories in Kabete had worked out a great deal about the wildebeest form of the disease, and shown it to be caused by a virus. The sheep-associated form was much less well understood. Hence the excitement.

CHAPTER 3

THE MZEE

*The official opening of the veterinary college at Kabete,
and some direct dealings with the president and his cattle.*

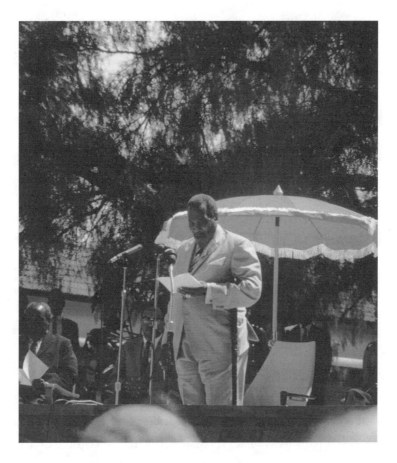

"Ladies and Gentlemen," Jomo Kenyatta, 1965.

A BIG SURPRISE WAS IN STORE for me when Paul Kinyanjui announced that one of our calls was to the president's farm at Dandora, a community on the other side of Nairobi. The president had several farms, all of them — except his main home base in Kiambu — having been the property of settlers who had departed.

Jomo Kenyatta had spent a number of years in England, arriving in 1929 and leaving after the Second World War. In his book *Mau Mau, An African Crucible*, Robert Edgerton writes, "Kenyatta's magnetic presence, his great, resonant voice, his riveting eyes and his masterful sense of showmanship quickly made him friends and supporters in left-wing circles." Edgerton also states that Kenyatta was a compelling speaker and had, during his time in Europe, traveled to Russia and Germany, and had become a charismatic figure, allegedly seducing numerous compliant women.

He obtained a degree at the London School of Economics, where acquaintances and classmates had included Elspeth Huxley, doyenne of

Kenyan authors, and Louis Leakey, the anthropologist. He had published his important text, *Facing Mount Kenya*, even married an English woman while over there, although he more or less abandoned her, pregnant with their second child, as soon as he had the chance to return to Kenya and fulfill what he must have seen, even then, as his political destiny. On his arrival at Mombassa in 1946 he was met by his first wife and their two children, now 25 and 18, and was mobbed by the dock workers, who more or less ignored the other passengers who disembarked after him.

As the Mau Mau rebellion gained momentum, he had been incarcerated in a remote prison in Kenya's north by the British administration. My godfather, Tony (later Sir Anthony) Swan, an Oxford chum and fellow K.A.R. officer of my father's, had remained in the country and risen through the administration to become the District Commissioner for Kiambu. It was he who had signed the papers for Kenyatta's arrest on October 20th in 1952. The State of Emergency was declared the next day.

In *Out in the Midday Sun*, one of her many books about her beloved Kenya, Elspeth Huxley wrote that "Kenyatta's period in prison gave him time for reflection away from the turmoil of politics"; "Just before his final release he said, half jokingly, 'We have been in a university. We learned more about politics there than we learnt outside.'"

Kenyatta's election to the presidency of the newly independent country had been a shoo-in, and even before the official handover he made strenuous efforts to placate the Europeans who chose to remain, assuring them that they too would have a part to play in the new situation, and promising them that he would let bygones be bygones, as long as they would do the same.

My first view of the president had come at the official opening of the new veterinary faculty buildings, soon after my arrival in Kenya. As the day had drawn closer, the excitement level had risen among the staff. Elma became the centre of operations, as sweepers searched in every nook and cranny, ferreting out bits of paper from under the prickly bougainvillaea. The ingrained dark red mud stains on the walls of the older buildings had been vigorously scrubbed, then given a lick of paint. The quadrangle at the veterinary college might have been specifically designed for the event: a raised bank at one end made a fine stage. On the morning of the big day dozens of chairs were put out by a team of blue-uniformed staff, and a table and six chairs were set up on the bank under the shade of a large pepper tree. Excitement rose as the appointed time of 2:00 p.m. approached, and all activity at both large and small animal clinics was suspended by 10:00 a.m.

A grim-visaged group of men in battle fatigues had inspected every inch of the grounds, and the doors and windows of the surrounding buildings had been locked by lunch time. No one could have entered, even in an emergency.

Elma had seen to the seating arrangements. As very junior members of staff, the interns were seated well back in the crowd, and our view was somewhat obscured by the array of ladies' hats that adorned the more important guests present. My own view was somewhat restricted by the bright pink gown and skull cap of a cleric from some Christian denomination sitting right in front of me.

Mzee Kenyatta, the President of the Republic of Kenya, "the" *Mzee* as most knew him, emerged from his Mercedes limousine about 20 minutes late. Already past middle age (he was never quite certain of his birth year, but it was thought to have been just before the turn of the century) by the time he took the reins of the country in 1963, he was still an imposing figure, slightly corpulent, but massively built. He carried his familiar fly whisk — a traditional symbol of power — like a badge.

The speeches were short and to the point. Political rhetoric was of course part of the package, but the newspapers would have a story to tell, and the donor agencies would have their pound of flesh.

Tea and biscuits followed the formal part of the proceedings, but by that time the *Mzee* had left and we had a chance to meet staff from other veterinary organizations that served the Kenyan public. These included the Veterinary Laboratories, also in Kabete, whence all the veterinary services of the nation were administered, the East African Veterinary Research Organization, based at Muguga, and the Animal Health and Industry Training Institute, located near the Vet Labs. The bull station of the Artificial Breeding Centre was also represented. Some of the people I already knew from evenings at tennis, but many were new faces whom I would come to know in the ensuing months and years. By next morning all signs of the event had disappeared, and it was back to work as usual.

■

As we drove into the farm yard, a large number of Friesian and Friesian-cross cattle crossed the road in front of the Land Rover. This was my first visit to the farm and no one had warned me what to expect. Paul Kinyanjui and I had come to see a lame cow. The farm manager was waiting for us in the office, and together we went into the milking shed to deal with the patient. About 40 dejected-looking beasts stood in their stalls, some chewing on small bunches of hay. All were in poor condition. Some looked like coat racks.

The cow had been lame for a few days and it was not difficult to determine that she had an advanced case of footrot, which would require some vigorous treatment after being cleaned up. I called for hot water and asked Paul to get the bag of Epsom salts from the Land Rover.

Between us Paul and I managed to control the cow's leg, which we hoisted with a rope tied to an overhead beam in order to prevent her from kicking. With a hoof knife, a scrubbing brush, and lots of clean water we were able to get to the root of the problem and clean out the infected area. By now the hot water had arrived and after Paul had dumped in a generous double handful of salts, and given the bucket a vigorous stir, we gingerly lowered the foot into the solution. At first the cow objected, but soon the soothing action of the warm water settled her down. I persuaded the manager to help out, and prepared a good dose of penicillin.

The immediate task over, I began to ask about the overall health of the herd. I was astonished to be told that the average milk yield was less than a quarter of a gallon. Many of the so-called milk cows gave nothing at all. It was not difficult to understand why the yield was so low when I learned that no extra feed was used, and occasionally, when available, some hay was given. The cows were expected to fend for themselves off the pasture.

As we stepped outside the barn I saw that there were cattle of all ages milling about in the muck, and that the paddock beyond was bereft of anything approaching grazing.

At that moment a large black Mercedes drove up, a beefy uniformed man jumped out of the front passenger seat and opened a rear door and out stepped the president. He had come to inspect his herd.

He had an astonishingly imposing presence. The hair on the back of my neck stood up as he greeted us. Whether this was due to the fact that I knew that he was the president, or simply something to do with the man's aura, I don't know. He was courteous and seemingly interested in the animals, but did not wish to discuss any management matters.

"Tell my manager, he will deal with it," he said firmly. He spent most of the short time that he was there greeting and chatting briefly with the large number of men and women that appeared from various quarters. They stood shyly, talking to him only after being greeted individually. Several small children, dressed in a variety of hand-me-down shirts and dresses, were running about. One baby with a runny nose was being carried by a young girl, no more than about eight years old herself. She had obviously had lots of practice as her left hip was thrust out, her arm holding the tot around his waist. Both were staring at me, rather than the president. I suppose that my white skin was more of a novelty to kids who had no concern with politics.

I started to write up the charges for the visit when I got back to Kabete.

"Don't waste your time," said Jimmy, smiling cynically. "No bills for the *Mzee*."

From my perspective, two years after he had become president, there was no apparent doubt about Kenyatta's grasp on power. Security was tight, and the press carried only positive stories about him. Hardly a day seemed to pass without some item about him in one of the two newspapers. This did not change throughout his presidency. He was widely respected, and no opposition was brooked. Once or twice, when traveling on the highways, one would see a group of uniformed motorcycle outriders spanning the entire road. With firm gestures they would indicate that one should head for the ditch, and woe betide anyone who was not quick to obey. Pretty soon afterwards a small cavalcade of black Mercedes limousines would sweep past, straddling the white line in the full knowledge that they owned the whole thing. Darkened glass obscured the occupants, but the flag fluttering on the wing told one who was who.

Another visit to Dandora, again for a lame cow, about two weeks later, again coincided with a visit from the *Mzee*. On this occasion I had been discussing with the manager the question of the dozens of uncastrated bulls of every age mixed in with the cows. I urged that he get rid of them at market in order to reduce stocking rates and improve feed quantity for the milking herd. Kenyatta, brandishing his fly whisk with characteristic vigour, would not even discuss the matter. He was there to ask after the welfare of his manager's family. I should have remembered that to get rid of bulls would be to fly in the face of African tradition. The number of cattle a man owns is a direct indication of his wealth and

status, his *heshima*; this involves prestige, pride, face, and dignity. To castrate the bulls would invade the personal space.

Others of us who had visited the farm during our field service rota-
tions had had similar experiences. Paul Sayer, who had graduated from
Glasgow one year ahead of me, had lived in Kenya most of his life. He had
completed his internship at Kabete and was now employed as a clinician.
He too had been out to the farm and struggled with the shambles that it
was. Jimmy, Paul and I broached the topic with Dean McIntyre, in the
hope that his exalted position in the hierarchy might earn a more sympa-
thetic hearing from the president and so change the conditions on the
farm and improve the lot of the virtually starving cattle. We heard the outcome of the short meeting a month or so later, as the dean recounted it.

"*Mzee*, my clinicians tell me that you have too many young bulls
breeding your cows," Dr. McIntyre had said. "You should get all of your
bull calves castrated. In that way we could be sure to get the best bulls for
breeding your cows. These young bulls will not improve the quality of
the herd."

Quick as a wink, Kenyatta had replied, "Why should I castrate them?
I enjoy a good jump myself now and again."

There the matter rested.

CHAPTER 4

19,000 FEET ABOVE SEA LEVEL

*A climb up Africa's highest mountain, a trip to the coast, a switch
to the small animal clinic, and a surprise when I deal with my
second wildlife case, a cheetah with a purr like a generator.*

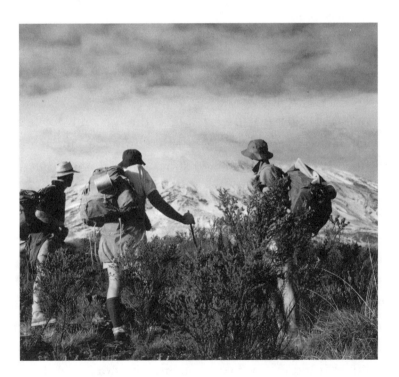

A pause at 14,000 feet on the Outward Bound route up Kilimanjaro.
The peak of Kibo in the background.

D URING A BRIEF HOLIDAY, I joined three friends for a trip up Mount Kilimanjaro. Most people know the mountain as the single, much-photographed snow-covered cone called Kibo, which rises to 19,340 feet. There are in fact two summits; the lesser-known Mawenzi, which is a jagged peak that rises to 16,900 feet, lies to the east of Kibo. Early European explorers were scoffed at when they claimed to have seen snow near the equator, but indeed, due to its altitude, the cone of the mountain does have a permanent white cap.

A popular myth, which I believed for years, has grown up to explain why Kilimanjaro lies in Tanzania, and why the border between Kenya (at the time British East Africa) and what was then German East Africa, has a decided kink in it just east of the mountain. The story goes that Queen Victoria "gave" the mountain to Kaiser Wilhelm II, her grandson, as a birthday gift. Colin Clarkson of Cambridge University put me straight.

"There is little to support the story that Queen Victoria gave away Kilimanjaro as a present to the Kaiser, her grandson. Wilhelm II did not come to the throne of Germany until 1888 and it is well known that the Queen's relations with her son-in-law, the German Emperor, were far from cordial. It is much more likely that she reacted strongly against any such suggestion."

The truth, according to one of Clarkson's many sources, seems to be much more prosaic. "It appears that the line skirting this mountain with, according to Gladstone (British Prime Minister at the time), an unrememberable name, was established as the result of compromise between the competing claims of treaties made by Britain and Gemany with tribal rulers in the late 19th century."

We climbed from the Kenya side, starting from the Outward Bound school at Oloitokitok, and crossing the Kenya-Tanzania border as we climbed. I remember taking a shower under a stream that ran over a rocky ledge when we stopped to camp in a cave at 14,000 feet. Cold hardly describes it. My painful schoolboy memories of mandatory early-morning cold baths at Sherborne were superseded by this experience.

I also vividly remember crawling up the final scree on the approach to the top. I was overcome by altitude sickness; my head was bursting and my breathing was becoming laboured. Luckily my companions made sure that I went no further, and sent me back to Top Hut.

I was lucky enough to avoid any clinic duties over the Christmas break, and so on Boxing Day I joined the Parklands hockey squads for a memorable trip to Mombasa. We took both a men's and women's team, and a crowd of about 30 of us, including spouses, supporters and significant others, boarded the train at dusk in Nairobi. After an excellent meal in the dining room, we settled down for the night.

At about four in the morning, the train stopped for a water fill at Voi, a town sited amidst vast acres of sisal plantations, only about 100 miles from our destination. Sisal had once been the cash crop of the region, used to make rope all over the world. Now it was being edged out by nylon, and many of the plantations had an unkempt appearance. The cessation of the rhythm of the wheels woke most of us up, and before I knew what was happening we were out on the platform playing an impromptu game of hockey, until the disappearance of the ball under the carriage brought the game to a halt.

As the train set off again there was no point in going back to sleep, and I sat by the window watching the miles and miles of thorn bush, occasional glimpses of the red murram road, and rocky outcrops. This was my first trip to the coast since childhood. My mother had shown me a grainy black-and-white print of myself, aged about two, standing with two equally naked little kids on the beach at Diani south of Mombasa, but I had no memory or preconception of what it would be like. Soon the landscape changed to palm trees, banana plants and thatched houses as we got nearer the coast, and we finally steamed into the station soon after six o'clock. Our hosts met us and we were whisked off to their homes in groups of two or three for breakfast, followed by a wonderful day at the Nyali Beach Hotel, a few miles out of Mombasa. We relaxed, caught some sun, and goofed off with an impromptu game of sand hockey.

After the proper game in the evening, a late, late night at the club, and another day in the sea and sun, we boarded the train for the return journey. There was little response to calls for another hockey game at Voi, and most of us retired early.

Karen Blixen, among others, had described seeing teeming thousands of animals on the Athi plains upon awakening at dawn in the train. By 1965, the numbers had dwindled to a few hundred. The vast herds of zebra, kongoni and gazelles had gone. But the view we woke up to — small groups of stately giraffe, some dozens of wildebeest and other plains game, a wheeling pair of eagles, and the light against the early morning sky — was spectacular enough.

No sooner had we returned than I was embroiled in preparation for the New Year's dance. I had foolishly volunteered to help with decorations for this fancy dress affair, which was to be based on the theme of "Cowboys and Indians." Given the nature of the Nairobi population and the club membership, we changed the name to "Cowboys and Red Indians," although this too would now be considered politically incorrect. Huge rolls of blank newssheet were taped to most of the walls of my flat. The task was to transfer the pots of powder paint to the paper in some recognizable form. After three days of hectic work, the other volunteers and I had enough colourful giant posters to decorate the Parklands club walls. For the pillars we made imitation totem poles. I knew nothing of the culture of North American Indians, and the mix of feathered head dresses, totem poles and cowboys in saloons was hardly true to the original. More likely it was built upon my Hollywood-learned misconceptions. Luckily no one else knew any better or took me to task.

The new year brought a change at the school. Paul Sayer went away on a short leave, and I moved to the small animal clinic where he had built a successful practice.

Most of my new routine consisted of vaccinations, worm treatments, minor surgical cases, neutering of both cats and dogs, and skin and ear problems. My inexperience was again a considerable worry to me, but I had the support of an experienced veterinary nurse, Diana Boxall, and technical assistants Lawrence Kahara and James Ngugi, both of whom had been at the college for several years. Ngugi was short and had a sort of surprised look most of the time. Lawrence was taller, and very slim. Both were Kikuyu, and therefore not far from home.

The words of the dean of the Glasgow Veterinary School surfaced to reassure me. As my classmates and I had stood in the hall at Bearsden, in our rented graduation robes, having all sworn the veterinary version of the Hippocratic oath, Professor (later Sir William) Weipers said, in his dry

Scots brogue, "Remember, animals will usually recover in spite of what you do to them."

When it came to some of the more severe parasitic diseases seen in Kenya, this rule did not always apply. I quickly learned that if an animal of any species had a fever, a blood smear was the essential first step. While cattle had their specific problems, dogs were very prone to a different form of tick fever.

■

"Good morning," said the smartly dressed lady as she led a small, mostly white terrier into the clinic.

"Hello, Mrs. Hughes. What seems to be the problem with Ginger this morning?" The receptionist, Mrs. Trendall, had dug out the patient's chart, and Lawrence had brought it to me. A quick glance had shown me the dog's name.

"Well, for the last two mornings he has refused his buttered toast crusts, and today he would not even look at his bacon. I think he may have tick fever."

The link was not immediately obvious to me, but I kept my mouth shut. We got him up on the table, and after letting him smell me and settle down, I looked at his gums, which were almost completely white, and took his temperature, which was a couple of degrees higher than it ought to have been. Mrs. Hughes was probably right.

Lawrence was ready, without being asked, with a fine gauge needle and a couple of glass slides. I clipped the very edge of Ginger's ear and cleaned it with a swab. A moment later I had pricked the ear and a tiny drop of rather watery-looking blood had been transferred to the slide. Lawrence took it to the counter and began the staining procedure.

As we waited, I quizzed Mrs. Hughes about the breakfast tidbits. She was an old Kenya hand and had far more experience than I of dogs in these conditions. Like many other observant owners, she had noted that a dog with tick fever will immediately go off fatty foods.

The slide was soon ready, and it was no challenge to see the numerous pear-shaped blue bodies inside the red blood cells. Another lesson for me in the importance of listening to experienced, if untrained, people.

As I prepared the injection, which had to be carefully measured against an accurate patient's weight because an overdose could be dangerous and an underdose might not do the job properly, Mrs. Hughes and I discussed the need to rest the dog and ensure that he had plenty of good food over the next while.

The daily breakfast of buttered toast and bacon had caused Ginger to lose the svelte shape that should go with his breed, but it had given his owner a vital, possibly life-saving, signal.

Becoming acquainted with the dog-owning public sometimes meant taking on public relations tasks. An important social activity for dog owners was the annual show at the East Africa Kennel Club show grounds at Jamhuri Park. I had been asked to provide two honorary vets for the show; Jimmy Duncan, who was finishing his tour and was about to leave the country, agreed to help me. I was unsure what duties and responsibilities the show might involve.

"Oh, it's nothing, really," explained the secretary, a large lady in a florid print dress. "Just check the dogs as they come in, make sure that they're not sick and that all the bits are there. Then hang around in case anything happens that needs your attention."

A couple of weeks later, early on Saturday, Jimmy and I found ourselves dressed in clean white coats, standing on either side of a table in a small office at the show grounds, as a long line-up of dogs of every imaginable breed, and their handlers, in an even greater variety of garb, snaked off around the corner out of sight.

It seemed easy enough. Check the eyes, lift the lip to check the teeth and gums, feel the coat for any obvious lumps, and feel under the belly to see if "all the bits were there." It would never do to have a show champion, however beautiful, unable to pass on his genes due to some prior surgical intervention.

In short order I discovered that "easy" is a relative term. I bent to introduce myself to a large Alsatian. He either took a personal dislike, or had a general hatred of men in white coats. His flashing teeth clamped on to my coat as I threw myself back against the table. He had missed the real me by inches. Luckily the secretary was present to record the entries and hand out ring badges. She had seen the whole thing, and the owner and his dog were on their way home.

Next came the question of "all the bits." A boxer, smart and glossy as he should be, and slobbering a bit like all his brethren, had something missing. In non-technical terms, he was a "one-stoner." My quiet announcement of this deficit to his owner produced a torrent of scorn. You would have thought that I had taken a page out of some book of insults, or suggested that the owner herself had dubious ancestry involving a pig.

"What do you mean young man? You don't know what you are talking about. I demand that someone competent examine my dog."

Jimmy was there just across the room, and he stepped up. We offered the lady a chance to return later for a re-check if she thought it worthwhile. As the secretary politely suggested that the lady could bring the dog next time, if the situation changed, she left with an attempt to repair her dignity by saying, to all within hearing, "Well, he had two this morning."

Difficult clients are often less pleasant, and less easy to deal with, than one's animal patients.

The Monday morning started much as usual: a couple of dogs to vaccinate against distemper, a poodle showing much discomfort and bum-dragging due to overfull anal glands, and a dachsund with itchy skin. When, as I was preparing to vaccinate a puppy, I glanced through the examining room window and saw a man come round the side of the building, it seemed odd to me that he was not bringing his pet into the waiting room via the usual route, but I thought no more of it. As I could only see his upper half, I didn't realize that I was about to have my next brush with something outside the usual range of domestic animal.

As the puppy left with the young couple who owned it, the man came through the door, walking a full-grown cheetah on a leash. As he stopped to chat at the reception desk, his sleek companion rubbed itself against his legs, and a loud noise started up. The cheetah was purring. In fact, one could hear him purring right across the reception area. He then jumped up on to the magazine table and stood there, looking out of the window, as pleased as Punch. Magazines, the day's newspapers, and the ashtray flew on to the floor.

From Mrs. Trendall's response, I guessed that this was not the man's first visit. She greeted him with a cheery, "Good morning, Mr. Bryant. Nothing more than the usual trouble, I hope?"

"Oh no, I don't think so," he replied, "but I thought I had better bring him in, just to be sure. I've brought the usual sample, so that we can run a check."

The usual sample turned out to be a small amount of feces in a plastic bag, and Lawrence, who had also obviously seen Mr. Bryant before, took it from him and disappeared into the back rooms where the laboratory was located. Taking my cue from the others, I tried to seem nonchalant as I asked Mr. Bryant to bring his pet into the examining room.

"What seems to be the problem?" I asked, in what I hoped was my best professional manner.

"Oh, he's lethargic and has gone off his food. His gums looked pale when I checked them this morning."

The examining table was not designed for such a large patient. As I had by now got over my initial surprise, and the cheetah was still rubbing himself against his owner's legs and purring loudly, I bent over to check him. His gums were indeed very pale. Almost white in fact, rather than the usual healthy pink colour that one would expect.

Still a trifle unsure of myself, I asked the owner whether a check of the patient's temperature was feasible. "No problem," he said. The temperature was normal.

I was not sure what else to look for. One of the first rules a young veterinary student is taught is that one must know the normal before one can deal with the abnormal. But there are no more normal cheetahs in Glasgow than there are giraffes, so I had no point of reference. The short springy hair on this fellow was unlike the fur on any tabby that I had ever seen, but Mr. Bryant assured me that the speckled coat was not its usual glossy self.

About this time, Lawrence quietly slipped into the examining room and told me that the sample was ready under the microscope. In the field of view, I could see dozens of characteristic hookworm eggs.

It was indeed the usual problem.

Hookworms have developed a cunning strategy to make their lives complete. The adults set up shop in the intestines of a mammal and lay their eggs. The eggs are excreted in due course and then hatch on the ground. The young larvae are specially adapted to burrow through skin — often, of course, through the soles of the feet. There are many species of hookworm; some live in humans, others in dogs and cats.

None of this would be too bad if it were not for the way that the worms feed, which is to puncture small vessels in the intestinal wall and use the blood as a constant food supply. If there are enough of them they can cause a serious loss of blood, which can have quite an effect upon the host. This is what was bothering the cheetah.

"Looking at his medical record, I see that this seems to happen fairly often," I said. "Why don't we get him treated with his usual tablets this time, and I'll give him an injection of iron and vitamins so that he can build up his strength quickly. Then you can take some more tablets home with you and give him routine treatments."

"How often should I treat him?"

"Well, according to his history, he seems to need a dose about every three to four months. Why don't we give you three complete doses, and you can try him at four-month intervals? You can easily bring us a fresh stool sample after, say, three months, to see how things are coming along."

CHAPTER 5

YEAR'S END

*Working with a living legend on another cheetah, a lucky horse
mixes with a car windshield, another mountain climb,
and an idyllic few days at the coast.*

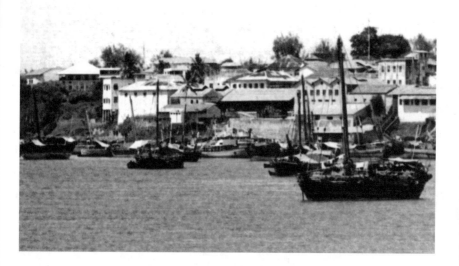

Mombasa harbour.

I SOON HAD ANOTHER CHEETAH to deal with. While I was checking an ancient spaniel's somewhat manky teeth, a phone call had come in from Dr. Toni Harthoorn concerning a young adult animal which had been brought to him by an out-of-town client. He needed to use the X-ray facilities and would arrive in about 20 minutes. Clinic hours were over, but we would be on the lookout for him.

Toni was already well known for his pioneering work on animal capture, and had done some impressive things with the rescue of rhinoceros and many other species that had become stranded when the Kariba dam filled up. In wildlife veterinary circles, he was considered *the* world authority. He was also head of the department of physiology at the university, and taught the junior veterinary and medical students at Chiromo.

He soon arrived, together with his wife Suzanne, who had worked with him on many wild animals. I had met him once, soon after arriving at Kabete, but did not expect him to remember me. Luckily Mrs. Trendall

made the introductions. Toni, all 6'3" or so of him, was carrying the cheetah in his arms, and took it straight into the X-ray unit where we had
made things ready.

"This animal is a pet whose owner feeds him raw meat most of the
time. This morning the cheetah was frightened by a strange animal getting up on top of his cage. He took a violent leap and I think he has
broken both his legs. Here, have a feel," he said to me.

Both hind legs were bent at an unusual angle at the hock joint or
heel. The cheetah did not seem to be in any pain, but he made no attempt
to stand. Suzanne was able to keep him quiet by stroking him, and he
even started to purr.

The X-rays told the story. Both heel bones were broken across the
middle at almost identical angles. For an animal built for speed, with long
hind legs that create huge leverage, the heel bones play a crucial role in
the final push for the sprint. One broken bone would be bad news. To
have both broken at once was a disaster. The X-ray also revealed the
probable reason for the breaks. The walls of all the bones in the legs were
paper-thin.

I knew that my limited experience was quite inadequate to repair this
sort of damage, and Toni too knew his limitations. He said to his wife,
"Sue, I wonder if we can persuade Mr. Griffiths to help us. He's an ortho-
pod with the Glasgow team at Kenyatta."

Being used to British ways I knew that human surgeons, once they
become specialists, change their titles from Doctor back to Mister. This is
a throwback to the early 19th century, the days of the barber surgeons.
The idea of calling on a human surgeon to help in such a case had never
occurred to me, but once voiced, it was an obvious solution. After all, the
principles are identical, and we could handle the "animal" side of things.

Two days later, as I administered the anesthetic, Mr. Griffiths inserted
long bone screws down the shaft of each broken end of the heel bones,
carefully lined the broken pieces up, and screwed them together. We

checked the alignments with another X-ray.

Because of the fragile state of all the bones, the surgeon felt that we could not simply leave the animal without support.

"We must cast both legs to support him until some healing occurs. Any athletic movements will almost certainly cause another break, probably over the screws. If that happens, the heel bones will be impossible to repair."

The solution was simple, although no doubt uncomfortable for the cheetah. We encased both lower legs in plaster of Paris for two months.

"I'll get after the owner about the need for roughage, especially calcium and phosphorous, in the cat's diet," said Toni. "The cat will also need supplements of bone-meal to help his bones regain their proper strength."

When the plaster came off the fractures had healed, and the X-rays showed overall signs of improvement in bone density.

None of us interns ever became a small or large animal specialist, because when one was "on" one had to deal with whatever came through the door or over the phone. One of the strangest cases I ever encountered came to me the latter way.

Over afternoon coffee one day, one of our field service clinicians explained that he had gone out that morning to see a client, Paddy Migdoll, about a horse.

"It happened like this. Mrs. Migdoll had sent out one of her mares, April First, who had just come out of training, in the care of a *syce* (groom). He had been instructed to keep her under control at the end of a long rope while she grazed. Well, she jumped away from him and pulled the rope out of his hands, and then took off through the coffee for home. She ran between two rows of bushes and up an embankment, jumped out on to the road, and landed plumb across the hood of a small car, one of those Fiat bubble jobs that you see here."

"Was anyone hurt?" I asked.

"That's the strangest thing. A lady was driving the car, taking her little daughter to school, and was suddenly confronted with a thousand pounds of horse smack in front of her on the windshield. By some miracle, both she and the child were uninjured. The car was totaled. The horse also suffered some pretty severe damage. They caught her up and took her back to the stables. I got the call, and Charlie drove me there. I wondered what on earth I was going to see."

"The horse was pretty badly shaken. I was able to get some of the biggest bits of glass from her hide, but you know how it is with these windshields. It had shattered into a thousand little pieces, each about the size of a ten-cent piece, and some were too small to find. The big ones consisted of several small fragments joined together. I reckon we'll have to see her again, and I asked Mrs. Migdoll to keep an eye on her."

Thinking no more about this bizarre tale, I set off after work for the Impala Club. The rugby season was underway, and there was a training session that evening. Under the whip-and-carrot approach of coach Duncan Brown, we engaged in arduous circuit training for about the first half of each 90-minute session, followed by a variety of drills, including ball-handling skills, that were more fun.

As the rapidly falling dusk settled in at five to seven, Duncan called for one last run up the pitch, practising scissor movements.

"Pair off, take a ball to each pair, and come up the pitch crossing every ten yards or so. Take no more than three strides with the ball in your hands."

This particular evening would be my last training session for a month, as a mistimed switch led to a trip and fall. In good light the fall would have been inconsequential. After all, falling is an integral part of the game. Unfortunately, this fall was followed instantly by a searing pain in my shoulder.

Duncan wasted no time in getting me to Nairobi hospital, my right arm cradled against my chest with my left hand holding my wrist. I suppose that neither of us smelt exactly as sweet as the roses, after 90 minutes of hard work in sweaty rugby jerseys, but the nurse in the casualty ward did not seem to mind.

"Right," she said. "We'll have to cut your right arm out of this sleeve, and then perhaps you can slip the rest of this thing over your head. Nasty rough game, you should have more sense," she added with half a smile.

I was too uncomfortable to reply.

She split the red shirt from wrist to shoulder and before I knew where I was she had it on the table beside me. After X-rays had been taken and we sat for a while in the examination room, she returned with a doctor who examined me and said, "Nothing broken. You look as if you've dislocated your collar-bone. Nurse here will fix you up with a figure-of-eight bandage. You should keep it on for two to three weeks, depending upon how you feel. Nurse, please give Mr. Haigh 100 mgs of Pethidine before you pack him off."

"Will I be able to wash at all with the bandage on?" I asked the nurse as she strapped me up, pulling back my shoulders into a military posture.

"Oh yes, just get someone to help you take it off before you bathe or shower. I expect you vets know how to put bandages on, don't you?" she said, this time with a proper grin.

Duncan had organized for my old car to be taken back to the college, and he delivered me, safe, sound, and a little woozy from the Pethidine, back to my flat. I had forgotten that I was to go on duty at eight o'clock, and was sitting in a sort of daze when, just as I was getting ready to go to bed, the phone rang.

"Hello, this is Paddy Migdoll. Can someone come out and look at my horse? Professor Aanes came here this morning, but the *syce* tells me she's pretty poorly."

Knowing that I was not exactly in good shape, I started to phone around, desperately trying to find a substitute. But everyone was either at the club, at the movies, or out to dinner. There was nothing for it but to set out, driving more or less one-handed, shifting gear with the left hand while holding one spoke of the wheel with the other in a gingerly fashion and hoping that no sudden turns would be needed. Mrs. Migdoll greeted me as I drove into the yard. We walked over to the stables together and she repeated the saga of the morning's events.

The thoroughbred's painkiller had worn off, and several more bits of glass had worked their way to the surface. In the inadequate lighting of the stable I stood and looked at the animal. The whole of her right hand side was scattered with a host of tiny and not-so-tiny puncture marks. There was also an interlacing mesh of scratches. She was visibly upset, and in quite some discomfort. Using a pair of fine forceps I was able to get out a couple of glass chips, but each time she flinched and struggled, and my painful shoulder and one-handed approach was no doubt making me nervous, a feeling that was almost certainly being picked up by the perceptive patient.

It was obvious that to continue I was going to have to sedate her. It was also obvious that this was not a true emergency, and that discretion would have been the better part of valour. A visit from a clinic colleague in the morning would have been the sensible course. Being either pig-headed or dulled from pain, I foolishly decided to try and carry on. Moving round to the front of the horse I said to the groom, "Put the twitch on her nose, and I'll give her an injection in the vein so that we can work."

The mare was having none of it. Objecting to the entire procedure, and no doubt fed up with all the interference, she reared up and struck out with her forelegs. A fit and alert human, familiar with danger signals being sent out by a patient, can often get out of the way in such situations. Although fit in the training sense, I was certainly not fit or alert in any other way. Inevitably, and in exact accordance with Murphy's Law, one of the striking hooves caught me right on the point of my recently dislocated collar-bone.

My next memory is of sitting in the house on a sofa being ministered to by Mrs. Migdoll. As I came round, her husband handed me a stiff brandy. It was quite some time before I was able to get back into the Land Rover and make my way home, all thoughts of doing any more calls for a few days entirely banished.

The horse's name was April First, but my condition was no joke.

All medical students are taught that disease conditions are a result of interaction between the patient, a disease agent and the environment. In this case there had been two patients. The animal patient was a thorough-bred racehorse, the disease agent was glass, and the environment was a coffee plantation next to a main road. The human patient was a vet func-tioning on about half strength, the environment was a stable, and the agent a hoof.

I took a couple of days off work, but with the resilience of youth and a fit constitution I was back in the small animal clinic by the end of the week, limited only slightly by the bandage.

■

A group of my Impala rugby teammates and I, sitting at the bar after practice one evening, decided it might be fun to climb Mount Kenya. Some of them had been up before. A couple of weeks later, we were grinding slowly up a rough mountain track in a 4-wheel drive Land Rover through bamboo and a host of huge lichen-covered trees. We stopped the vehicle at the forest edge and made our way up on to the moorland. The first day we had to contend with the so-called vertical bog, and most of us fell in up to our crutches at least once.

As I paused to recover my breath, I looked back over the forest from an altitude of about 11,000 feet. An incredible vista lay before us. Away on our left the Aberdare mountains pushed up through a ring of cloud. In front was a vast plain, mainly pale brown in colour, but threaded with green where the Naro Moru river and several other small water courses wended their ways across the Laikipia plains. They joined the Ewaso

Ngiro, which flowed north and then east before it petered out in the Habaswein swamp.

The first night's rest at the Teleki hut, at about 13,000 feet, was most welcome. Several rock hyraxes turned up to greet us. These attractive little animals look like rodents, but are nothing of the sort. They are supposed to be the closest living relatives to elephants, based upon some anatomical features which certainly don't include size — they're about as big as a house cat. The ones that lived among the rocks near the camping hut had become completely habituated to climbers over the years, and they stood around hoping for handouts of food. We sat and marveled at the array of peaks around us and the giant lobelia and groundsel plants growing on the sides of the valley. I was reminded of Felice Benuzzi's description of the view, in his classic mountaineering tale *No Picnic on Mount Kenya*: "And then I saw it: an ethereal mountain emerging from a tossing sea of clouds. A massive blue-black tooth of sheer rock inlaid with azure glaciers, austere yet floating fairy-like on the near horizon."

By the time we reached top hut, at an elevation of about 15,000 feet, we were puffing and blowing. We found packets of rice and porridge oats stacked on the joists, opened, but almost unused. This was soon explained. It proved impossible to cook the stuff at this altitude. The water boiled, and boiled, and boiled. We had initially planned to have rice with our first course of tinned meat. It was still rock hard after 30 minutes of boiling. We decided to turn it into a dessert dish, but this, too, was a failure. It still had the consistency of rock chips after a full hour and a half of cooking. Porridge in the morning created the same problem.

The climb up the side of the Lewis Glacier in the dawn light to Point Lenana, the third highest peak, and reachable by non-technical climbers, was truly spectacular. The golds, reds and oranges of the sunrise glazed the underside of a carpet of cloud, a second carpet beneath reflecting the lustrous colours. The whole wall of Nelion, to our left as we climbed, seemed like beaten, jagged, burnished bronze sprinkled with talcum powder.

My year in Kenya was drawing to a close. When my contract ended, I had no need to rush back to Scotland, at least not until my money ran out. My brief trip to the coast at Christmas had given me the yen to go back again. I had gone to the southern coast at Diani Beach with a girlfriend for three days at Easter, but this had only whetted my appetite further.

I had been offered a bed in Mombasa, but I had to find some way of getting there. My meagre intern's salary had not matched the cost of running my car, and so I had sold it. Fortunately, I was able to borrow a 50-cc motorized bicycle, full frame size, with the tiny engine beneath the seat, from a friend at Kabete. With the machine in the luggage compartment, I set off on the train.

As I boarded, I remembered an anecdote my father had told me about the Mombasa train and Nairobi station. It dated back to the pre-war days, and the Happy Valley set. My father had heard the story this way: "A man thrashed another man with a horsewhip on the platform at Nairobi one Friday night. The two of them had been playing high-stakes poker in Thompson's Falls, and one, having been cleaned out of his money, had put up a dirty weekend in Mombasa with his wife as his bet. He lost. Then he turned up at the station as the couple were heading out, and attacked the bet's winner. The intriguing thing was that he was promptly ostracized by all and sundry."

"Why?" I asked.

"Oh, that's simple," Dad had replied. "He had reneged on his bet."

He made no comment on the wife's implicit compliance. As far as he was concerned, it had been an example of the tired one-liner, "Are you married, or do you live in Kenya?"

The borrowed scooter was an ancient one, and a new spring for the carburetor, vital for efficient running, had been unobtainable in Nairobi. If I was going to be able to explore the old town and the neighbouring coast thoroughly, I had to find a solution. My host suggested a backstreet where spares could often be found. The thatched shop, with its hand-painted sign, had a front of no more than about ten feet. Outside lay the rusting remains of Vespas and numerous pedal bikes. With little confidence I showed my problem to the proprietor, who turned to a teenager nearby and spoke to him in a tongue I did not recognize. The boy beckoned me to enter, and behind the banana leaf facade I saw several large piles of mixed wheels, chains and other unidentifiable bits of machinery. He took a brief look at the carburetor in my hand and stuck his arm into one of the piles. After a few minutes of grunting and puffing, his hand emerged holding the same type of carburetor, with its spring intact inside. So much for written ledgers and inventory checks.

The revamped bike gave me lots of freedom to explore. On the first day, avoiding the more touristy areas, I puttered around the old town, with its narrow streets and curbside coffee emporiums. I visited Fort Jesus, with its tangled history of conquerors and rogues that included Arab, Portuguese and British invaders. I didn't have much spending money, but it cost nothing to look at some beautiful carpets almost buried in the bowels of a dark shop with heavily shaded windows. I drove under the huge artificial tusks that meet above four lanes of traffic in what was then Kilindini Road. I passed the Konzi mosque, a corner of which jutted out a yard or so into the traffic lane on what's now Digo Road — the mosque predates the tarred road and naturally takes precedence.

I boarded the ferry at Likoni, on Mombasa Island's south side. Muslim women clothed from head to foot in black *bui-buis*, and others more gaily dressed and carrying large loads upon their heads, babies in cloth slings behind their backs, or both, chattered cheerily. Battered old trucks massively overloaded with produce and several bicycles wheeled by slim men all poured off the ferry at once. A young man with a portable radio perched on his shoulder made sure that the volume was turned up high enough so that everyone would take a look at him and his status symbol. The smooth tones of the late Jim Reeves, still hugely popular at the time, were an odd contrast to the chatter of other languages. A roadside hawker tried to lure passersby behind a hastily erected screen to view a two-headed calf.

Later that day, near the old Arab town, I found my way to the water's edge and sat watching the ships in the harbour. An *ngalawa*, a small out-riggered *dhow*, moved across the water's surface, creating ripples as it went.

Next morning I went looking for a more secluded spot and headed north past the Nyali Beach hotel. Quite soon I found a small beach-side restaurant hidden among the trees, which was just right, as I needed a con-genial spot to relax on the beach and keep my fluid levels up in the heat. The fluid was mostly delicious fresh fruit juices. Big moist slices of paw paw (papaya) with a squeeze of lemon juice across them were another treat. I spent most of the day in an indolent half snooze; occasional dips in the almost bath-water warm Indian ocean broke the monotony. Every now and again another human would appear on the white beach with its fringe of coconut palm and casuarina, but most of the time it was deserted and pristine. The rising tide had washed away the footprints of all previous visitors.

And so my time was up. It had been a fabulous year, but I had to get back to the UK, see my family, and look to my future. Little did I realize that after a very few months I would be back again, this time for a much longer stint, and that my future held many wild animal cases and much co-operative work with a certain medical doctor.

CHAPTER 6

A POSTING TO MERU

After a short stay in Britain, a return to Kenya, a new job, a new circle of friends, and a meeting with a dedicated hunter.

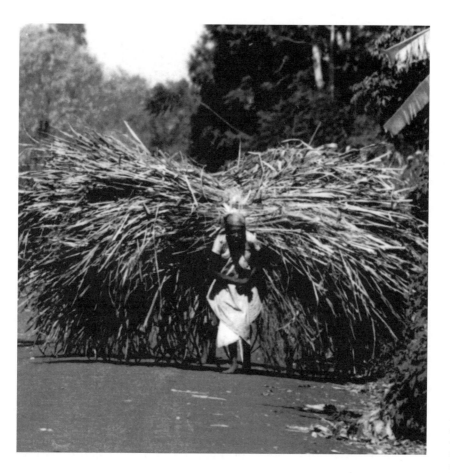

On the road to Chuka; bringing home the thatch.

M Y RETURN TO KENYA AFTER six months of England and Scotland was less dramatic than the previous one, which had followed a gap of almost 18 years. This time I had a two-year contract with the British Ministry of Overseas Development in my hand, and no idea of where I might end up in the government veterinary service. Paul Sayer, my flatmate from internship days, had picked me up and arranged for me to stay with him until I received my posting.

"Jerry, it's good to see you back," he said with his characteristic chuckle as we shook hands in the crowded airport.

As we drove along Uhuru highway, I said, "Gosh it's beautiful. I'd forgotten the range of colours of the bougainvillaea. I'd mostly remembered the purple, but there's an orange, some white there, and of course the red."

We returned to Paul's Kabete house. That evening I had dinner with him and his fiancée Elma, whom I had known in Glasgow and who had helped so much in my internship year, and I gave them news of what I had been up to. This had been a mixture of family visits and some locum jobs in England to earn much needed cash. The locums had been in mixed practice. One of them had been a three-month position in Wallingford; on my Wednesday afternoons off, and the odd Saturday, I'd driven up to London to spend time with my sister Brigid and her flatmates. They were all dancers, Brigid and Nuffy with the Tiller Girls, Foxy with the Royal Ballet. They lived in a somewhat dowdy flat in Rowland Gardens, in the Kensington area, and all three shared one bedroom. By September I knew that Kenya still held me in its sway. I interviewed for a posting with the Ministry, which allowed me to return there just after Christmas.

Within a couple of days, I visited the headquarters of the Veterinary Department at Kabete to meet the Deputy Director, Dr. Marcus Durand, and his boss Dr. Murithi. From there I went to the Ministry of Agriculture on Kenyatta Avenue to sign a pile of forms. I also purchased a second-hand Peugeot 403 from Joginder Singh, whose main claim to fame was that he had won the East African Safari in a second-hand Volvo, beating out more fancied rivals in cars supported by teams of technicians brought in by the car's manufacturers.

Dr. Murithi, the Director of Veterinary Services, had assigned me to the district veterinary office in Meru, and I asked some of the other senior staff at Kabete about the workings of the bureaucratic system, and what was expected of a District Veterinary Officer (commonly known as DVO). All I knew about Meru was that it was about 50 miles from Nanyuki on the northeastern slopes of Mount Kenya.

At dinner, I asked, "Paul, have you got a map I can look at? I want to see what is the best way to get to Meru." A map was produced, and studying it, I saw that there were two main possibilities. I decided to try the route via Embu.

The next morning, armed with nothing more in the way of veterinary equipment than a few instruments and a stethoscope, I set off for what was to be my home for over four years.

Past Thika and its huge coffee and pineapple plantations, the route turned left at a T junction towards Fort Hall. Pretty soon I was winding along through a series of bends, admiring the very fertile country on either side of me and trying to avoid the worst of the dust-cloud that enveloped me every time a car passed the other way. Much worse was the occasional cloud that I came upon from behind. It meant that something moving slower than me was ahead. Extra caution was needed, not only to avoid rear-ending somebody, but to ensure that anything coming against me would know I was there. Overtaking was something of a lottery, unless there happened to be a crosswind right at the point of passing, so that the plume of red powder was wafted to the side, away from the oncoming traffic.

I passed groves of banana, coffee, and the occasional roadside flat-topped thorn. After Embu the road turned to sand and gravel, dry and dusty but luckily fairly wide. Having learned from others the previous year, I instinctively put my hand on the windshield each time an approaching car came past. This was supposed to prevent the glass from shattering if hit by a flying stone, although I am not sure how effective it really was, as I was never hit. I had opted to take the low road, as the alternative through Chuka had a fearsome reputation for its hundreds of hairpin bends, and I had had enough of eating dust around curves for one day.

Here, there was nothing in the way of agriculture except a few straggly native pea plants alongside the two or three rivers that were crossed by the road. Every now and again I would pass a herd of gaunt humped cattle, and once a group of zebra exploded in a cloud of dust as I surprised them round a bend. There was little traffic, but after about an hour I was almost pushed off the road by a heavily overloaded Land Rover driving at breakneck speed, bearing nothing but bundles of green leaves.

After passing the yellow-and-black sign marking the equator, I arrived in Meru at about tea-time. From the bridge over the Kazita River

I saw the sign to my hotel. The Ministry had booked me in for a ten-day stay at the Pig and Whistle.

I pulled up alongside a long wooden bungalow with its pale brown *mabati* (corrugated iron) roof, the rails on the verandah needing a new coat of white paint. Stiff from the three-and-a-half-hour drive, I climbed the rather rickety steps towards a sign that said Reception. As I reached the top step, a dapper Asian man whom I had not noticed sat up in his armchair and said, "Good afternoon. How may I be helping?"

"Hello. I hope you have a room for me. My name is Jerry Haigh. I'm the new District Veterinary Officer."

"Oh yes indeed. I'm Sadru Din. Call me Sadru. We thought you would be here in the morning. You are most welcome. Your room is over there, cabin number six." He pointed to a dark-coloured cabin across a flower bed full of roses in several colours and garish yellow and red canna lilies. The bed was surrounded by whitewashed stones that made up a roundabout in front of the main building.

"If you care to park your car over there I will send someone to help you unload. After a while we will be having tea here on the verandah. Water is hot if you are needing shower."

The Pig and Whistle had been a well-known Kenya watering spot before and during the war years, but had fallen on hard times during the Mau Mau emergency years in the fifties. Sadru had bought it, reputedly for a song, and had refurbished the interior, leaving the character of the buildings intact. The main building housed a few rooms and the bar and dining room. In a semi-circle with their backs to the river stood the half dozen wooden guest cabins. The gardens were full of bougainvillaea, several colours of canna lilies, and moonflower. Huge trees, remainders of the forest that had stood before the town was developed, stood guard away from the road. Poinsettias provided their gaudy colours around the buildings, and there were jacarandas, bottle brushes, and even a lofty palm. One tall tree near the entrance was almost lost in a blaze of magenta where a bougainvillaea had climbed up at least 40 feet and was slowly taking over.

"You have picked a good day to arrive," said Sadru at tea-time. "Tonight is a club night. After tennis there will be many people coming and you can meet them."

We sat in peaceful repose, listening to the sounds of the river as it crashed through the narrow gorge just above the bridge, and the various bird noises from all around us. Most striking was the cooing of a dove whose repetitive sound reminded me of nothing more than its distant cousin, the wood pigeon of Europe. It was strange to think that I had been flighting them into a small wood of oaks in the Scottish border country just north of Lockerbie only a few days before.

I decided to miss out on the tennis, and instead try to wash off the layers of red road dust that had crept into every crease of my skin, as well as what hair I had. After that, ten minutes before dusk was due to make its usual brief appearance before full tropical dark, Sadru and I headed about three hundred yards up the hill and turned into a gravel lot where several cars were parked.

Four hardy souls were still hitting the ball about on the nearer of the two red murram courts, and I could hear the muffled cracks of a squash ball hitting a wall, interspersed with the squeak of shoes as the players moved around. There were about 20 people in the main room, which had a bar in the corner, and a snooker table on the left. The tennis players followed us in through the glass doors.

The usual introductions were made, most of the names flying by in a blur. I knew that I would have to go at the task of memorizing them more slowly. Sadru demanded a membership form from the barman and proceeded to fill it out after he had ordered up four bottles of Tusker: one for me, one for himself, one for a slim gangly Englishman with a slight squint whom he introduced as Tim Roberts, and the last for a shorter, dark-haired man, Jim Black.

"Tim is a livestock officer. He is staying at the Mulika Coffee Hotel until he finds accommodation. Jim is with the forestry department, he lives in the Forestry Officer's house."

"Hello Tim, Jim. Good to meet you both. It seems we're in the same line of work, Tim. I'm the new veterinary officer."

"Good to meet you Jerry," he replied, a trace of an English west country burr in his accent. "How did you get to Meru?"

"Oh, I did an internship at Kabete last year, and then I went to the ODA in the UK and applied to come back. They posted me here from headquarters."

"Sorry, I didn't mean how in that sense. I meant which road did you take?"

"Oh, I'm sorry. I took the bottom road out of Embu. I was nearly pushed off the road by a Land Rover going full tilt near a place called Mitungu. It had a huge pile of green leaves in the back — they looked like banana leaves."

"Oh, that's almost certainly a truck load of *mira'a* heading for Nairobi. They wrap the bundles of leaf in banana leaves for transportation. You want to watch out for those fellows, they're worse than the *matatus* (local taxis). Only last week a child was killed by one just below town here."

"*Mira'a*, what's that?" I asked

"It's a crop that grows on the north slopes of the Nyambeni hills, out thataway," he said, pointing out of the window into the now-dark sky. "It's also called *quatt* in some countries. Those who own trees can get rich quickly. They fight feuds about single trees when someone dies. The freshly cut twigs, with their few leaves, are chewed by people all over the Middle East, Ethiopia, and Somalia, creating all sorts of problems as addicts lose any sense of responsibility. The leaves are apparently no good unless fresh, and so twice a week a mass of vehicles leave Meru for Nairobi. The drivers take no account of other traffic, or even pedestrians. The airport is their sole goal."

Tim's words proved prophetic. Four years later, when I was away from Meru on leave, a *mira'a* driver smashed into the back of his Land Rover at high speed. Tim ended up in Meru hospital, his food being brought to him over rough roads by a friend, as the hospital did not provide any meals.

After a couple of beers I headed down the hill for some supper.

There was another white man staying at hotel, but he seemed rather distant, only nodding as I walked into the dining room. He and the woman with him were elegantly, although casually, dressed and both wore expensive silk scarves, his as a cravat, hers around her shoulders and held with a clasp that looked very much like a cluster of diamonds. Later Sadru told that he was an Austrian count named Frans-Joseph Windisch-Grätz, who had a house in Langata and who had come to Meru every year for several years.

"He comes up just after Christmas to shoot the green pigeons that fly every morning and evening to and from their roosting sites and the wild olives trees lower down the slopes. He stands in the bushes at the roadside and shoots them as they fly over. The lady is his sister-in-law."

Sadru managed to put the "sister-in-law" in discreet quotations, with a slight raising of his eyebrows.

I chatted with the couple a few evenings later as we drank an after-dinner coffee in the lounge.

"It is most annoying," said Windisch-Grätz. "One of my Purdeys has developed a fault, so I will have to use the Holland and Hollands for the next few days. The season is almost over so it will not be a great hardship." Somewhat akin to exchanging the Rolls Royce for the Daimler, I thought to myself.

At our next encounter he said, "This year I have only shot 6,001 pigeons."

Trying to hide my surprise, I asked, "How do you know the total so exactly?"

"Oh, I employ several small boys to pick up each bird and put it in a drum. Then I count the birds to see that they have picked them all up. I know what I have killed because I count them as I shoot."

"Are they any good to eat?" I asked.

"I do not know, I have never tried one," he said in his slightly stilted English.

Later I heard that he had been discovered some years prior somewhere in the Northern Frontier District by George Adamson, then game warden at Isiolo, with a huge pile of sand grouse, which he had killed in a one-hour period as they flighted into the water holes in a *lugga* (stream bed, normally dry most of the time). George had successfully brought charges of overhunting against him, and a limit of 25 sand grouse had then been instituted. Windisch-Grätz (Windy-scratch as we called him) used to go directly from Meru to Arusha in Tanzania for the sole purpose of shooting sand grouse there. Perhaps they did not have a limit.

Another story about him emerged later. One year he had had trouble finding enough pigeons, so he had tried his hand at dove shooting high up on the slopes above Timau. One afternoon had been enough. His success rate had fallen below his usual 90% or so, and he had not returned.

Even stranger, over 30 years later I saw a photo of him, standing in a typical gun-in-hand pose, at the entrance to three rooms dedicated to his collection of African big game trophies in a Hungarian castle. Apart from the considerable variety of species involved, I was struck by the total head count. There was evidence of half a dozen rhino that had fallen to his gun, as well as several specimens of each of the big cats. Strangest of all, and a testament to his mania for sheer numbers were the horns and skulls of at least a couple of dozen Grant's gazelles, and a similar number of Thomson's gazelles.

There have been examples of rapacious hunters throughout the ages on many continents, most of them gaining in killing efficiency as weapons and technology improved. Some had commercial or political motives, such as ivory hunters in Africa, or bison hunters in North

America, who killed millions of animals for their tongues (sold to restaurants), bones, or, reportedly, to deprive native people of their resources. I had never met or heard of a hunter who seemed to see shooting simply as a numbers game.

CHAPTER 7

THE LUCKY VET

*My first case in the new district is a success. I begin to learn
the names of local villages and attend a meeting where the slow
pace of translation proves to be a boon.*

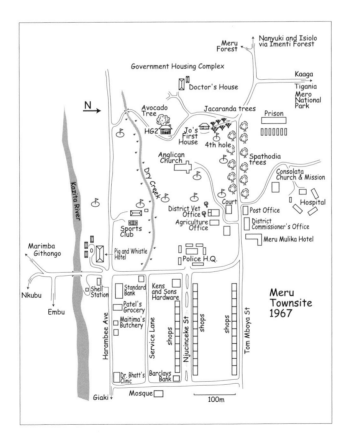

I HAD NOT EVEN HAD TIME TO meet my new staff when my first client turned up. A short, slightly tubby, very efficient laboratory technician, whose name I soon found out was Vitalis Kirimania, had the task of greeting clients and hearing their concerns. He knocked, stepped into my office and said, "Excuse me sir, but this farmer, Mr. Ntima, has a sick cow. He needs help."

"What's the problem?" I asked. Vitalis turned to the farmer, who stood behind him in the waiting room, and said something in Kimeru — the local language, which I had not yet learned.

"*Jambo mzee*," I said to Mr. Ntima, and repeated my question in Swahili.

"*Jambo bwana*," he responded, following with a long stream of more Kimeru directed at Vitalis.

"Say it in Swahili," I interjected when he paused.

"My cow gave birth yesterday and then fell down after the calf had sucked. I think she wants to die. Can you come and see?"

"Mr. Ntima, wait a little. I will find some drugs and we will come in the Land Rover."

Vitalis told me that there were a variety of drugs available in the store and that the official driver was free to take me to the farm. We put whatever equipment we had into the Land Rover with its Government of Kenya plates, GK 881, and the driver in his beige uniform got up behind the wheel. Land Rover seats are fairly high off the ground, and he was a short, rotund man, so for him it was a bit of a climb. The farmer piled into the back among the equipment.

The driver's Swahili had a different sound than that of either Vitalis or the farmer, and when he introduced himself I knew that he was not from Meru.

"Jambo bwana," he said. "I am called Kipsiele. Kipsiele arap Kurgat." He emphasized the "r" in the third part just like a Scot would.

By the name, I knew him to a member of the Kalenjin group of tribes from western Kenya. Many men from these tribes had served with my father in the King's African Rifles during the war. Here was a chance to put some more phrases from Dad's foolscap sheet into practice. I still had it in my luggage, although I had not often referred to it as my Swahili had improved. One of the phrases that he had remembered had been a greeting in Kipsigis, the language of one of the Kalenjin tribes.

"Ajamage mising," I responded. This is roughly equivalent to an enthusiastic "Howdy."

We quickly established that this was virtually the limit of my knowledge of his tongue, but the ice had been broken. He later taught me how to say goodbye in Kipsigis: *Sai sere.* Kipsiele was from the same tribe as Kipchoge Keino, who was the first and most famous of the phenomenal string of famous Kenyan long- and middle-distance runners who have won athletic medals all over the world. Kip Keino, as he was known, was the first Kenyan to win an Olympic gold medal, and set the standards for all those who followed. Kipsiele, however, was no Kip Keino. About 5' 6", round as a barrel, and quite unlikely to be seen running anywhere, he was the most cheerful person I have ever worked with.

The farm was no great distance from the office, and the history that I had obtained from the farmer had already given me a strong inkling as to what might be wrong. Once I saw that the cow was a Guernsey, I felt even more sure that the diagnosis was probably a condition called milk fever. This occurs when the demands of producing milk suddenly deprive the blood of its calcium. Without calcium the muscles cannot work, and the nervous system shuts down. The Channel Island breeds are particularly susceptible.

As I examined the cow, I became convinced. Her ears, lower legs, and feet were quite cold.

The problem was the length of time that the cow had been down. My education in Glasgow, and experience as an intern, had taught me that milk fever is a genuine emergency requiring treatment within an hour or two. This cow had calved the previous day and had been down since early afternoon. The elapsed time was about 20 hours. Not only were her extremities cold, but her pulse was exceedingly slow, and her eyes unresponsive to touch.

Forgetting for the moment that fools rush in where angels fear to tread, and realizing that, like many of his neighbours, this man had only a very small number of cows, and much of his wealth tied up in them, I decided to try the standard treatment: a calcium injection. Normally this injection would be given slowly, directly into the jugular vein, and the cow could be expected to be up and about very quickly. However, this was far from a normal case. The risks of a sudden return towards normal calcium levels in the blood were considerable. A slow rise would make more sense.

"I'm going to give the cow two injections. The first one will go under the skin, and we'll see what happens. Then I'll give another one into her neck if she needs it," I told the farmer.

The first injection took about 15 minutes, and a grapefruit-sized bulge appeared under the skin behind her shoulder. The cow showed no visible response. However, her pulse rate increased very slightly, and I fancied, perhaps with wishful thinking, that the sounds of her heart through the stethoscope were slightly louder. The second bottle went into the vein, also very slowly. After this I had to turn my attention back to her shoulder, where the fluid from the first injection had not completely disappeared. To get rid of the lump I used the empty bottle as a rolling pin. Calcium salts sting rather sharply. The cow had by now decided that she was going to wake up. The pain that I was inflicting in her side caused her to kick. With a couple of thrashes she rolled onto her belly, took one look at me, and decided that enough was enough. Up she got, starting to graze almost at once.

It would be hard to gauge who was more delighted, the farmer for this apparent miracle, or the newly arrived veterinary officer. What luck to have such a case as a first challenge in a new district!

Kibirichia, Githongo, Nkubu, Kithirune, Kirua, Kaaga, Michimukuru, Karienne. The names, spoken in the musical tones of Kimeru the local language, trip from the tongue like tinkling bells. At first, they meant no more to me than words on the large-scale district map, but soon they began to develop real identities.

I traveled around the district almost every day for medical emergencies, routine visits and farmer's *barazzas* (meetings). The first *barazza* I attended took place in the village of Kirua and I really had no idea what to expect.

Kipsiele and I traveled up the bumpy road together in GK 881. Daniel Gatururu, the animal health technician for the area, had told us to be there at ten o'clock.

"Where are all the people?" I asked him in Swahili as he emerged from the coffee shop in the middle of a row of the stores that stood around three sides of the market square. I had forgotten about the difference between "real" time and "African" time.

"They're late. Come for some tea." Without voicing it we established that my Swahili was better than his English, so we continued in that language.

We entered the cafe, passing behind a partition that screened out the scene of the market-place, and found ourselves in a small room painted eggshell blue to waist height, and what had probably once been white, but was now spotted cream, above. Two life-size human figures, a man and a woman, had been boldly drawn on the white, giving the whole place a cheerful look. Although the style could only be called raw, it was distinctly African, a sort of modern version of Gauguin, without the softly muted shading.

A young man appeared and, in Kimeru, Gatururu ordered something. I recognized the words *chai*, meaning tea, and *samosa*, the delicious spiced pastry of Indian origin. In fact both words are from the Hindi, as are many in Swahili. These two had made the jump from Swahili to yet another language. Like English, with its lexicon borrowed from dozens of languages, Kiswahili is a "mongrel" language, created over time as Arab merchants met Bantu-speaking Africans of the Swahili people on the continent's eastern coast. The language changes as one travels inland through Kenya and Uganda. By the time one reaches Rwanda, Burundi, and the eastern parts of countries in the basin of the Congo river, elements of other languages, even Portuguese, have displaced words used on the coast.

The refreshments came, the *samosas* as expected, the tea hardly recognizable. It had been made by boiling a few leaves with both milk and water. Kipsiele and Gatururu ladled generous dollops of sugar into theirs.

"When will people come?" I asked Gatururu. "What about the chief?"

"Soon," he replied.

"At what time?" I asked, well aware that "soon," like "not far," was a typically evasive response that could be used with great flexibility. It all depended upon what the informant thought one wanted to hear. This didn't seem to be meant as a deception so much as a matter of courtesy, a way of saying something positive instead of the expressive *sijui*, meaning "I don't know."

"By eleven or eleven-thirty."

I was not amused, but there was little I could do. We fell to discussing the weather and the chances for a good crop. Farmers the world over have the same concerns. Half an hour later, I stood and looked out of the door. There still seemed to be no organized gathering, but the number of people in the square had substantially increased. Then Gatururu greeted a small group of men as they approached the restaurant. Switching to Swahili, he told me, *"Bwana*, this is Chief John. He is the chief of Kirua location and he says that we can start the meeting."

"Good morning, Chief," I said. "What news?"

He in turn introduced half a dozen other men as deputy chiefs and similar officers. The names went by too quickly for me, but a handshake and a formal *"Jambo mzee"* seemed sufficient.

We walked over to a row of chairs that had been set out on the grass and sat down, the chief in the middle, me on his immediate right. There were already about 60 people sitting facing the chairs, and the milling group in the square soon moved over and joined us. One or two of them came up to the front and joined us as more chairs were quickly found. One I recognized as Bernard, who was the animal health technician of the neighbouring village of Kibirichia. Then came the introductions, all in Kimeru. I understood only the polite clapping after each name was announced.

Gatururu acted as master of ceremonies and also interpreter. This was definitely a veterinary department *barazza*.

At first things were slow, as we explained the artificial breeding program that was being extended to the area and the farmers haggled over the most convenient time for the service to be carried out. Much of the discussion was again in Kimeru, and I wondered why I had been asked to attend. The answer was not long in coming. As I sat in a bit of a daze, not really concentrating on the proceedings, I suddenly realized that I was being addressed in Swahili.

"The government is going to send motorcycles to the crushes to service our cows," said a tall man who stood about halfway back in the crowd. "This is good, but how will we know that we have not missed them when we bring our cattle? Surely we should be allowed to keep a bull, so that if we miss the man at the crush we can still be sure that our cattle get pregnant."

Before I could respond, Gatururu said to me, "*Bwana*, there are some people who do not speak Swahili here, so I think I should translate to Kimeru." I nodded.

Choosing to ignore the fact that the motorcycles would not actually be doing the inseminations, I told the tall man, "There are two things to answer here. First, the matter of the time. We will instruct the" — I struggled to find a Swahili word for "inseminator," but failed — "the man who serves the cows that he will have to be at each crush until a certain time. He will not leave until that time has been reached." I paused to let the translation go ahead, then continued. "If the time for the crush below Kirua is ten o'clock in the morning, then even if he arrives at nine o'clock and finds no cattle present, he must wait until ten o'clock. In that way you will know how things will be, and you can leave home with your cow that is on heat in plenty of time. Now are there any questions about that matter?"

"What happens if a cow comes on heat just after the inseminator has passed?" a woman sitting near the front asked in Kimeru. Again the pause as the words were translated for me.

"Then the cow must be brought on the next day. It is better to serve a cow after she has been on heat for at least half a day, so if your cow comes in heat in the afternoon she should be served next morning."

After this was translated, I looked around the crowd and went on, "The matter of the bulls is a matter of the County Council laws. It is illegal to have a bull with his testicles present if he is over six months of age in areas where there are grade cattle. This ensures that only good semen will be used. Think how you would feel if you were taking your cow that wants a bull to the crush and a *shenzi* bull jumped her. You would be very cross." *Shenzi* is a most useful word which means "of low quality," and can be applied to almost anything.

Other important subjects were disposed of, particularly the matter of tick control, and then Gatururu asked if anyone had specific questions for the new *daktari* (direct from the English "doctor"). The first two, concerning lame animals, were easy. I made appointments to call at specific crushes over the next few days. Then a woman in the front row caused a slow chuckle in the crowd as she asked about a problem cow. Gatururu translated the Kimeru for me.

"She has a cow that keeps running away. It breaks her fence. She has tried improving the fence around her *shamba* (small farm). She has even made a wooden yoke around the animal's neck. Still it gets out almost daily and eats the vegetables in her neighbour's farms. What should she do?"

As the question was rendered sentence by sentence into Kimeru, I had the chance to do some thinking. There didn't seem to be any obvious magic solution.

"Tell her to buy a long rope," I began.

Gatururu translated this, and before I could go any further, the chuckle in the crowd turned into a happy laugh, led by the questioner. Sometimes the slow pace of translation can be a real boon. I was reminded of my response on many later occasions when I visited the area.

CHAPTER 8

HG2

*A new old house, a kindred fisherman soul, a sick pig,
and a life-altering meeting.*

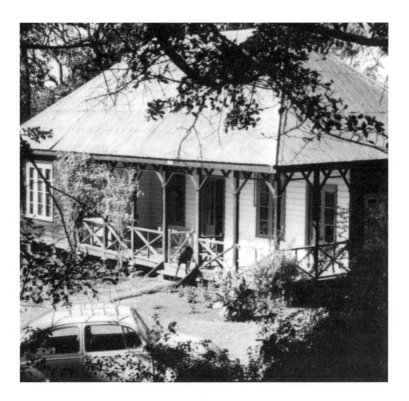

HG2, home for two years for two bachelors.

WITHIN A WEEK I WAS informed by the District Commissioner that there was no house available for me unless I was willing to share accommodation. Fortunately, by then Tim and I had discovered that we had enough in common to become friends. At the club, over a game of snooker, we agreed to double up.

Tim moved out of the coffee hotel, and I moved up from the Pig and Whistle. We were assigned an old dark-stained, tin-roofed wooden house, prosaically named HG2 (presumably it was the second government house built in the compound); this was painted on a board near the gate. The main feature of the house was an enormous avocado-pear tree that towered over it and seemed to produce fruit almost non-stop.

A slight, brown-skinned African bearing a somewhat sweat-stained letter appeared like a wraith at the gate within a day of our arrival. We had not advertised that we were searching for a cook, but the word had got out, and since the letter stated that Stanley Thambura had worked as the writer's houseboy for three years, we took him on. He proved well able to deal with the needs of a couple of bachelors.

One evening, as Tim and I sat on the verandah enjoying the last of the light, a stranger walked into the garden.

"Good evening. Would either of you be Jerry Haigh at all?"

His accent at once identified him as an Irishman. He was slim, with graying hair, no more than about five foot eight inches tall, and his metal-rimmed glasses framed a pair of piercing pale blue eyes.

"You must be Dr. O'Callaghan the new medical officer. Sadru told me about you. Good evening."

"Call me Fin, short for Finbar. Nobody uses the full handle, unless it's Lorna, my wife, when she's cross with me. When might you be free to do a little fishing? I understand you know the local spots."

"I'm free most evenings after work. Usually about five o'clock. Would tomorrow or the next day suit you?"

"Tomorrow would be fine, but I don't usually get away from the hospital until after five-thirty. Is that still feasible?"

"Yes, I don't see why not. I'll wait for you here."

We headed up the road to a spot on a government farm called Marimba where the river had been dammed and some administrator from times past, obviously a kindred soul, had stocked trout. I had made some spectacular catches there, including a four-pound rainbow. The most amazing time to be there was between six-forty and five to seven in the evening. As the light disappeared behind the rounded hill above the farm, the water looked as if it was beginning to boil. There seemed to be six fish rising at any one moment. Even in the dark, the sound of rising fish could still be heard.

When we got back to town, Fin showed me a new and much improved method of examining the food items of our quarry.

"You cut open the stomach and put the contents in a glass of water. Then pour the water off very carefully and put the last drops together with the contents on to a piece of blotting paper, or failing that the edge of a newspaper," he said as he demonstrated over his kitchen sink, while Lorna looked on with raised eyebrows, but no comment. No doubt she had acquired the thick skin needed to deal with avid fishermen.

We had many successful trips to the dams over the next couple of years. I learned that Fin was a medical graduate from County Cork, and a classic Irishman: loquacious, enthusiastic, entertaining, and seemingly inexhaustible. If one was to believe every one of his fishing anecdotes, one would have had to wonder how he ever got into medical school, let alone graduated. His stories were by no means limited to fishing. Once, he recounted that years earlier, in the office of an older practitioner from whom he was learning his skills, there had been a sign posted that read: "Examinations sixpence, use of the tubes, sixpence extra." As the proto-type instrument was invented by French physician Rene Laënnec in 1781, this sign must have been kept by Fin's boss as a relic of times gone by. No doubt the MRI of its day, the stethoscope must have been the latest gizmo to reach the rural County Cork when the sign went up.

Some mornings, as I walked into the office early, a farmer would be there ahead of me waiting under the pepper tree that threw its shade over the building. This morning there were two.

"*Hamjambo wazee.*" ("Good morning old men" — the plural form of the universal polite greeting.) "What's the news?"

"Good morning Doctor. The news is good. But my pig is sick," said the shorter of the two.

"What sickness?" I asked.

"She is not eating, and her skin is red."

"We'll come and see her. Wait a little until we get things ready and we will go together." Turning to the other man I asked, "What is your problem?"

"I gave my cow her medicine for bad milk this morning and she became sick straightaway. She is a bit better now, but I saw my neighbour Frederick" — he gestured to the first man with his chin — "coming with a taxi and we decided to come together." The second farmer was named Erasto Twerandu.

At that moment Tim came round the corner, greeted Frederick and asked after his farm. Tim explained that Frederick had just won the Agricultural Department's annual competition for best farmer in Kibirichia for the second straight year. His reward had been an abandoned neighbouring property, which had increased his single holding to about 20 acres, double the average for the area.

We piled into the Land Rover about half an hour later, and after a bumpy 40-minute ride, stood looking over the stall at a large, unhappy pig. Red splotches about the size of a playing card were scattered all over its body, and the tips of its ears were bright red. The feed in its trough had not been touched. I climbed into the pen after Frederick assured me it was a quiet animal. The temperature was elevated, and the skin hot to the touch. It looked like a classic case of diamond disease, or by its Sunday name, erysipelas.

"I'm going to give this pig an injection, and I'll leave *dawa* with you for more injections for the next four days. Even if the pig gets better quickly, every injection must be given. Tell Bernard that I've said this, so that he can come each day and give the injections."

Now there was time to admire the farm. There were three large sows in a pen together, and one on her own with her piglets. The rest of the property resembled half a bowl. The upper parts were steeply sloped and the contour terracing had been carefully maintained. A small herd of Guernseys was grazing contentedly up on the slope, and many rows of neatly weeded vegetables were laid between: cabbages, onions, potatoes, peas. These were cash crops, and brought a steady income when shipped to market. Napier grass was flourishing along all the contour ridges, and a young man was cutting bunches of it and bringing them down to the dairy. A hedge of large, bright yellow, daisy-like flowers indicated the boundary. On the newly acquired plot a crop of pyrethrum was just coming into flower, and half-grown maize stalks covered a couple of acres. Frederick was one of the many Kenyans entering the new "middle class."

Next on the agenda was a cup of tea, which it would have been churlish to refuse, and during this break Bernard, the animal health technician (AHT) for the area, walked in. I explained to him about his responsibilities with the pig and asked him to keep an eye on the other pigs in case they showed anything like the same signs. I also mentioned that the germ that caused the red patches might also make people sick, and stressed the importance of hygiene and keeping children away from the sick animal.

Turning to Frederick as we walked back to the car, I said, "When the pig is better, you should clean out her pen. Dig up all the dirt, leave the pen empty, with the sun shining on the ground for a week before you put any animals in there. Use the manure for cabbages. Don't put it on the Napier grass or anyplace where the cattle will be eating."

We left Frederick and his family after a sackful of carrots, cabbage, and potatoes, which he insisted we accept, had been placed in the back of the Land Rover. This generosity was typical. It had nothing to do with the fee, and there was no implied bribery or pressure to return. We proceeded up a narrow track to the next farm. Half a dozen mixed-breed cows were grazing contentedly. Erasto pointed out the black-and-brown Jersey cross that had been the problem early that morning.

"Her milk went bad last year, and I went to the office and got some of this *dawa*," he said, showing me a used tube of intramammary penicillin. *Dawa* is an all-important word understood in Swahili and virtually all tribal languages. It means medicine, whether for animals or people. It can even be applied to crop spray or topical substances used to control pests.

"She got better, but when she gave birth this year her milk was bad again. I got the same *dawa* from Vitalis and gave it to her yesterday. Almost at once she started to breathe very fast and all her hair stood up on end. What should I do? The milk is still bad."

Although penicillin allergy is a common enough problem in people, I had never heard of it in cattle. However, one is always learning, and the solution seemed simple. I exchanged his remaining tubes of mastitis ointment for a different type, but more importantly, at his request, I wrote him a note explaining the problem. As he pointed out, I might be transferred long before his cow died, and he wanted a record to show to any future doctors or Animal Health Technicians.

We were only about five miles from Marania. At a recent rugby practice I'd met Frank Douglas, manager of the first large-scale farm on the way to Nanyuki, and he had generously invited me to drop by, so Kipsiele and I set off *pole pole* (slow, or slowly) up the hill. Frank was standing in the driveway next to another veterinary department vehicle. From the passenger seat stepped a short, red-haired man dressed in khaki shorts and a golf shirt. Frank introduced him as Kieran Kane, the District Veterinary Officer for Nanyuki district, who was there to respond to a call about a sick bull. They had just finished dealing with the patient and were moving off up to Frank's house for a bite of lunch. With typical rural Kenyan hospitality, they invited us to join them; afterwards, we dropped back down to the yards and met Frank's employers, George and Irralie Murray.

Several large dogs ran up to greet us; one in particular caught my eye. Her head had a savage scar from the eye backwards over the skull. I stroked it, asking her, as one foolishly does, "Hello my girl, what happened to you?"

"Oh," responded George, "that's Carrah, she's got quite a story. She was stupid enough to run under the whirring prop of my plane about two months ago, and it caught her. Knocked her cold. I bundled her into the back of the pick-up, got Irralie to radio to Nanyuki, and took her to Kieran."

Kieran picked up the tale, his Irish brogue not as thick as Fin's. "She arrived in my office still unconscious. I clipped back the hair, cleaned out the bone chips and discovered that the dura" — for Irralie's benefit he added, "the delicate membrane surrounding the brain" — "had not been damaged. The right eye was utterly destroyed. There was only one thing to try. I cleaned up the skin edges, put some antibiotic into the wound, and stitched it back together as best as I could. I never gave her any anesthetic and she slept on for about four hours before recovering. I kept her in overnight, and sent her home."

"She's never looked back," said Irralie, "but she's no smarter around machinery."

In a small community like Meru, there was not much chance to meet new people. Being a bachelor had its downside, unless one was inclined to visit the fleshpots of Nairobi in search of a much more active social life. A pretty face was always likely to cause heads to turn. One morning while walking to the municipal offices to settle our water bill, I ran into Fin's wife Lorna. With her was an attractive brunette, her hair in a ponytail.

"Good morning Jerry," said Lorna. "Beautiful day again. I'd like you to meet Joanne van de Riet. She's just arrived as a new medical officer to help Fin and Subash at the hospital. Jo, this is Jerry, the district veterinary officer."

"Well that's good to hear. How do you do? Welcome to Meru."

"We were just trying to get Joanne organized in her new house. It's the newish brick one just above the fourth green. We're here hoping to get them to open up the water supply so that she can move in."

"Will we see you at the club this evening?" I asked Joanne. "If you play tennis, we have a mix-in. One set, first to six games, and then change partners."

"Oh thank you, that would be fun. What time?" she asked.

"'Bout five."

"Why don't you come and have a bite to eat with us after tennis?" said Lorna, perhaps sensing a spark. "Then you can have a bit more of a chat."

On and off through the day, I tried to figure out where Joanne might be from. Her accent was a bit of a puzzle. It was almost completely devoid of any of the characteristic lilts or phrases of any of the European countries, and only after listening for a while could one detect that it was not a BBC English. It had none of the hard edges of an Afrikaner accent, although her name might be South African.

At dinner, for which she had changed into a smart tartan dress and put her hair up in a French roll, accentuating her slim features, I learned more of Jo's history. The accent was soon explained, although only after she had kept us guessing for a while with an impish smile.

"Well, I was born in Poona (now Pune), India. My parents are Dutch. My dad went out to India in 1935 with Philips. I did all my high schooling in India, and went to medical college at Vellore Christian Medical College. After that I went to Holland for a year and began to study in paediatrics, and then had a year in Zambia as a rotating intern."

"How did you get to Kenya?" I asked.

"Just stopped in at Nairobi, as I had been told it was worth a visit. Then I took a tour bus organized by the hotelier."

Being by that point broke, and having particularly enjoyed Nairobi National Park, she walked into the Ministry on the Monday morning and made herself known. Within a week she was squeezed in between two staff members in the front of a government Land Rover, on her way to Meru to join Fin at the district hospital.

CHAPTER 9

MOBILE CROCKERY

*A blossoming romance, perceptive cooks, an unusual way
to lose a needle, and my first rhino case.*

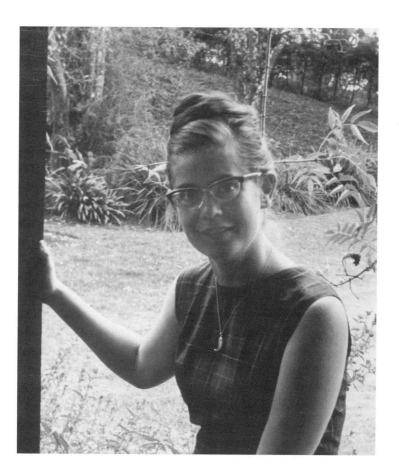

A favourite portrait. Jo on the verandah at HG2.

UNLIKE ME, JO WAS SOON granted a house on her own. However, having arrived in Kenya with only 40 pounds of luggage, the limit permitted by the airline, she had no crockery, cooking pots, or anything of the kind. A government clerk allowed her to borrow the bare necessities from stores — a battered collection of plastic and cheap china bits and pieces of varying sizes and a couple of dented aluminum saucepans. The dull-green plates and cups had no visible pattern, other than old tea stains and cigarette burn marks.

Jo and I often met at the weekly Tuesday night tennis mix-ins, and at the post office, and other places around town. She would greet me from the front garden of her house as we putted out on the fourth green. As we got to know each other, she also made trips to Marimba and even tried her hand with the fly rod.

Others in the community must have seen what was happening even before we did. One evening, at dinner in her house, I noticed that she had acquired a new floral water jug.

"Funny," I said, picking up and turning it to get a better look, "did you get that water jug here in town? I don't remember it from last time. We've got one just like it."

"I don't know, the cook just put it on the table," she replied.

A couple of nights later this conversation was repeated, this time because there was a matching set of china plates and bowls on the table that resembled those in HG2. The occasion was a local celebration of the Dutch Queen's official birthday, so other Hollanders were present and I had been made an honorary Dutchman for the evening. Henk Faberij de Jonge, a trim dark-haired volunteer with a Laughing Cavalier beard and a cheery temperament to match his appearance, was naturally a fellow guest. He turned one of the dishes over and said, "Jerry, these plates are like yours. I wonder from where they are coming." As Juma, Jo's cook, came in with the main course I asked him, in Swahili, which Jo had yet to master, about the new bits and pieces.

"Oh *bwana*, it's easy. I went to your cook and borrowed them when I heard that the *memsahib* had invited you to dinner. They are much smarter than the old *shenzi* green ones that she got from that Hindi clerk. I knew you wouldn't need them, as you were eating here, and so Stanley brought them down from your house this afternoon. Don't worry, I'll return them in the morning."

Another person who had some inkling of what was going on was Jo's father. Shortly after the dinner party, she wrote to him in Holland recounting the evening and her other current news, and mentioned in passing that there had been one non-Dutch guest: "a fortyish bald Scottish vet." He told us later how he had turned to Jo's mother and remarked that there might be something in the wind with Jopie (with a soft J), as she was known to her family. As it had during my early forays into African veterinary medicine and *barazzas* with farmers, where the cult of the young man had gained virtually no foothold, my bald head again served me well. When she wrote that letter, Jo had not yet discovered that I was only 28.

Upon his return from leave, Tim also noticed an unexpected change in the contents of our pantry at HG2. Formerly the only drinks present had been a couple of cases of Tusker, but now there were bottles of Fanta orange juice and a case of pop.

■

Jo's experience in India and Zambia stood her in good stead, but the caseload was heavy, with only three doctors to deal with up to eight hundred patients a day. A system had developed in which clinical assistants acted as front line troops and filtered out all the common complaints. If a patient obviously needed a direct referral beyond the first examination, or returned to the clinical assistants a number of times with the same complaint, they would eventually refer him for an afternoon appointment with the doctor. Malaria was rife in the district, and the symptoms described by the patients included intermittent fevers, chills, headaches, and general malaise.

One day Jo and I were discussing the apparently recidivist malaria patients who would keep coming back, the chloroquine that they had been given proving ineffective. "Even when they are fevered, we can't find any parasites in the blood smears," said Jo.

"The symptoms sound awfully like undulant fever. It seems to me that medical schools are a bit lax when it comes to zoonotic diseases — those transmitted from animals to man. Brucellosis is quite common in cattle round here; that's one reason why we boil our milk. Why don't you send some blood samples off to the lab to test for brucella?" I suggested.

The first two came back positive, so now Jo could try a course of antibiotics as a treatment when blood smears proved negative.

■

Jo and I began spending many weekends together, often going off together to see friends. We paid several visits to Peter Gamble, District

Veterinary Officer at Isiolo, and his wife Judi. Pete was about my height, but much less heavily built, and had two immediately noticeable characteristics. First, he was constantly pushing his glasses back onto the bridge of his nose, and second, his virtually complete lack of a backside made the impending and potentially indecorous descent of his trousers a constant risk. This was most evident when he broke into a canter on the Nyeri cricket ground as he ran in to bowl, with his shirt-tail flapping like a comet streak, and the top three inches of his bum-crack evident for all who cared to look.

Pete and Judi had come to Africa after the disastrous 1967 foot-and-mouth disease outbreak in the UK. Pete had been drafted right out of veterinary school into the control campaign, and after that was over the couple had suddenly found themselves in the vastly different world of Isiolo, gateway to Kenya's Northern Frontier District. One man, Johnson Mutiso, had rescued the greenhorns.

"That man just about saved our lives," Judi told us. "We arrived here after dark at about nine at night, having spent hours in town looking for directions. We'd only been in Africa about four days, and we were broke. Johnson let us into the house, and all there was were two filthy mattresses on the floor and a broken chair. Not another thing! The place was an absolute pigsty. A wood stove without a chimney pipe sat in the kitchen alcove, and the entire place was covered in a thick layer of black soot and grease. Johnson took one look and said, 'You'd better stay with us until we can get something done about this.'

"Within two days he had drafted about 45 herdsmen into a complete clean-up crew and had found enough paint for them re-do the whole house. He took us down to the government stores in town and stayed with us until they produced beds, chairs, tables, a new chimney pipe, and everything else we needed. He seemed to know what we were entitled to in a three-bedroom house, and didn't let the clerk give us the runaround. He even had herdsmen tidying up the garden, such as it is, and putting whitewash on the stones. He organized loads of firewood from the veterinary quarantine for both the kitchen and the water heater. Within five days you wouldn't have recognized the place."

On our first visit to the Gambles we arrived in time for a late tea, and then Pete said, "I've got to go up to a crush about five miles into the quarantine area before dark. The herdsman has reported a sick cow, so we could all go together for a bit of drive if you fancy it."

None of us needed a second invitation, although Judi, an attractive, petite Scottish border country blonde, was near the end of her first pregnancy and might find the bumpy road a trifle uncomfortable. We set off into the quarantine area, some 110,000 acres that lay behind the house and up into the hills to the west of the town. Although we were well outside any national park, we saw many giraffe, as well as zebras, and several mobs of impala, both as bachelor sets and in breeding groups dominated by a rutting buck. Most intriguing for Jo and Judi were the several pairs of tiny dik dik that peeked out at us from under thorn bushes before running off to disappear in the long grass. I was also much impressed by the very large numbers of both yellow-necked spur fowl and guinea fowl. The latter were vulturine guinea-fowl, whose bald heads were circled by a narrow ring of brown curly feathers that looked almost like a monk's tonsure. The brilliant blue of their breast feathers and the blue-and-white capes that flowed from mid-neck over their shoulders were quite magnificent.

We arrived at the crush, where a Boran herdsman had gathered a group of about 50 humped cattle. Pete asked me to request that he bring in the sick one, so after the usual greetings we were faced with a dun-coloured cow standing dejectedly at the front on the cattle crush. She was certainly sick. Her temperature was a sky-high 105.4, the pinkish membranes in her mouth and eyes were spotted with numerous red splashes, indicating a blood clotting deficit, and the lymph nodes in front of her shoulders and on her flanks were the size and consistency of large, slightly over-ripe mangoes. Normally these can barely be detected, and feel like hard little chipolata-sausage-sized lumps under the thick hide.

"This looks just like East Coast Fever, Pete. Have you got some slides?"

"I'm not so sure. It could be something else. It's possible, but as you say, let's take a couple of slides and we'll stain them back at the lab. Can you tell this fella what we're doing, and that we'll come back in the morning and see the cow? Ask him to keep the cattle nearby."

We made the slides by nicking the cow's ear and catching a drop of blood on the glass, and by grasping one of the large nodes through the skin and punching a wide-bore needle into the soft meaty part of it. A squeeze of the lump, and some bloody fluid emerged from the hub of the needle. A finger over the end, out with the needle, and we had enough material to make thin smears on several glass slides.

Later, a look at the slides proved Pete right. There was no sign of east coast fever, but there were at least half a dozen little spindle-shaped pale purple objects in each field under the high-powered lens of the microscope: Trypanosomes, the scourge of many parts of Africa. Some of the types of this parasite, usually spread by tsetse flies, cause sleeping sickness in humans and used to kill thousands of people in some parts of the continent every year, but this one was a little different. The species *Trypanosoma vivax* had adapted itself to transmission, not by the tsetse, but by several kinds of biting flies known collectively as horseflies.

The treatment was fortunately easy and likely to be effective, so it was a much better situation than if it had been a case of East Coast Fever. A single dose of a German drug called Berenil, a yellow powder mixed up in sterile water, would do the trick.

Several months passed, during which Jo and I spent many evenings, and most weekends, together. We fished at Marimba together, traveled together, talked medicine together, and made friends together. Curiosity had turned to respect. Sex appeal had been there from early on. Respect had remained but been enhanced by enchantment, which had turned to love. I could no longer contain myself, and after tennis on the evening of my birthday, I popped the question.

Jo thought for a moment, and said "I'll tell you on my birthday," which meant that I had to wait 19 days. I agreed to pick her up at lunch time on the day, and steeled myself to keep quiet and not pester her with repeats.

Late on the morning of Jo's birthday, a farmer arrived at the office with my old acquaintance Ntima, whose cow had made a dramatic recovery from milk fever a year before. This farmer's cow had developed signs of the same thing, and when Ntima had told him of the "miracle cure," he came immediately. We hopped into the Land Rover and drove the six miles to his farm. It was indeed a case of milk fever, which was soon remedied with a standard calcium injection, but the call had made me 20 minutes late for my all-important lunch date.

Jo was chatting to the hospital administrator, a Goan named Reuben Thomas, as I pulled up in the car. She got in, and sat in the passenger seat, not saying a thing. "Well?" I said nervously as we headed back along towards the post office.

"What happened?" she asked. I explained the situation and apologized.

"No wonder you were late. Yes, let's get married, but not until after I go to Holland to see my Mum and Dad."

When I asked her over dinner what had made her decide to take the plunge, she said, "I realized that I missed you." That case of milk fever may have played an important part in our future.

Mr. Thomas, when he heard of the engagement, said in his sing-song lilt, his head nodding from side to side, "It is karma. Marriages are surely made in heaven. Dr. Riet, you came from India, and you met your future husband-to-be in Meru of all places. Who would have thought it possible?"

The heady euphoria of our engagement was somewhat tempered by the fact that Jo had promised to go home to Holland in September to see her parents. The surprise for them was that she would not be returning to Rotterdam to complete her paediatrics specialty, but would instead be coming back to Kenya.

Setting a wedding date was another challenge. The most logical time seemed to be at the end of my current contract in January, and so we picked the 25th. Robbie Burns Night: appropriate enough for an ex-pat from Glasgow, whose father had served for years in the Highland Light Infantry. I would have no excuse in future for forgetting the anniversary.

Meanwhile there were routine cases, and more unusual ones. The routine could bring surprises. The artificial insemination scheme that we had started up at that first meeting almost two years ago in Kirua had blossomed. We were serving many cattle farmers around the district and we had a team of eight motorcycle riders, all on 100-cc bikes, heading out each morning to their designated cattle crushes to inseminate cattle. Naturally, we had to check accounts on a regular basis, as each insemination cost the farmer five shillings. Our figures seemed to be out of whack. Mr. Richard Muhoma, the livestock officer in charge of the day-to-day running of the scheme, had little trouble sorting out the discrepancy. One of our technicians had been pocketing his funds, instead of passing them on each week.

We sat over coffee and tried to decide on the best course of action. Mr. Muhoma was from western Kenya, and had the elegant good looks and the very dark skin of many of his Luo tribesmen.

"It looks as if Jonathan has taken 650 shillings for himself over the last three weeks. I don't know how he thought he would get away with it," he said.

"What do you suggest we do?"

"Of course what he has done is a criminal offence, and we would have no trouble proving it. However, I think you should have a word with him. His salary is just over two hundred a month, and we might be able to deal with it internally. He supports several brothers and sisters, as well as his mother, and his father is dead."

"OK," I said, "I'll see what I can do. You interview him first and confirm if what we have found is correct."

Next morning I called Jonathan into my office and made sure that all the doors were shut. He was tall and slim, with a receding hairline, unusual in a young Meru, and had dark brown, rather than black skin. He was understandably uncomfortable, and twisted an old bush hat in his hands as he stood in front of my desk. His English was good enough that we could stick to that language.

"Jonathan, I think you know what this is about. Why did you do something so foolish? You must have known you would be caught."

"I don't know, sir. I needed some money for my family, and I wasn't thinking."

"Well, what are we going to do with you? I should call the police, but Mr. Muhoma tells me that you are a good worker, and are also willing to pay the money back quickly. Is that right?"

"Yes sir."

"Jonathan, you will pay the whole sum back in six months. I'll cover for you by paying it into the books, and you will have to live on half salary. I will deduct the sum from your paycheck at the end of each month when I do the pay-outs. Mr. Muhoma and I have seriously considered charging you at the police station, but we have decided to give you one more chance. Don't betray our trust."

"Yes sir." He seemed dumbstruck. Perhaps he could not believe his good luck.

That evening I told Jo about the scene and she related a similar situation at the hospital. "Today we caught a male nurse diluting penicillin. He seemed to divide each vial into about ten doses and make off with the surplus that he accumulates."

"How did you catch him?" I enquired.

"Oh, Mr. Thomas found an imbalance in the stocks, and we made some enquiries in the male ward. We checked the nurse's coat when he went for lunch and found about 15 vials in his pocket. No wonder some of our infected patients don't seem to get better. They're only receiving minute doses."

"It's even worse than that. There must be all sort of resistant bacteria now," I responded.

Perhaps the male nurse was moonlighting on the side or selling his ill-gotten products to others. A newspaper headline a few years later caught our eyes: DOCTOR IN BEER HALL DRAMA. The story concerned a scene that could have come from a Keystone Cops movie. A man in a bar in Nkubu, a small town some ten miles south of Meru, had sought the services of an unlicensed medical practitioner. Based on a tip-off, a police raid had occurred as the patient was receiving his injection. The ensuing scene must have been chaotic and the dry tones of the article hardly did it credit. The "doctor" took off like a long dog and managed to get away. The patient ran out of the bar, forgetting that his trousers were at half-mast. He tripped and was easily apprehended, the syringe standing out as the highest point on his body.

One day, both Jo and I received lessons in the value of observation, keeping an eye out for unusual signs that could help in making a diagnosis.

That afternoon, Kipsiele and I were at the cattle crush at Githongo when a battered old Peugeot 404 van, in service as a taxi, pulled up on the roadside. The most unusual thing about the taxi was that there seemed to be only one passenger. It was more normal to see such a vehicle disgorge 15 or 20 people from its rear compartment, and three or four more from the front seat. I always wondered how the drivers of these wrecks had any control over the steering; with all the weight in the back, the front wheels seemed to be in the air.

The passenger, a stout woman wearing a well-worn bright cotton print dress and a head scarf, came through the gate, approached Kipsiele, and broke into a stream of Kimeru. I recognized the formal greeting of *"Muga,"* equivalent to the Swahili *"Jambo,"* and his response of *"Muga meukuru"* (Good morning old woman). Before she could go on he gestured to a nearby farmer and continued in Swahili.

"I do not speak enough Kimeru to help you. If you cannot speak Swahili perhaps this old man will help us."

Between us, we managed to sort out the fact that the woman had a valuable Guernsey cow that she was worried about.

"When it tries to walk it grunts with every step," she said, and demonstrated, deliberately placing one foot in front of the other. "Ugh! Ugh! Ugh! It seems to be in great pain. Yesterday it gave two gallons of milk, but this morning it gave no milk at all."

"You're in luck, we have just finished here and we can come with you. Where do you live?" I asked.

"Near Nkubu, just above the mission hospital."

"Good. We can go now. You can travel with us in the Land Rover. I do have one question. How did you find us?"

"I went to Meru town and they told me that you had gone to Githongo, so I got the taxi to bring me."

We cut across the path of the main arterial roads and dropped down to the winding hairpin-corner route between Meru and Nkubu. Most of the homes we passed were made from mud and wattle, and had grass-thatched roofs. An occasional sign of affluence was evident where *mabati*, corrugated iron sheeting, replaced the thatch.

There was only one cow at the farm. She was standing, looking thoroughly dejected, in a small corral made of twisted bits of lumber rather loosely attached to several crooked poles sunk at irregular intervals in the ground. A small calf with a rope around its neck was tethered nearby.

"Try and get her to enter the crush, so that I can examine her," I said.

A couple of minutes later I had taken her temperature, which was slightly elevated, and was examining her chest and abdomen. The heart sounds were muffled, and more rapid than they should have been. The normal gurgles and squeaks that one should hear from the two compartments of the stomach on the left-hand side were simply absent. Not a sound. Same on the right. The entire intestinal tract had gone on strike.

I placed my hand high up on the backbone above her shoulders and squeezed. Normally a cow will buckle slightly when this test is applied. This patient not only buckled, but let out a grunt of pain. My suspicions aroused, I asked the owner to bring a pole, about six feet in length, and told Kipsiele to hold one end of it as we passed it under her body just behind the front legs.

"Now lift when I say," I told him. "Ready? Lift."

The cow let out an even louder grunt.

I turned to the woman.

"I think your cow has eaten a nail, or a piece of wire. It has gone through the wall of her stomach and is hurting her. I think I can do an operation and try to find the nail. What do you want me to do?"

"How much will it cost?" she asked.

"About a hundred shillings," I told her.

"That's good. Do you need anything?"

"Yes, please. While I get the cow ready for the operation, please can you put some water in this pot and boil it. My instruments are in it and I need the water to boil for ten minutes."

I administered local anesthetic to the nerves on the left side of the cow's stomach and skin, and then proceeded to shave the skin as best I could, using half a safety razor blade with a pair of forceps as a handle. Next came a vigorous scrub with soap and disinfectant.

The surgery itself was relatively simple. A cut down through skin and the layers underneath it allowed the stomach wall, or more properly the wall of the rumen, or second stomach, to appear at the surface. Next, I gently ran my hand down beside and to the front of the rumen to search for damage. Right up near the diaphragm, I could feel an area of rough tissue joining the rumen to adjacent structures. Now I knew that my tentative diagnosis was almost certainly correct. The trick would be to find the nail.

"Kipsiele, please pass me one of those plastic gloves after I cut the stomach here. Don't touch my arm, but slide the glove over my hand and pull it up as high as you can."

After cutting through the wall of the rumen and sliding on the glove I groped forward and downward towards the first stomach. Very soon, a sharp pain in the ball of my thumb indicated that I had found the foreign body. I grabbed it and pulled it out. It was a very sharp six-inch darning needle, large enough to be used for sacking. About four feet of dark blue heavy-duty thread was attached.

As I held it up, the woman's eyes opened wide.

"I was wrong. It's not a nail, but it's a big needle," I said.

"I wondered where that needle had gone," she said. "I was using it to repair my daughter's school uniform. Then we could not find it."

I stitched everything back together, and after I had given the cow a generous dose of penicillin, we were on our way. As luck would have it the farm was only about 500 yards from one of our AI crushes, so I told the woman that the inseminator would call every day for the next five days and give the cow further injections.

That evening, as we sat at dinner in Jo's house, she smiled at my account of the darning needle story and said, "That reminds me of another bit of observation that has me foxed. Today Stanley, one of the clinical assistants, brought me the third case of ectopic pregnancy that I've seen in two weeks. As we went into the theatre to operate, he told me which side it was on, and how he confirmed the diagnosis. 'Naturally there is abdominal pain,' he explained, 'but on top of that I always know because the tip of the patient's nose is cold.' I still can't figure out how he knows that — or how he always seems to know which side it's on."

Soon Jo was on her way to see her family. She also faced the daunting task of traveling alone to Scotland to meet my parents, her future in-laws, surely not an easy thing to do. A couple of weeks later, I wrote my fourth letter to Holland:

> "On Tuesday last I had a strange experience. The warden in Meru Park called me down to look at a sick rhino, one of the white rhino that came up from South Africa last year. (Of course we're not allowed to say South Africa, so the animals are said to have come from Lesotho.) Apparently this animal, a female, had been on heat, and a male had begun to court it. I didn't know this before, but a rhino's courting is a rather rough affair. The male had attacked the female and at one point had run her into a pepper tree after more or less picking her up on the end of his horn. The little old guard who tends the animals showed me the tree. Anyway, I tried to listen to its heart and lungs. If you thought a cow would be more difficult to hear than one of your patients, just imagine this. I couldn't hear much, but the rhino was obviously uncomfortable.

> "What to do? I took a blood slide, but there was nothing visible next day. I was foxed. I decided to give her a large dose of penicillin and trust to luck. The injection posed a problem. Luckily I had taken along some of my four-inch needles. I thumped her on the backside a few times, just as if I was giving her a friendly pat, and then turned my wrist over and drove in the needle. She took virtually no notice. I then attached the end of the syringe and started to inject. About halfway through the process, she realized

that everything was not quite as it should be. She started to walk off, no doubt to get away from whatever it was that was causing the pain. I had to finish the injection at a dog trot!

"Yesterday, I heard indirectly that the rhino died a couple of days later. Apparently they found that she had some broken ribs, and the end of one of them had punctured her liver. Imagine the force that the male must have exerted!"

CHAPTER 10

THE ADAMSONS
AND THEIR CATS

Paul and Elma Sayer join me in a visit to Meru National Park, where we spend time enjoying the lush scenery and the remarkable diversity of wild animals, as well as paying a social call on George Adamson and a professional call on his wife Joy.

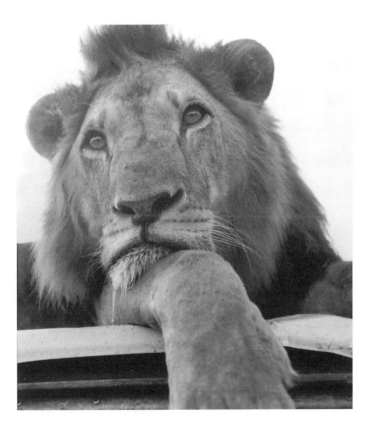

Film star Boy sunning himself on George's Land Rover.

TIME DRAGGED WHILE JO was away, although daily life in Meru was as enjoyable as ever, with evening fishing trips, tennis, golf, snooker, and the odd glass of Tusker. Paul and Elma Sayer (now married) visited for a weekend. Early that Saturday morning, we set off for Meru National Park. Paul had an open invitation to visit George Adamson at Mughwango, where he had his lion camp. George's godson, Jonny Baxendale, who was acting as his assistant and whom I had met in camp on a previous visit, had used HG2 as a staging post between the park and Nairobi. Tall, blond, personable, and good-looking, he used his visits to the city to give him a break from the isolation, as well as to do some socializing and to visit his family near Limuru. Jonny had made it clear that George would welcome a visit from us.

The clear atmosphere allowed us spectacular views over the Northern Frontier District as we headed round the north side of the Nyambenis among the small farms with their patchy tea plots. A quarter of a mile past the park gates, we got lucky. Elma spotted a small group of cheetahs moving slowly through the yellow grass. Then they seemed to vanish, although there was nothing to obstruct our view except the grass itself. We decided to investigate.

The reason for their disappearance was soon obvious. They had chosen to lie down in the shade of a thorn tree.

"It looks as if they've eaten recently," said Paul. As we drove up to within five yards, we could plainly see the animals' swollen bellies. In turn they stood, stretched, and walked over to the Toyota, where they again flopped down, no doubt attracted by the more complete shade available. We stayed with them for over half an hour before we spotted a mixed group of reticulated giraffe and zebras, which we decided to try to capture on film.

By mid-morning, when the temperature was beginning to climb, we arrived at the park headquarters and paid our respects to Peter Jenkins, the warden, who had picked up where the previous warden, Ted Goss, had been forced to leave off after being trampled by a partially drugged elephant. Between them they had done a huge amount to make the park an attractive place to visit. Years had been spent building a road system that blended with the environment and allowed visitors to drive amongst all the types of vegetation that grew in the area.

"Morning, Peter," I said. "Sorry to hear about that rhino. I hope everything else is OK. I'd like you to meet Paul and Elma Sayer. Paul works at the small animal clinic at Kabete. He's done quite a bit with Toni Harthoorn."

"Oh right," said Peter, holding his inevitable pipe in his hand. "Morning, Jerry, Paul, Elma. Glad to see you here. Can I offer you guys a coffee?"

"No thanks Peter. We are off to see George, and shouldn't arrive too late."

"All right. Oh, by the way, Joy says there's something wrong with one of her cheetahs. If you get a chance, call in and see her."

George lived in a simple camp near a rocky outcrop called Mughwango. He had been permitted to stay in the park in order to try and rehabilitate some tame lions. Not only did he have Ugas, the one-eyed lion upon which Toni Harthoorn had successfully operated, but also some animals that had featured in the film *Born Free*, a huge hit that had done much to kindle an awareness of conservation needs among the general public.

George emerged from the shade of his thatched lean-to, wearing, as usual, only his patched and faded khaki shorts, and a pair of the leather sandals known as chaplis. His frame, thickened by middle age, but hardened by many miles of walking, carried not an ounce of extra fat, while his thin white hair, beard, and wrinkled skin spoke of years of exposure to the equatorial sun. We spent a delightful hour or so with him and his brother Terence, who happened to be visiting, discussing a wide range of topics, from wildlife to the latest political scandal in England. At one time George and Terence had owned the Pig and Whistle, which these days was my occasional watering hole and source of Sunday night chicken biryani, but the story goes that Terence's views on alcohol consumption had inevitably driven customers away. He would harangue anyone who ordered a second tot on the evils of drink. Not exactly the best way to run a pub!

On a previous visit I had found out that George was a fascinating character, full of anecdotes of life in the bush, and a charming host. I had also found out that he seemed to have only two basic requirements in life. These were Legation tobacco for his pipe, and White Horse whisky. The latter was evident because he used to take the little plastic tags of a prancing horse from the bottles and add them to a wire in his mess hut, so our gift of a bottle of Scotch went down well. As we sat inside the 12-foot-high chicken wire compound, shaded under the open-sided hut that had been thatched with palm leaves, drinking instant coffee from tin mugs, he enthralled us with stories of his early days as a game warden.

A lioness came to check us out. She rubbed up against the wire, and George scratched her and made soft noises.

"That's Girl, isn't it?" I asked. George half-grunted a yes. "Do you remember my last visit, about four months ago, when I brought that Scottish surgeon and his wife and small daughter down? Girl was more than a little interested in the kid. It was a bit spooky."

"Yes, I suppose they must have viewed humans as handy prey at one time. The child was probably no more than a bite-sized morsel," he replied.

George has written two successful and entertaining autobiographies. The first, *Bwana Game*, starts as an account of his early days in Kenya, then evolves into the beginning of the saga of his fascination with lions. Both show some interesting omissions about "his" lions. In the second one, *My Pride and Joy*, he admits to having shot the resident adult male, whom he named Black Mane, near Mughwango, after it killed one of his charges and became a threat to his program. If the warden had known of this at the time he might not have taken very kindly to it. Both books attest to the fact that although he could tell a marvelous story, he was never willing to grasp the inevitable risks attached to attempted rehabilitation of something as large, powerful, and essentially carnivorous as a lion. Starting with the mauling of Peter and Sarah Jenkins' son Mark, right there near Mughwango, and continuing through the two books, there are scattered stories of attacks, and even killings, by lions of humans. To my mind George never seemed to deal with this subject adequately, even after he had himself been the victim of an attack.

Mark Jenkins had had a close call. The lad, almost four at the time, had been bitten on the shoulder by Boy, of movie fame, as he sat between his parents in the middle seat of a Land Cruiser. Only the quick thinking of his parents had prevented him from being dragged out of the cab. Worse yet, a doctor at the nearby mission hospital had made the mistake of stitching the wound, which had gone septic in short order. With nowhere for the pus to drain, his arm had swollen up to a frightening size before the stitches were taken out and he recovered.

I have since seen big cats in captive settings, even cheetahs, react in a very distinct manner when small children come near their enclosures. Their ears prick up, they suddenly look alert, for all the world as if they are checking out a herd of something tasty, and their body language and gait both change.

We sat and listened to George's accounts of early days, when he and Terence were free spirits having a string of adventures. After a while he said, "Would you like to see my youngsters? I got them as cubs a couple of years ago."

We walked with him to a white dombeya tree about four hundred yards from the compound, passing a couple of impressive termite mounds as we went. The tree was about 14 feet tall. It had large roundish leaves, about three inches across, and a mass of pink-tinged snowy white flowers. Looking at us with an inquisitive expression from a fork about ten feet off the ground was a young male lion, his mane just beginning to show. Various bits of lion anatomy could be seen flopped over other branches.

"They fed last night, so they're resting up just now," said George.

"Isn't it rather unusual to see lions up a tree?" I asked. "I know that the ones in Lake Manyara are famous for climbing, but I didn't know that one saw it anywhere else."

"Oh, I think it's more common than people realize," he responded.

We returned to the shelter and took the hint when George said, "Can you please call in on my wife as you go back? She has a lame cheetah."

After a leisurely and luxurious picnic lunch in the shade of a thick mass of trees by the Rojewero River, we had a brief snooze and then drove to Joy's camp, which was handily set up under two magnificent tamarind trees that bore signs, as she wrote, of once having been rubbing posts for some large creature. Joy's books about the lions, the first of which was called *Born Free*, had led to the making of the film. She no longer lived with George, but there was some sort of non-aggressive relationship between them which I could not fathom. She continued working with and writing about wild cats. She had made technically fine paintings of Kenya's plants, and her astonishing portraits of tribesmen and women, called "The Peoples of Kenya," were important historical records of times that had more or less passed.

It took us a moment to establish our credentials as Joy emerged from her tent, dressed in faded military green shorts and a cross-over halter top. She looked trim and fit but her wrinkled skin, like George's, owed much to the effects of the sun. She brusquely greeted us in her thick Austrian accent. Once this was done there were none of the niceties or friendly atmosphere that we had enjoyed with George. A female assistant emerged from another tent, but no introductions were made. I later found out from Jonny that she was American and that her name was Netta Pfeifer. She was very involved with the Elsa Trust in the U.S.A., and had offered to help Joy in camp for a period.

"As George told you my cheetah, Pippa, is lame. She has hurt ze front leg. I will take you to see if we can find her, but she is very nervous and frightened of strangers. Only vun of you can come viz me. The uzzer two moost stay back in ze Land Rover viz my assistant. At least a hundred yards."

As Paul had recently passed his British Royal College Fellowship exams with a specialty in orthopaedics, the decision on who should examine the patient was easy.

"Fine, Joy, Elma and I will go in the second vehicle. You take Dr. Sayer," I said. "But tell me, how will you be able to get up close to the animal for Paul to examine it?"

"Zat is easy. I vill get some goat meat from ze fridge and she vill come for it. I have not fed her for two days, so she should be hungry."

With that she turned and shouted, in a crude Swahili dialect almost of her own invention, at a man standing no more than five yards away, for him to bring some goat meat from the fridge. It became apparent, as we waited to get organized, that this was the only form of communication with her staff that she knew. Perhaps, like the cartoon Britisher, she had decided that if a foreigner could not understand English, one could persuade him to do so by speaking louder and louder. Certainly, her Swahili owed little to book learning, and paid no attention whatever to grammar or syntax.

"Where do you get the goat meat?" I asked.

"Zat is easy. I go up to ze village just outside ze park and buy animals on market days. I bring ze goats back in ze Land Rover and slaughter zem as I need zem."

"You mean Athiru Rujine?"

"Is zat it? I don't know. It's just about five miles from ze park. Ze first one you come to on ze road to Maua. I can often get vegetables zere as well."

We drove back towards the park gate, and with a sense of *déjà vu* ended up within a hundred yards of where the three of us had seen the cheetah group only about six hours previously. In fact Elma, Netta, and I used the shade of the same tree that had been chosen by the animals when we first saw them that morning.

We watched as Joy got out of the vehicle and called Pippa. The cheetah rose lazily from her resting place near the cubs and walked over to the Land Rover, where Paul was leaning out of the passenger window. For the next half hour or so Joy petted Pippa, stroking the animal's leg in a haphazard fashion as she chewed half-heartedly on a lump of meat.

Then Paul emerged and went over to Pippa. He gently ran his hand up and down the right foreleg, and then moved to the left. After a minute or two the cheetah winced as he manipulated the joint about six inches above the foot.

"That's her carpal joint," I told the others. "She seems to react when he moves it."

We returned to Joy's camp by the river. Under the shade of the tamarind trees we discussed the case.

"I gather you've been feeding raw meat to her," said Paul. "Does she get any offal or hide?"

"Oh no. She prefers ze meat. I always give her ze best bits, usually cuts from ze hind end."

"Does she kill for herself?" I asked.

"Sometimes. She has been teaching ze cubs, and I saw her on an impala only three days ago."

"Why do you continue to feed her?"

"I like to maintain contact, and she always comes when I call."

"How often do you feed her goat's meat, and how much?" asked Paul.

"I try to give some every day. Usually two or three pounds if she vill eat it."

"Well, both Dr. Haigh and I have seen bone problems in cheetahs fed raw meat without offal or skin. They get a condition called metabolic bone disease, or osteomalacia. Sort of like rickets in young animals. In fact it's a common problem in all cats, and even large dogs here in Kenya if they are not fed enough calcium and phosphorous. It makes the bones very weak, and can easily lead to breaks if not treated. I suggest that you either stop feeding raw meat, which is extremely low in calcium, or if that does not suit, then you should get a sack of bone-meal and always feed it with the meat."

"How much?" she asked.

"We advise at least a large tablespoonful every day for Alsatians, so I would think that Pippa should get at least that much. You could dust it on the meat before you give it to her."

"It is difficult for me to get bone-meal here in ze park."

"I can arrange to order some for you and have it delivered to my office in Meru, if that helps," I offered.

As the Sayers and I sat on the verandah of our *banda* (cabin) at Leopard Rock camp that evening, we revisited the day.

"You know, the interesting thing about Joy is that she really doesn't want to let her animals go. She dotes on them, but if they were self-sufficient she'd have no reason to be here, and of course she couldn't write a book about them," said Elma.

"It was also interesting that she let you get up close," I said to Paul. "How come it took so long to examine the animal?"

"At first she insisted that I stay in the Land Rover. She said she would follow my instructions if I talked to her from the window. She's a bit clueless. I asked her to run her hand up and down the leg and then start to palpate the various joints. When I asked her to press on the shoulder she had no idea where it was. I did notice that the animal winced a bit every time she ran past the carpal joint, but Joy couldn't seem to manage a proper exam, so after a while I suggested that she let me make the examination directly. You saw what happened. Pippa didn't seem the least bit bothered with me."

"There's another thing," I added. "You heard how she talked of getting goats from the market every week. Right now, the district is under a foot-and-mouth quarantine. That means that absolutely no live animal movement of hoofstock is allowed without a permit from my office. I know that she has never applied for one, but I also know that she is far too well-connected politically for me to make any waves. From a practical point of view it makes no difference, as the animals are destined for the chop anyway."

Years later I was intrigued to read Joy's own account of her attitude to the cheetahs and the incident with the injured Pippa. She named the cubs Mbili, Tatu, and Whity. In her book *The Spotted Sphinx* she states, "I was so happy at being again with Mbili that, not knowing when I might see my favourite little clown again, I dragged out the time we spent with her as long as I could."

There is also a description of our visit (I'm referred to as "another vet") in which she changes Paul's diagnosis to one of a sprain and states that he prescribed Butazolidin. At least she was right in naming a drug that might have helped for her own diagnosis.

One can only speculate about the sad events that followed almost two years later. Joy maintained her connection with the cheetahs. On the 21st of September 1970, she found Pippa with a broken leg. Attempts at repair did not work, and eventually the cheetah had to be put to sleep. I have always wondered how much goat's meat Joy continued to use, and whether she used any more bone-meal after we sent the first sack down to the park. She never ordered any more through me.

■

A major thread of both George and Joy's books, and indeed the ostensible *raison d'être* of the last part of both of their lives, was that big cats, especially lions, that have been held in captivity need to be gradually reintroduced into the wild if they are to be able to independently make a living and kill prey. Certainly they will come out on the short end of competition if other established predators are present at the release site, but the suggestion that they may not be able to hunt does not stand up well under the harsh light of reality. After all, the most domesticated of all cats, the house cat, is a highly successful predator. It has been estimated that in Britain alone, house cats kill 275 million small birds, small mammals, and reptiles every year. In Australia, an unfortunate consequence of European immigration has been that settlers' pet cats, and their feral descendants, have become a major threat to native species, who had never met predators quite as efficient.

Another slice of evidence that cats need no instruction in hunting from humans comes from the experiences of John and Ros Poulton, who managed the Ol Pejeta ranch near Nanyuki, which was owned successively by millionaires Court Parfet, Adnand Keshoggi, and Lonrho's Tiny Rowland.

Quite by chance a single lioness was acquired by the ranch. She was fenced inside an eight-foot-high electrified *boma* and fed cattle carcasses. Later a young male was added to the *boma* at the insistence of Mr. Keshoggi. Biological imperatives being what they are, five cubs arrived in due course. It did not take long for the seven lions to become 26, all of them fed on either dead cattle (the 130,000-acre ranch held over 12,000 head) or the carcasses of zebra culled from the large herds that were perceived to be cutting in on the cattle's grazing.

Meanwhile, outside the enclosure, which had by now been increased to about ten acres, wild game, including a small herd of huge old buffalo bulls, continued to mix with the cattle.

The inevitable happened. After five lions escaped one night, and were quickly enticed back in with a carcass tied to the back bumper of the Land Rover, the whole lot got out.

When John and Ros went out in the early morning after an *askari* alerted them, they found no less than five of the buffalo lying dead, and the lions enjoying a good feed.

Any student of Africa knows how cantankerous and dangerous a buffalo can be. These lions, which had never hunted in their entire lives, had had no trouble dispatching over 10,000 pounds of live and very powerful prey in a single night.

CHAPTER 11

GREATER THAN KINGS

*Help for a small boy with a dramatic case of poisoning is found
in a veterinary textbook; a disease moves from an animal to a man;
the newsboy, a wedding, and a honeymoon.*

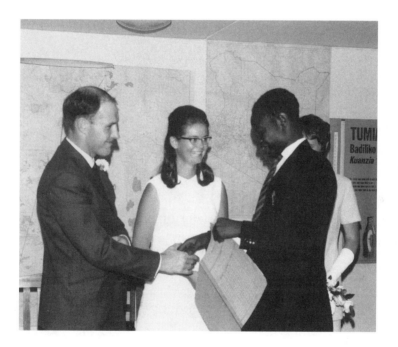

Meru District Commissioner's office, January 25, 1969.

J O RETURNED BEFORE CHRISTMAS and was almost at once thrown into the medical deep end. Within a week our joint medical educations were put to the test.

After dinner we went for a short moonlight walk down the avenue of jacaranda trees beside Jo's house, and shuffled through the carpet of pale blue petals that had fallen from the trees above as the flowering season came to an end. I drove back to HG2 and an early night. Only a couple of pages into my novel, as I found my eyes closing, and my mind unable to grasp anything that I had read, I turned off the bedside light.

I don't usually dream much, but this one was vivid. There was a car chase, and then the honking of horns. Suddenly I realized that the horn noise was real, and as I struggled up through the layers of sleep I could hear someone pounding on the glass of the front door. I rolled out of bed, checked my *kikoi* to make sure that I was decent and walked blearily out to the verandah. Tim emerged from his room with a sort of strangled grunt.

"What's going on?"

"I'll see," I said.

"Doctor," said a man in a khaki uniform, "Doctor Riet asked me to give you this letter."

"What time is it?" asked Tim.

I looked at my watch. "Three-fifteen."

The letter was a note scribbled slantwise and obviously in some haste on the back of a prescription sheet.

> *Jerry,*
>
> *I have a kid here who has swallowed something called* KUPATOX. *It's in a yellow tin, about 1/4 pint. Pic of a cow on it. He's convulsing and we can't control it. Have you got a text book or anything on this stuff? Can you bring it?*
>
> *Jopie*

"Tell the doctor I will come as soon as I can," I said to the driver. "I must go to my office to get a book."

Tim grunted again and shambled back to his room.

I arrived at the hospital about ten minutes later, my copy of Garner's Veterinary Toxicology in hand. The active ingredient of Kupatox is a synthetic substance called toxaphene. It was one of the most effective chemicals used for prevention of tick-borne diseases in cattle. These diseases were and are the scourge of cattle owners throughout much of East Africa, and owners had to apply the chemicals as often as twice a week to keep the ticks, and the fatal diseases that they carried, at bay.

Jo's patient was creating quite a stir among the hospital staff. Even Lily Mwenda, on duty in the maternity ward, had been co-opted to help and was not her usual bubbly self. The child was a chubby three-year-old, who had found the interesting-looking yellow tin at home. It wasn't hard to imagine what had gone through his mind: "Tin . . . got some fluid in it. . .

drinks come from tins . . . drink some." Fortunately, the distraught father had had the presence of mind to bring along the tin. Every couple of minutes the little boy would go into a violent convulsion. His whole body would arch up and no human strength could hold him. He was unaware of his surroundings, and while arching his breathing came to an abrupt stop. Three nurses and the boy's father were unable to hold him still.

"Have you got anything?" Jo asked as I walked in. Just then the child arched again and she tried to soothe him.

"Hello love. Let me look, I know it's here, because I've had to use it myself for three or four dogs. The signs you're seeing are just like those in the last one I saw."

I opened the text at the appropriate page, and as Jo struggled with the child I read out and paraphrased, in staccato bites, the relevant passages. *Toxaphene is a chlorinated hydrocarbon . . . dogs seem to be particularly susceptible to it . . . these things are diffuse stimulants of the central nervous system . . . main expression neuro-muscular . . . may be explosive . . . speed of onset depends upon dose . . . occasional maniacal seizure.*

"Seems to fit," I said. "Here's the treatment section."
Treatment aims at controlling convulsions by means of central nervous system depressants.

I passed the book across to Jo, open at the correct page, and she read it to herself.

"I think it's a bit risky giving barbiturates, the way this little fellow is throwing fits. If he jerks the needle out we'll have all kinds of trouble."

The next challenge for her was to select the right drug. She decided on paraldehyde. It had to go into the bloodstream for maximum effect. After a syringe had been filled another problem became evident. The boy's convulsions were so violent that it was impossible for the nursing staff to hold him still. Jo's experience in paediatrics in Holland, and all her work with babies in India and Zambia, had refined her natural talents so that getting sharp needles into tiny veins held no terrors. However, in this case, every time the needle got into a vein, a twist or turn would tear it through the wall of the vessel, and another potential injection site would be lost. Eventually, in desperation, Jo took a longer needle and felt for the pulse in the lad's groin. The needle went straight into the vein, which is large and lies next to the artery that she could feel thumping under her fingers. The drug went into his body, and his convulsions stopped as if by magic.

Twice more during the night she had to return to the hospital to administer further doses, but each time the movements were less violent, and recovery was obviously very likely. By the next day the worst was over. The boy recovered completely, and tests showed that his liver had suffered no permanent damage. Within a couple of days he had gone home. Great news for the parents and family, and a lesson in the common thread of medicine for both of us.

We soon settled back into our usual routine, eating supper at one or other of our houses most nights of the week. By now she had a proper set of cutlery and dinnerware, and there was no need for Stanley and her cook to be exchanging visits and materials.

One evening, as she walked past me on her way to the kitchen, she noticed me scratching the top of my head. She stopped and had a close look.

"That's a funny-looking rash you've got there," she said. "It looks red and itchy. Did you bang yourself?"

"Not that I can recall," I replied.

A couple of evenings later, when the rash seemed to have spread, and was now itching most of the time, I said, "Jope, could you have another look at my head? I've a nasty feeling that it might be mites. I saw a case of severe mange in some pigs about a week ago. I even confirmed it with a skin scraping — we saw Sarcoptes mites, and I wonder if I didn't inadvertently transfer something to my head."

She looked down her nose at the top of my head. Her eyeglass prescription needed renewing and for close-up work she sometimes took them off altogether.

"Hmm. It certainly could be. Have you got any slides in the car? I could make a scraping."

Five minutes later she had taken a scalpel blade out of her medical bag, put a drop of liquid paraffin on it, and scraped a small piece of skin and scab, plus a few scraggly hairs, from the top of my bald pate. We headed for the veterinary lab. It took no time to confirm the presence of the unwelcome guests. Right in the centre of the microscope lens was an almost circular mite, lying on its back so that it was easy to count all its stubby legs and identify it with certainty.

"Well, that's easy. Now for some treatment. I'll get you some medicated shampoo from the hospital tomorrow and that should fix it."

Our wedding had a couple of unusual features. We still have Jo's letter to her parents, written on the 26th on letterhead from the Mount Kenya Safari Club. It is pasted into the wedding scrapbook and nicely sums up the process of a civil wedding in a country where polygamy is legal.

"Pam did my hair. Mrs. Haigh made my bouquet from yellow and white roses and white jasmine-like flowers. Very nice. Tim Roberts (the best man) came and collected Pam (my bridesmaid) and Judi at 12:00 & Fin O'Callaghan collected Mrs. Haigh. So, there I was left to await Jerry's arrival. Jerry & the cook took photos of us & then off at 12:27 to the D.C.'s office. D.C. was sick so Gitau [a district officer] married us. I had to stand up & he spoke so badly, & there was so much noise from outside that I stuttered and stumbled through the statements that to the best of my knowledge and belief I was not married by native law! Jerry didn't have to swear to anything. In fact he didn't have to say a thing all the way through."

What she did not mention was the extraordinary interruption of a newspaper vendor. As Mr. Gitau was reading the ceremony, there was a knock at the door. We were offered either the *Daily Nation* or the *East African Standard*. Mark Twain summed it up in his *A Connecticut Yankee in King Arthur's Court*: "One greater than kings had arrived — the newsboy."

We had a small party in Meru, just salad and a glass of champagne, and then headed for Nanyuki where we gathered with friends at the Sports Club. I don't suppose that my mother could have dreamt that 25 years after managing the place for a few months she would be attending her son's wedding there. A December 1944 painting that hangs in our house today shows the main club buildings and the lawn besides a guest *rondavel* (round cabin) where we held the reception. To honour her Indian background Jo wore a beautiful cream-coloured Benares silk sari as a going-away dress.

The next morning, as we lay in a sort of semi-daze with the sun reflecting off the mountain above our honeymoon suite at the Mount Kenya Safari Club, the phone beside our bed pealed. I wondered if it was some sort of prank. Six-fifteen a.m. was not exactly the time to be expecting a call on the first morning of a new marriage. Hardly anyone knew that we were there, as I had done my best to avoid any potential shenanigans by wedding guests. I had parked our old Peugeot 403 behind the club in the staff parking lot. This turned out to be a wise move. A gang led by Kieran Kane had turned up with the intent of disturbing our evening. They had had no luck.

The phone call was no prank.

"Dr. Haigh? It's Jenny Burroughs. My husband Brian is the manager here. Sorry to disturb you so early, but our little bitch is having pups and seems to be in some trouble. I can't get hold of anyone else to help. Can you come down?"

The little bitch turned out to be a beautiful long-haired, russet red miniature dachshund. I asked a few questions about how long she had been in labour, and then bent to examine her. A pup was on its way, but its head was slightly turned back, and it was making no progress. A little help, with my finger hooked under the jaw, and it soon popped out onto the blanket. The mother at once started to lick it. As I cleaned up at the sink another one appeared and again the mother started her instinctive behaviour.

"Jenny, I'll leave you to it now. If there are any more problems, let us know. We'll probably be down for breakfast at about half-past eight. I'll check then to see how things are going."

By breakfast time, things were going fine. Five little masses of hair were wriggling in the basket, and their mother was lying contentedly on her side. Three of the pups were already searching for the milk bar.

We went to settle up. I took out my wallet and the clerk said something I did not catch. "How much do we owe you?" I asked.

"Nothing," said Brian as he appeared round the corner.

I tried again.

"Nothing," he repeated. "Just a little thank you for your help. Also, we've got something to show you."

Jo and I stepped round the counter and headed into the back office. Jenny was there holding an official-looking piece of paper.

"This is Honey's pedigree. She was bred to a show champion from Nairobi. We'd like you to have one of her pups as a wedding gift. Of course they won't be ready for about six weeks, so you can pick it up later."

"That's marvelous. Very many thanks," we said, almost in unison.

"There is one small problem," I continued. "We're off on honeymoon to South Africa, and then we're going to Europe to see friends and family in Britain and Holland. I don't think we'll be back until about early April. Can you look after it for us until then?"

"That's no problem at all. Of course we will. Would you like a bitch or a dog?" said Jenny.

"Oh, whatever's free."

"As there is only one bitch in the litter, we'll make it a boy. There is one thing we'd ask of you."

"What's that?"

"Will you please take him to a puppy class show in Nairobi at the end of the year? Reputation and pedigree is very important to us and showing is all a part of that business."

Of course, we happily agreed. We left the club after lunch, and headed for Nairobi and thence south.

In South Africa, things were very different from what we were used to. At the time the apartheid policy was in full swing, and was gaining ever-increasing attention in the world media. The first indication of this happened right at the immigration desk. When we explained that we were only visitors, and would be returning to Kenya, the official promptly got out two pieces of paper, stamped them, signed his name, and tucked them into our passports.

"We don't want you having South African stamps in your passports. You might not be allowed back into Kenya if immigration there saw them," he said, in the characteristic Afrikaner accent. I had heard it before, in the Earl's Court area of London, when I used to visit my sister in her flat, and in the Eldoret area of Kenya, where many South Africans had ended up after trekking all the way north in the early part of the century.

We traveled by several methods of transport. First to Cape Town by air, thence to George by train. From there to the coastal resort of Knysna by bus. It was everything that a honeymoon is supposed to be, but so far we had not really met a single South African socially, other than spending a wonderful day with my godfather in Cape Town. After ten days at the Leisure Isle hotel, where we had the best food I have ever had in a hotel, we decided to try another method of getting around: hitch-hiking.

This was the age of the mini-skirt. I even took a photo of Jo standing in front of a dry-cleaning store. The sign said, "Mini-skirts dry-cleaned. One cent per inch."

As we waited by the roadside for a lift, Jo's thumb sticking out as the cars came past, I tried to seem inconspicuous in the background. We covered a couple of thousand kilometres without trouble and for free with this strategy. We did run into one more thing that made us aware of the divides in the country. Just outside Pietermaritsburg we got a lift from the driver of a vw minibus. He and his passengers were all church ministers. One of them was a black man. They explained that they were probably taking a serious risk in traveling to Johannesburg together. This was at a time when park benches that we sat on were clearly marked "WHITES ONLY" in both English and Afrikaans.

After South Africa we went to Holland, had another wedding reception and spent time with Dutch relatives. Thence to England. Another reception among London friends, and then finally to Scotland where Jo met my folks again, this time as a married woman.

On about our third day there, while I was out running some errands for my mother, Dad broached a topic that had been bothering him.

"Tell me Jo," he said. "Have you sorted out your financial arrangements? How much allowance will Jeremy be giving you?"

As we sat in bed that night and laughed about it, I asked her, "And what did you say?"

"Oh, I told him that I had my own bank account and had been independent for two years already. He had nothing to say after that."

I suppose that my father, the product of an Edwardian upbringing and a British military career, had not even imagined such an answer.

CHAPTER 12

CAESAREAN SECTIONS

*Two Caesarean sections under very different circumstances,
and Glasgow on the equator.*

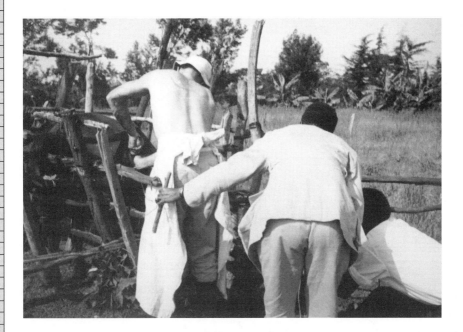

Everything set for a safe delivery after the feet have been straightened out.

U PON RETURNING FROM OUR honeymoon, Jo and I were assigned the former medical officer's house. Although it did not have the rustic charm of HG2, or a giant avocado tree like the one that had fed Tim, me, our dogs, and our steady stream of guests for two years, it did have a sheltered verandah that faced the setting sun and looked out towards the Kazita River where we had both walked and I had waded after trout. Beautiful fuchsias grew just outside the dining room window, and several species of brightly coloured sunbird would flit in and around the blooms seeking the nectar.

Stanley, who had looked after Tim and me in HG2, moved up the hill with us. He was somewhat reluctantly getting used to catering for a *mem-sahib* for the first time in his life. I suspect that life with a couple of bachelors who were often away on safari had been much easier for him.

Tim had looked after our dogs, Pie (Greek π) and Rinty, and we agreed to take one each. Jo and I took Rinty, who had mellowed into a real old gentleman, and we picked up our new pup, whom we named Muffin, at the Safari Club. They soon settled in together, the ten-year-old quite tolerant of the youngster. Both would greet us with great enthusi-asm each day as we returned from work. By standing on his hind legs, and bouncing up and down like a coiled spring, Muffin made sure of get-ting his full share of attention.

The first seven months of work in the government hospital before our wedding had been an enlightening experience for Jo. The caseload had been varied and fascinating; the need to be able to turn her hand to almost anything made for stimulating and endlessly challenging work.

As she and her colleagues sat around the coffee table on Jo's first morning back, Lily, always a bundle of energy and a source of endless laughter said, "Oh, Dr. Riet" — she pronounced it Riot, just for the fun of it — "it is good to see you back. We have missed you so much. I'm sure we will get you working hard again pretty soon."

"Did anything interesting happen while I was away?" asked Jo.

"We did see one interesting case," said Anna Nkabu the Matron. "A man from Kianjai came in with his wife and we had to do some emer-gency repairs after he had operated on her."

"You mean he did an operation himself?" said Jo.

"In our Meru culture a woman who dies in childbirth cannot be buried together with the baby. They must be separated before burial. This man cut open his wife when she seemed to die while trying to give birth. He removed the baby, which was dead, and then his wife woke up. He stitched her stomach using some string and then brought her in here in a *matatatu*. We, Erastus and I, did an operation. We put her under anes-thesia and cleaned her up."

"Had he stitched up the uterus?" queried Jo.

"No, we had to do that after we had taken the string out. At any rate, the woman recovered and we sent her home."

"Imagine," said Jo to me that evening. "That took some guts."

"He hadn't much choice."

My own first Caesarean after we got back was nothing like as dramatic, but had its moments. Nothing in the final year of the veterinary curriculum in Glasgow could have prepared me for the local conditions under which this life-saving surgical intervention took place on a Kenyan small holding.

One Sunday, a farmer walked up the drive and called *"Hodi?"* which is the Swahili equivalent of "Anyone there, may I come in?" After the usual courtesies of the ritual greeting, I said, "What is your name, and where is your farm?"

"My name is Thambura. My farm is near Githongo."

"What is the problem?"

"My cow has been trying to give birth since early morning, but she is beaten. She is lying down and cannot get up. Can you help?"

"Yes, I can try to help, but it is Sunday, so I will have to bring my own vehicle, so you will have to pay mileage because I cannot bring the government Land Rover. You say that your farm is near Githongo. Where do you mean by near?"

"You turn at the coffee factory, just after the cattle crush, and go up about two miles. The farm is near the forest."

Soon afterwards Thambura, Jo, who was off-duty, and I piled into our own Toyota Land Cruiser. It was a good thing that we had the 4-wheel drive option, considering the road conditions and the fact that we would be on rural tracks. I knew the "road" by the coffee factory only too well.

It was the season of the long rains. The rain had turned trickles into rivulets, the drainage system had broken down, and the rivulets had turned into small streams. The water cascading down the roads had eroded them even further and car-eating ditches of irregular size were evident almost anywhere. Steering became almost a question of guesswork. In one place the abandoned carcass of a bus, whose driver had miscalculated going downhill, had slid several yards and become inextricably mired in a drainage gully. Even where water was not running, the road resembled a mud bath. And we hadn't even reached Githongo yet. Forward progress was sometimes also sideways progress. Our 4-wheel drive allowed us to negotiate past the abandoned bus and luckily no one else had ventured out.

The previous weekend had been Easter, and Jo and I had worked one of the check stations for the East African Safari Rally, which took place over that weekend every year. The filthy, mud-spattered cars roared through Meru and out again onto the infamous stretch between Meru and Chuka, which was said to have more hairpin bends than it did miles. The cars slithered to a stop just long enough to let the navigators get to us to stamp the time sheets.

The top Safari Rally drivers are superbly skilled at driving in such conditions, but even they got stuck occasionally. The previous year had seen only seven crews finish from a starting line-up of 93. They had rightly been named The Unsinkable Seven. Two years prior to that, heavy rains had also reduced the starters to a mere seven crews. They had been named The Magnificent Seven.

About ten miles from home, and at least 2,000 feet higher up the slopes of the Mount Kenya, we arrived at the little farm, which was about eight acres in size, lush grass growing around a thatched hut, corn cobs stored in a shed set above the ground to discourage rats and chickens, and a couple of acres of freshly dug ground with the first tiny shoots of the next maize crop just showing. Thambura's family were all standing by the door of the house, from which smoke seeped out through the peak, as, typically, there was no chimney. His slim wife was carrying a tiny sleeping baby in a sling on her back. Another tot, of about four or five, was wandering about dressed in nothing more than a T shirt about two sizes too small for him, which reached about three inches above his belly button. He had some sort of food smeared round his mouth, and his mother quickly grabbed a cloth to wipe him as the strange white man emerged from the vehicle. An older girl, who looked to be about eight, and was dressed in a much-used cotton print dress, had a two-year-old child on her hip. She came over and took the half-naked little boy by the hand. They both stared at Jo, probably the first white woman they had ever seen.

A cross-bred Guernsey cow was lying exhausted in the middle of the paddock. A rope, low down around one foreleg, extended to a peg in the ground. One small foot could be seen protruding from her vulva, but there seemed to be an air of resignation about her. A few more questions elicited the information that her waters had burst about 7:30 that morning, and she had stopped trying to give birth about noon.

It was by now about 5:30 p.m. and I knew that I had to get on with things if we were to have any luck. In order to keep my clothes clean and dry I stripped down, donned a protective plastic sleeve and examined things. It was quickly apparent that the calf was tortuously twisted inside the uterus. Furthermore, it was dead. There was no chance of a delivery by the normal route. The only choices were to cut up the calf piece by piece and extract it, or to do a Caesarean section. With everything so dry inside her, the latter seemed to be the best option.

I got out the cooking pot that did duty as a sterilizing tray and turned to Thambura's wife. She seemed to be quite unfazed at being addressed by a half-dressed *mzungu*.

"Please put water in this pot and get it boiling," I said. I then selected the necessary instruments from my kit and put them in the pot. I had discovered that if I did this job right away, and then proceeded to prepare the patient, the instruments would get their obligatory 20 minutes' boil before being used.

Next, some local anesthetic around the proposed incision site for the cow. She was in such poor shape that a sedative would have been too risky.

Ideally the next step would have been a meticulous clipping of the hair over her side, but there was no electricity for a fancy shave here. Using the broken edge of a safety razor blade clasped in a pair of forceps, I cleaned the hair off an area about 18 inches wide and two feet long on the cow's left side.

"Jo, please give this a scrub with the Betadine soap, while I scrub up myself. It'll save quite some time. Then if you can take a sterile 18-gauge needle and prick her skin we'll know if the local has taken effect."

"I think that's enough," she said after a while. "Have you got any alcohol for a final cleansing?"

The alcohol was soon applied, both to the patient and my arms. Now came the easy part of any Caesarean section: first a long straight cut through the skin, then another through the underlying muscles, and the bulging uterus appeared. Another careful cut through the uterus and the calf came to hand. With this little guy dead, all my forces could be concentrated on putting everything back together again and trying to save the cow.

By now the evening was drawing in. Much worse, a massive head of clouds had loomed over the shoulder of Ithanguni, the hill above. Githongo is at the edge of the tea and coffee growing country. It is an area that gets about 50 inches of rain a year, and it felt as if about half of this fell in the next ten minutes. I was soaking wet within seconds. Everyone else retired to the house and watched through the cascade of water that fell over the eaves as a bedraggled, nearly naked European, wearing only black rubber boots and soaking wet underpants, went about his business. Looking up briefly, I saw that the little girl was getting over her shyness; she began feeling the material of Jo's skirt, and then tentatively reached up and held her hand.

My lack of hair ensured that there was no forelock to interfere with my vision, but the water cascading down my shiny forehead presented its own problems. Stitching the uterus with one long mattress suture, followed by another on top for insurance, was no problem. Even stitching the muscles was not too bad, but took a little longer as my body began to chill. A sharp needle and little resistance in the tissues made for fairly easy going.

But now I was in some trouble because the deluge was not only wet, it was cold. Numbing, in fact. By the time I started to stitch the skin my hands were not really functioning. Stitching cow's skin is not as easy as the deeper layers. When one cannot feel one's instruments, things are even worse. As my teeth began to chatter, and my knees to knock, it occurred to me that I was never going to get this job done alone.

At this point Jo, who had been making fitful conversation with Thambura's wife but was awake to the situation, called, "Jerry, why don't you get into the warm and let me take over?"

I don't normally take sugar in my tea. In fact I rather dislike it, but never has the mixture of tea, milk, and sugar, all boiled together for a prolonged period, tasted better. It took quite some time for me to begin to thaw. I stood outside and watched, a smoky-smelling blanket draped around my shoulders. By now the rain had stopped, but it was still quite cold.

Jo was obviously going through some novel experiences. As she told me later, she had never realized how incredibly tough it was to stitch through a third of an inch of skin. A few stitches in human skin over an inch or two was no problem. Trying to close an 18-inch gap in a piece of hide was quite another. Not something for which her medical training had prepared her! She finished, but not without some difficulty.

Luckily Thambura's wife produced another cup of her magic tea and a blanket for Jo, and we slithered off home down the hill once the exhausted cow had begun to show signs of recovery from her ordeal.

A few weeks later, after the rains had finished, Thambura returned to the office, once again asking for help with a cow that could not deliver her calf. This time the drive up was easy, and Kipsiele was available to do the driving.

With the farmer perched among the drug boxes in the back of the Land Rover, guiding us along the lanes and pathways, we were soon back at Githongo. Thambura had obviously learned from his last experience. The cow had only been trying to calve for about three hours. An examination told me that the legs were not positioned quite as they ought to be, and so with some contortions on my part, and the calf kicking and making my job much easier, it took only about 20 minutes to sort out the muddle and deliver a soggy brown heifer onto the ground. Thambura and his wife were delighted. A cup of tea was on the go, and, as the cow cleaned off her new baby, Kipsiele and I were each presented with a live chicken tied by the legs and thrown into the back of the vehicle, as well as several ears of the now ripe corn and two enormous cabbages.

As we prepared to leave, Thambura came up to the passenger window.

"Doctor," he said, "what is the name of the town in *ulaya* where you come from?" *Ulaya* had originally meant England, where early explorers and administrators had originated, but had come to mean anywhere other than Kenya where a white person might come from.

"I was born in Nairobi, but I studied animal doctoring in Glasgow," I responded.

I did not think any more about this conversation until about a year later when I saw Thambura, who told me that his heifer named Glasgow was doing really well and would soon be big enough to be taken to the AI station for breeding. A little corner of Scotland on the slopes of Mt. Kenya!

CHAPTER 13

POPULATION CONTROL

Cattle breeds for courses; a loan is repaid; a new way to tenderize chicken; of birth control and condoms from Ethiopia to Meru.

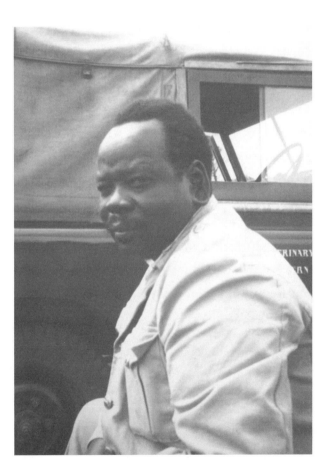

Kipsiele arap Kurgat.

BEFORE JO AND I HAD MARRIED, Kipsiele had asked me to help him buy a *shamba* in Bomet, about 20 miles from Kericho, in the tea-growing country of Western Kenya where his Kipsigis tribe was based. We worked out a deal, and I loaned him enough to make the purchase. The repayment schedule that he suggested seemed very harsh to me — he had insisted on giving up half his monthly salary for three years — but he said that he could manage it.

On the day of my second visit to Thambura, Kipsiele's repayment obligations were past the half-way mark, and he updated me on the progress of his *shamba*.

"I have been paid tea money from my crop, and last month I bought another cow."

"How many cows do you have now?"

"Only three, but two of them are pregnant, and should calve soon."

"What breed?"

"Guernseys, like the ones at Marimba. I remembered what you said about these Friesians that are coming in here, and I decided not to have any if I could find Guernseys."

He was referring to an unfortunate situation that I had seen develop in Meru. When I had first arrived, the bulk of the dairy cattle had been of Channel Island breeds, predominantly Guernseys. Then an artificial insemination scheme had developed, funded by Swedish aid money. Swedish experts had arrived at the bull station at Lower Kabete. The Swedes soon convinced the powers that be in the Veterinary Department that the high butter-fat, low-yielding Guernseys were *passé*. High-yielding, lower butter-fat black-and-white Friesians became the flavour of the day. I imagine some of them had strong Swedish bloodlines.

In all the excitement about higher milk yields someone forgot an essential truth. The Friesian, or Holstein as it is called in some parts of the world, is much larger than the Guernsey, and requires more food. A lot more food, especially if it is to produce those extra volumes of milk. The average small holding in rural Kenya, only a few acres in size, is not geared to such an appetite, unless of course the farmer reduces the number of cows that he owns. Such a notion flies in the face of long-held cultural traditions about the importance of cattle.

I was in no position to do much about the change, but when asked, I would advise farmers to stick to what they knew, and stay away from the idea that "big is beautiful."

Later that day, as Jo and I were enjoying our usual cup of tea and discussing the day's events, Stanley the cook came silently on to the verandah. He always seemed more comfortable speaking to me than to Jo.

"*Bwana*, can I have some gin from the bottle? Just a spoonful."

"What for?" I asked.

"You know that chicken you brought home today? I think it is very old, and will be difficult to cook well. I want to give it some gin and then kill it after while, when it is relaxed."

I looked at Jo and smiled. "Don't know if it'll work," I said, "but it may be worth watching."

Half an hour later we watched Stanley give brief chase to an erratic chicken and then administer a *coup de grâce*. That evening we ate a fat-free chicken. It was not exactly tender, but at least it wasn't stringy, as chickens that have spent their lives running after whatever scraps they can scrounge tend to be. Whether that was due to Stanley's prescription, or his excellent touch in the kitchen, was an open question.

An eight-foot moonflower tree stood beside our house. As dusk approached, the bell-shaped, cream-coloured blooms would begin to put out their distinctive heady scent. We began adding to and working on the house's lovely garden as soon as we moved in, and I soon discovered that Jo had a green thumb. Moreover, she had a fund of knowledge about plants and knew the names of dozens of them. As the rains abated and time passed, we began to see the fruits of her efforts. An array of daisies, sunflowers, marigolds, and roses emerged from the fertile ground. Tomato plants began to climb the small branches that we had cut as support sticks, and beans, peas, *nchugu* (a local pea), and lettuce began to appear. Even asparagus sprouted, although a friend asked us if we really thought we'd be staying long enough to get an edible crop.

Some far-sighted administrator had once had a complex series of irrigation furrows dug throughout the area where houses were built on the hill above the golf-course. No doubt he had arranged for inmates from the town gaol to dig the furrows and one of the tasks of the current crop of prisoners, clad in off-white calico vests and shorts and guarded by a single man carrying an ancient Lee-Enfield rifle, was to keep the furrows open. If the nearby District Commissioner's house had the best furrows around, who were we to complain? The furrows derived from a single trench that left the Kazita river about a mile upstream. Each householder had a certain amount of time each day during which the furrows could be tapped as a water supply for the garden. So fertile was the soil that even the tomato support sticks took root and sprouted young leaves.

Soon after we got back from Europe, Jo was approached by the folks from the International Planned Parenthood Federation (IPPF). Would she be interested in helping them in their family planning drive by providing IUD coils to women who did not want to conceive?

The Foundation was attempting to make a pre-emptive move to help the Kenyan population from growing at the furious pace that was already becoming a potential problem and would, within a few years, place it at the head of the world pack in terms of annual growth rate.

In 1985 Elspeth Huxley, who had known Kenya all her long life, and written extensively about it, noted that "Kenya's birthrate is now the highest in the world; the average family size is eight and a half children. This flood of babies is drowning the resources of the country, over-population has become the greatest threat to the nation's stability."

A telling example of the tendency towards large families is provided by farmer, soldier, politician and author Michael Blundell, who tells the story of Corporal Henry Ouma, who fought under him in the Ethiopian campaign. Thirty years later, Ouma wrote to Blundell seeking help with employment for his well-educated son. Blundell did what was requested, and records his pleasure at being thanked with a letter, but adds, "my heart sank when he mentioned that he had 17 more sons, all of whom would want work!" No mention of any daughters.

Later in the same book Blundell states that 55% of Kenya's population is under the age of 18. That figure doesn't mean much until one computes it into over 12 million youngsters who will, in the not very distant future, produce children of their own.

In the late '60s the shantytown around Nairobi was already growing at an alarming rate as rural people, with no land, no income, and virtually no hope, were migrating to the city on the chance of finding work. Within a few years similar shanty towns, lacking even the basics of decent living conditions, would start to appear in other towns around the country.

Jo was happy to try to help the IPPF, and she set up clinics every Wednesday afternoon. After a month, she told me, "At first it was very hard to get anyone interested, but after a while the nurses began to help, and we now have a steady stream of ladies. I do about ten every time."

But some time later, she said, "It's strange. These women are starting to come back to have the coils removed. It seems that they are quite happy to stop having babies for a while, and obtain some sort of control over their husbands, but then they decide to try and have a baby after all."

The IPPF team arrived from Nairobi the following week to see how Jo was doing, and we invited them over for dinner.

"I'm very interested to hear about your work," said the boss to me. "You say that you interact with farmers daily and meet them at cattle crushes. Do you think you could help us with the family planning scheme?"

I should have seen the trap, but didn't.

"I can try. What did you have in mind?"

"Well, I wondered if you could take contraceptives with you on your rounds and persuade the men to use them. It would greatly help our program."

I foolishly agreed, and within a week two large cardboard boxes of condoms had arrived by bus.

It was soon apparent that the whole thing was a bad idea. I discussed it with Kipsiele, my sounding board for local matters, and he was extremely skeptical when I tried to describe the function and use of "a rubber sheath for preventing children" as I clumsily put it, in the absence of a Swahili word for condom in either my vocabulary or my dictionary. Perhaps there wasn't such a word at that time.

I am no salesman. At any rate, not a single condom found its intended use. I was reminded of my father's attempts at distributing condoms to his soldiers in Ethiopia 25 years ago. One evening back in Scotland, as Dad and I had sipped glasses of Black and White and he'd instinctively picked up and carefully arranged the 50-odd hairs that he used as a token cover over his bald head, he had told me, "The commanding officer issued a standing order when we were camped at Addis. Translating from the official lingo, the order decreed that it was be a court martial offence for any officer to get the clap. The girls in Addis are stunningly beautiful, but they have a very virulent form of vd. All that there was for treatment was M and B tablets, and they didn't do the trick. It was my job to issue French letters to the guard post and to try and ensure that the troops took them along when they went out on passes. The task was quite hopeless. In all the time we camped there, only one FL was ever taken."

He finished with a graphic, if brief, bit of guidance: "Just be careful where you dip your wick."

One morning at Kibirichia, I did have cause to silently thank the IPPF for their generosity. At the communal cattle crush I was presented with a cow whose udder was covered in blood.

"What happened?"

"She is on heat, and was trying to find a bull. She tried to jump the fence. Her teat caught on the barbed wire and she has cut it. It is very bad," said the owner.

I asked Bernard, the local animal health technician, for water, and washed off the udder. The action of the washing caused it to start bleeding again, and it was now plain to see that there was a nasty three-inch cut down the length of right front teat.

"I shall have to stitch this up," I told the farmer and Bernard. "Bernard, please get some rope from the car, and get a fire going so that we can boil my instruments. I'm going to give her an injection above the cut, so she won't feel the pain of the stitches and will stand still while I work."

Fifteen minutes later we were ready to proceed.

"Tie the rope around her body just in front of the hip bones and the udder and pull it tight," I said, gesturing to her prominent pelvic bones. The cow arched her back as Bernard cinched down on the rope and tied it off. Theoretically she could not kick now.

The stitching itself was a bit fiddly. I had to try to seal the delicate lining of the teat so that milk would not leak through. This required the use of a strand of fine catgut, a suture material that would dissolve after the cut had healed in a few days. The next task was to close the torn skin on the outside. The jagged rent caused by the barbed wire further complicated the matter. After what seemed like ages, as my aching back rebelled at the constant crouch halfway under the cow, I placed the last stitch.

"Now I'm going to put this little tap in the opening of her teat. Make sure that you pull off the cap twice a day and keep it clean. Put it back on when the milk has come out. Each day put in a new tube after you have given her some *dawa* to prevent mastitis."

I dug five tubes of mastitis ointment out of my medical box and handed them to Bernard.

"You'll have to visit this cow every day to give her one of these. She will also need an injection of penicillin every day for five days."

Then I had an inspiration.

I pulled out a condom from the unused box beside the passenger seat, cut off the tip, and rolled the rubber up the teat so that it covered the wound.

"Try to keep that on for a few hours. It will help keep the wound clean until you can get her home and into a clean *boma* and off the muddy road. Take it off tonight when you open the milk tube."

I gave the cow her first injection of penicillin and sorted out the matter of a fee with the farmer.

The condoms languished in our house. Jo and I had decided that it was time to try and start a family of our own, so they were of no direct use to us. Eventually I shipped them back to Nairobi.

It is not everyone that can say that they stored 10,000 condoms under their bed for several months. Or even 9,999.

CHAPTER 14

THE FOUR-GALLON ENEMA

Jo resigns from the government hospital and becomes the first doctor at a nearby mission. Our daughter Karen arrives fit & healthy. Wilfred Thesiger, noted walker and author, pays a visit but gets limited satisfaction. I treat a white rhino that has suffered spousal abuse.

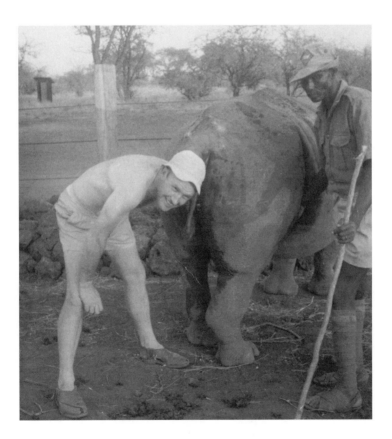

Rhino medicine *al fresco*.

O VER THE NEXT YEAR, IN LATE 1969 AND EARLY 1970, some important changes occurred in our lives.

After a few more months working in the government hospital, Jo's enthusiasm for medicine began to wane. At first she would get cross, but then she became disillusioned about some of the things that she saw. Discipline seemed to be non-existent. Overcrowding was ridiculous, and cleanliness was, in some areas, only a pipe dream.

One night, after handling an after-hours emergency, she came home fuming. Although it was two in the morning, she obviously wanted to vent her feelings. "It was almost unbelievable," she told me. "I needed to speak to the night nurse in the children's ward, and I couldn't find him. After several minutes of futile searching, I decided to open the linen closet in order to get some sheets for a little girl that I'd just admitted. I was nearly knocked over by the nurse. He rolled off the top shelf! He was so drunk I couldn't even get him to stand up. He was incapable of speech, and he stank of beer and urine."

There was not much I could say. Of course, Jo reported the nurse to the provincial medical office. This was the same man who had been caught diluting penicillin with water, dividing a single vial into as many as ten doses. For this second offense he was transferred to a government hospital in another district. Would that have taught him a lesson? Chances are that he would have been up to his tricks in no time at all, possibly with even less supervision.

After five months, when Jo was almost ready to become a lady of leisure rather than continue to put up with the daily aggravation, an amazing opportunity arose. It came up through our acquaintance with Andrew Botta, whom we knew as Father Botta, and who infrequently dropped into the Meru club for a beer and perhaps a game of snooker. He was the priest at the Tigania Catholic mission, about 20 miles away, part of the country-wide Consolata group. Andrew carried, in his slight frame and stoop, an incredible zest for life, a mischievous grin on his Punch-like face and a virtually unquenchable energy.

As Andrew saw it, his duties extended well beyond the religious. One of his major secular achievements had been to encourage the local people to get involved in a building co-operative. Not only did the members help one another to build solid stone homes of excellent quality, something that Andrew knew a great deal about, but they eventually built an office and went into business as a profit-making enterprise.

One day, during a chat with Andrew, the subject of his mission health centre came up. He had been running the centre for several years with the help of an excellent staff of nurses who had come out from Italy. Most, like the diminutive and feisty Sister Nunzia, who was in charge of the maternity ward, were fully trained. Others, like Terasina and Rosanna, were volunteers with basic training. There was also a group of staff from the local area.

"Do you need a doctor at the mission?" asked Jo.

"Of course, yes, but we have no money for salary so we could not afford."

"What about a volunteer?"

"Oh sure, that would be fantastic," said Andrew, beginning to get the drift of the conversation.

"Let us think about it and see what can be done. Perhaps you could also think about it and see what could be done about transport."

An agreement was soon reached. Jo resigned from her government post, and Andrew found a battered old Renault 4L, with its peculiar push-me-pull-me gear stick in the middle of the dashboard. This had been on its second-last legs when passed to Jo. The rutted roads and daily grind soon removed this set of legs, and the old car began to give more trouble than was reasonable. As a replacement Andrew provided a smart, almost new, Volkswagen Beetle.

Meanwhile, Jo and I were soon expecting our first child. When she was three months pregnant, Jo was exposed to German measles, giving us a bit of a scare. The disease is normally fairly harmless, but exposure during pregnancy can cause the developing baby to be born deaf, or worse. Following the sage advice of her obstetrician, a Scot named Donald Gebbie, she was injected with a huge 17-cc dose of gamma globulin — a volume more commonly associated with cattle than humans — and this gave us comfort, although her backside bore the bruises for a couple of weeks afterwards. Our daughter Karen arrived safe and sound in November.

Soon afterwards, another important member of the household also joined us. We had been searching for an *ayah* (nanny) for some time, and shortly before Jo headed for Nairobi and her delivery, friends told us of an experienced woman from the Nandi tribe. Her name was Ester. When we met, and I asked her for another name, she just said, "Ester. That's enough."

Many of the families in the Nanyuki and Timau area had *ayahs* of Nandi origin. Ester was tall, about five foot nine, large, and very motherly. Her duties were almost exclusively related to Karen's well-being, and she did everything possible for the little girl. Karen was soothed to sleep after lunch with Nandi lullabies, and cosseted in every way. Perhaps this was why Jo and I had trouble getting her off to sleep in the evenings, after Ester had gone off duty. At least, we had trouble until our Rugby playing American Peace Corps friend Wilber James lent us a copy of his Beach Boys tape. We soon discovered that it only took about two songs from our portable tape deck to settle her down and get her to drop off.

As we sat on the verandah one Thursday evening listening to the sounds of California Surfin' music coming from the nursery, a strange and somewhat dilapidated Land Rover drove into the yard. Out stepped a European who looked as if he had been around the block more than once. His heavily lined face and aquiline appearance gave evidence of plenty of exposure to the wind and sun.

"Good evening," he said in the cultured tones of an English gentleman. "Is this the home of Doctor Haigh?"

"Which Doctor Haigh?"

"Oh, I didn't realize that there were two. I'm looking for a medical doctor." His heavy eyebrows expressed themselves almost as independent bodies.

"Then you've come to the right place. This is my wife, Jo. She is the medic, I'm a vet. Can we offer you a drink? Come on in."

"Thank you. I'm Wilfred Thesiger. I'm leaving tomorrow on a walk from Maralal via Lake Rudolph and up across the Chalbi desert, and I need some medical supplies for my staff in case of emergency."

This seemed to us to be rather a prodigious walk, but as we sat and chatted about the Northern Frontier District we realized that the projected trip was to be a rather tame affair compared to ones that had gone before. We had neither of us ever heard of Thesiger, so his stories of the empty quarter of Arabia and the Iraqi marshes were fascinating. He also mentioned the possession of a house in London's fashionable, and very expensive, Cheyne Walk.

We later found copies of some of his books, and realized that he not only wrote with compelling style, but was an unusual explorer, and liked nothing better than to walk huge distances in tropical regions under extreme conditions accompanied by a small crew of locals and perhaps a few camels. An ascetic if ever there was one, although not totally dedicated to that lifestyle, as his occasional jaunts into civilization revealed.

Before long he had agreed to stay not only for dinner, but even to take advantage of the chance to stop for the night. Luckily there was room in our staff quarters for his Samburu companion, who had already made himself comfortable with Stanley and had had some tea and a bowl of maize meal.

Fortunately we happened to have arranged for Stanley to prepare a leg of the delicious fat-tailed sheep that provided our main variation from fillet steak, so there was no shortage of food. I cracked a bottle of Beaujolais. After almost, but not quite, declining a glass our guest proceeded to do it considerable justice.

During dinner the conversation again returned to his need for medical supplies.

"What exactly do you need for this kind of trip? How long are you going for?" asked Jo.

"I have a lot of the basic first aid stuff, so all I really need is some antibiotics and a dozen vials of morphine, in case anyone gets injured," he responded.

"Antibiotics I can let you have. I suggest some tetracycline and a couple of courses of ampicillin. I assume that you have a good supply of chloroquine for malaria, but the morphine is a problem. I don't have any here, and we are running short in Tigania. In fact, we are waiting on an order."

This was a bit of a white lie. As she said in bed that night, there was no way she was going to give morphine to a perfect stranger, whoever he said he was.

Next morning, soon after we had seen our guest on his way, Jo headed for Tigania in the Beetle, leaving baby Karen with Ester, and I left for the office, and the dubious delight of my Friday duties — completing a monthly report, paying staff, and generally playing the bureaucrat.

It seemed to be a quiet day. Just reams of paperwork, a steady stream of people coming in to pick up their pay and sign for its receipt. Kipsiele took his packet and, as usual, promptly divided it in half and handed over 200 shillings and some change. "Only three more months to go, and then the debt is settled," he said, smiling.

By about lunch time I was on top of most of the paper-pushing work, when the phone rang. It was a radio call, but at an unusual time.

"Good morning Jerry. Peter Jenkins here from the park. Over."

"Morning Peter, what can I do for you? All well? Over."

"Oh, pretty good, but we do have one problem that I think needs your attention. A white rhino has been injured. Can you get down here this afternoon? Over."

"How badly injured? Will I need to sedate it? Over."

"Possibly. It's been in a fight, and has a very swollen rear end. The *askari* (guard) tells me that it has not passed water or feces for over two days. It's now off its feed. Over."

"Right Peter, I'll see what I can organize here. It'll take me a couple of hours to reach you, and I can't get away right away, but I should be with you before dark. I hope that's OK. Over."

"Fine Jerry. We'll look for you. Have the guard at the gate radio me when you get there. Over and out."

"OK. Over and out."

I organized my drug boxes, trying to think of all the things that I might need for this unusual patient. I had treated one rhino previously, but that one had died, and I did not have much idea of the "normal animal" when it came to white rhino.

It seemed that I might be able to combine work and pleasure. When I got back to the house Jo had just returned, and was soon organizing

Karen's paraphernalia for a visit to our favourite game park. As always, it seemed to take three times as much luggage to travel with a small baby as with an adult.

We set off down the dusty road, back past Tigania, the Nyambeni hills to our right. In Kianjai we had to slow down for a group of roadside donkeys that showed no concern for us. They seemed to be pretty savvy, but how they avoided being killed by greed-crazed *mira'a* transporters was a mystery. Karen stayed asleep, the rattling of the Toyota being as good a soporific as could be wished for. After the village of Kangeta we climbed up again through a pass in the hills at about 6,500 feet. *Mira'a* trees stood out against the skyline, and on the higher slopes small patches of tea, growing near the lower limit of their optimum climate, dotted the *shambas*. Thatched mud-and-wattle houses showed how small each *shamba* actually was, a few acres at the most. The tea bushes grew within a couple of yards of each building, leaving little space for anything else. The road dropped sharply down, and became not much more than a track. Eight-foot-tall hedges full of large, bright yellow, daisy-like flowers bordered the road.

At the park entrance the ranger contacted Peter on the radio-phone, and he was waiting for us at headquarters. He stood just under six feet tall, and wore standard field dress: a pair of khaki shorts, and a meticulously ironed, jungle-green bush jacket which had been sun-bleached to a greyish tone. The *chaplis* (leather sandals) on his feet looked polished by wear, as they gleamed through the layers of fine dust. The lock of hair swept over the top of his balding head gave little or no shade to his pate.

The rhino *askari* explained the problem. The animal, a female, had come into heat on Monday. The aggressive male had started to show lots of interest in her condition. On Tuesday they had begun to get serious. The male had of course tried to get behind the female. She had played hard to get and kept spinning around and threatening him. The *askari* demonstrated by dropping his head and throwing up his nose. As he weighed about 120 pounds, and stood no more than about 5'4", it might have not been convincing, but his natural talent as an actor made it seem real.

Eventually the frustrated male managed to get in a couple of vigorous horn thrusts from directly behind the cow. The enormous force generated had all been concentrated at the end of his three-foot-long horn. The damage that he had done was plain to see.

The dejected patient stood under a scrawny thorn tree in the middle of the *boma*. The whole area under her tail was swollen. A couple of deep puncture wounds below her vulva were weeping a clear fluid, and her anus had almost disappeared in folds of swollen skin.

I checked my history again. "When did she last urinate or pass manure?" I asked.

"On Tuesday evening. Since Wednesday morning she has passed nothing."

"And eating?"

"She ate a little bit of hay on Tuesday, also some grass." He pointed to the flake of lucerne that lay untouched on the ground beside her. "She ate some hay yesterday, but nothing at all today. She has also not taken any water today."

I had read that foreplay and mating in rhino is a pretty energetic affair, but I had not realized that it could get this violent.

There was only one thing for it, although I knew I was charting new ground for myself. I had acquired a new kind of drug for capturing animals, but only had a small supply. I had no real clue as to the rhino's size, although "enormous" fitted. I estimated her at about two-and-a-half draft horses, and hazarded a dose based on that.

Things did not go as smoothly as I might have wished. Four top-up doses and 45 minutes later, she finally condescended to stop against a small tree. Every time I had tried to approach her from behind or touch her tender rear end before this, she had simply walked away. After the third dose she started to walk in a circle. The circle got smaller and smaller. The fourth dose seemed to do the trick. Best of all, she did not fall over.

The next hour was a steady stream of hard work. I soaked my arm with lots of soap and water, as well as a slippery lubricant, and proceeded to empty out the rear end of the patient. At first it was like breaking concrete, not an easy thing to do with one's fingers. By the time I had reached in up to my shoulder, and changed arms a couple of time to rest my hand, my fingers were bruised and tender.

It was time to take a different course. The rhino was showing signs of waking up, and I had no notion of what to give in the way of a further top-up dose. Calling over my shoulder to Jo, who was holding Karen in her arms, I said, "Can you make me up an enema, Jope? I'll probably need at least four gallons." I asked the *askari* to bring a bucket, and turning to Peter I said, "Can you find me about six feet of hose, and a large funnel? I'm going to try and get as much soap and water into this beast as I can."

He turned to one of the several staff members who had gathered to watch the proceedings, and taking his straight-stemmed pipe from his mouth he gave orders in Swahili. He was one of the old school of game warden. No formal education in resource management, but a wealth of practical experience and a vision of what he felt a well-run park should be.

While the various bits and pieces were gathered I prepared a couple of injections. First, large doses of antibiotic. Much larger than I was used to, and only one chance to administer them. A short-acting drug to attack the infection that was already starting to show in the deep wounds, and another to hopefully last two or three days and ensure a safe recovery. Then another injection to help reduce the swelling. My emptying of the rectum would hopefully have helped, but she still needed to empty her bladder.

We administered the enema in the deepening dusk, which comes quickly at the equator. In 15 minutes it went from daylight to dark.

Back then to Peter's house. As Jo sat chatting with Sarah, Peter's attractive blond wife, and dealt with a glass of fresh juice, I headed for the shower and a much-needed clean-up. Karen was a magnet for three-year-old Siana, Peter and Sarah's little girl, although their son Mark showed little interest in her. We listened to the night sounds, led by a chorus of cicadas, and I sipped a cold beer.

Jo shuddered as Sarah recounted the terrifying story of Mark's close run-in with the lion. Recalling the incident with what was obvious terrifying clarity, she recounted how his arm had swollen up and how the removal of the stitches had saved the day. She was still having nightmares about the whole thing two years later.

After supper we spent the night in the park's guest house, only 30 yards or so from the Jenkins's beautiful thatched home. In the morning we admired the small vegetable garden which Peter and Sarah had planted along the stream bank in front of their home, and Jo commiserated with our hosts on the problems caused for the would-be horticulturist by a variety of wild animals that enjoyed green things as much as any human. While it was feasible to fence out various bucks and hoofed animals, wandering elephants were another matter. Electric fences for elephant control had not been developed, and so most gardening efforts were doomed to frustration. The elephants knew when things were ready to harvest, just as well as did the people.

After breakfast we returned to the rhino *boma*. The *askari* greeted us with a happy grin. "She is much better," he said. "She has passed a lot of manure." To demonstrate he took us into the *boma*.

My only regret is that I failed to take a photo of the results of the enema. We do have a grainy old black-and-white print of me standing in sandals and shorts, my arm out of sight up a rhino's backside. A follow-up picture of the manure pile would have made a fitting end to the story.

After breakfast Jo and I took Karen with us on a sightseeing run. For the first couple of hours we skirted the various rivers that ran eastwards down from the Nyambenis to join the Tana, which in turn coursed to the Indian Ocean south of Lamu. It was like a piece of paradise. Hundreds of head of hoofed animals. Reticulated giraffe browsing among the treetops. Herds of zebra, showing little concern for the Toyota. A huge herd of buffalo moving through the bush ahead. As we drove round a corner they suddenly took fright, but not at us. They streamed across the road in front of us, kicking up clouds of dust as they went. We never saw what spooked them. A lone bull elephant idly plucking at the fruits on a sausage tree growing next to the Rojiwero river, and a crocodile slowly submerging as we stopped in the middle of a concrete causeway across the river to watch.

Hundreds of birds of many species. A group of ostrich chicks running behind a dark and stately male, the female nearby. Guinea fowl clucking and rushing about as they competed for some unseen food item. A mass of moving yellow dots as we passed under a tree full of dozens of weavers, all industriously building and checking nests. A gorgeous lilac-breasted roller sitting on a tree stump by the track, the sun catching the blues on his belly and wings.

We ended up with a picnic lunch on the banks of the Tana, just below Adamson's Falls. As we sat in the generous shade of a huge old fig tree we watched a large school of about 40 hippos in the pool below the cataracts. The noises they made accompanied the sound of the rushing water. Mainly snorts as the hippos surfaced and blew to clear their nostrils, and occasionally a loud series of grunts as they expressed their feelings.

It was difficult to imagine anywhere we'd rather be.

CHAPTER 15

ISIOLO INTERLUDES

*A temporary posting at Isiolo has its advantages, which
include trips into the semi-arid desert of the Northern Frontier
District, a camping trip with a Kenya veteran, and an unusual
breakfast. It also has its disadvantages, such as dealing
with bureaucrats and white tribalists.*

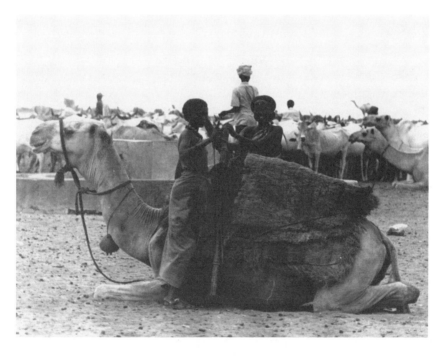

Camels, cattle, and their Boran herders. Wajir, Northern Frontier District.

PETER GAMBLE, DISTRICT VETERINARY OFFICER at Isiolo was transferred to Nanyuki. He and his wife Judi were good friends of ours, and we knew they had mixed feelings about heading for a much more social life and a new set of duties.

Soon after Pete's transfer, I received an unexpected call from Kabete. It was the deputy director of Veterinary Services, Marcus Durand. "How would you like to take on the duties of DVO Isiolo for a while, on top of your work at Meru? At least until we find a replacement for Pete."

"It sounds interesting. What would my responsibilities be?"

"You should probably attend meetings and try to get down to the District Commissioner's office about one day a week. If there's anything important in the way of sales you should also try to get to those, and of course keep an eye on the quarantine if there's anything there. The job may tie in nicely with your Meru duties; there is that longish boundary between the two districts."

I accepted, and soon discovered that there were some perks to the new position. Isiolo, although only 35 miles away, was considered a "hardship" posting. This meant that I could buy some things at duty free prices. These included brandy, so the luxury of an occasional after-dinner snifter became a reality.

The frequent trips to Isiolo also meant I could get to know the Carn family better. Tony Carn was the game warden for the entire district. He and Velia, and their daughter Sala, had been the Gambles' neighbours; they lived in the game warden's house, near the veterinary house. Tony, a keen outdoorsman, was away on safari a good deal of the time.

His slight frame and rapid, determined walk, leaning forward slightly, suggested a man who could accumulate mile after mile under his belt. His English background was confirmed when I discovered that his sister was Evelyn Home, the "agony aunt" of the well-known magazine, *Woman*. Velia, on the other hand, was a second-generation Kenyan. Her dark good looks and slim figure, as well as her expressive temperament, confirmed her Italian ancestry. They had been transferred to Isiolo in 1968, and stayed until the position was "Africanized" in 1972. Their daughter Lorian was born a month before our Karen. Two months before Lorian's arrival, just after Tony and Velia returned from a weekend at Maralal, the house burned to the ground. Juma, their cook, had been surreptitiously cooking on Velia's stove, instead of his own, while they had been away. He must have forgotten to turn off the gas properly. As Velia explained to me, "When I went to light the gas fridge and cooker there was a whoosh of flame, and the whole building was engulfed in an instant." She demonstrated with an upward and outward fling of her hands.

They had lost almost everything: family silver, linen, furniture, and their much-loved bull terrier Tiwi, who had been locked in a back room. Skitters, the cat, had made his escape. The only things that they saved were family photos and passports, which had been in a trunk. Wilfred Thesiger turned up unexpectedly and helped them sift through the ashes. One more treasure emerged: a jade lion had survived the heat.

About a month later Velia received an unexpected call from the

British High Commission: "We want to come up and visit you next week," the official told her. "I hope that will be satisfactory." It was less a request than an ultimatum. The visit was a scouting trip to prepare the way for a VIP visitor. Six months after the fire, when a new house had been built, but by no means furnished, Prince Charles arrived with an equerry. He was on safari and getting away from the media.

"They were just like all men," said Velia, recalling the visit with an exasperated smile. "Bedroom a shambles, clothes left on the floor."

The opportunity for an interesting work-related safari soon arose. The government cattle buyer, who worked for the Livestock Marketing Division, and had been dealing with the people of the Northern Frontier District for many years, was Hector Douglas. He called in at the Meru office on his way back from the north.

"I'm going up to Laisamis in two weeks' time. The Samburu are having an auction up there and I need to get some cattle for shipment to the Mombasa abattoir. Can you come along and do the health checks?"

"I'll need to organize some things here. How long will we be gone?"

"Oh, not long. No more than two or three days in all. I will be going on up to Moyale, but you will be able to get back after the sale. Don't bother with cutlery and stuff. I will supply tents and just about everything except bedding. Bring your own sheets, and a blanket, as it can get nippy at night. Make sure you bring your gun: there's good sand grouse shooting at Laisamis."

Pete had warned me about certain elements of traveling with Hector.

"Hector is a fascinating man," he said. "He always goes on safari with a full set of china and glasses. The plates are packed in specially made boxes with racks for each item. He likes to camp in comfort. He will also drink about three quarters of a bottle of Johnnie Walker each night, and he will definitely not offer to share it. If you want some booze, take your own. He's also a marvelous story teller, so be prepared for an interesting time."

As we sat by the fire that first evening I got a glimpse of Hector's earlier life. My own tipple was tea, and later a Tusker, but in the East African tradition of the "sundowner" he nursed his whisky from soon after six o'clock. In the gathering dusk, the sun setting blood red against a backdrop of gradually darkening blue, stars beginning to emerge one by one as the blue turned from pale to royal to blue-black, we began to chat. More precisely, he did most of the talking, and I acted as a blotting paper and occasionally prompted him.

"First, the morning. There's no need to rush. The birds come in at almost exactly eight o'clock. You can more or less set your watch by them. They finish after an hour or so. We probably won't need to shoot that long, as there's only you and I and the camp staff to feed. We'll have a late breakfast of fried sand-grouse breasts at about nine-thirty and then move across the *lugga* to the auction yards. Will a cup of tea at seven suit you?"

It was more a statement than a question. I nodded.

During the course of the evening, as the level in the bottle gradually dropped, he recounted stories from the war time. At one time he and a companion, the only Britishers on Marsabit mountain, kept an Italian force away for two whole days by moving around and letting off the occasional round in the general direction of the enemy.

"Later on I had the awkward situation of dealing with a whole Eye-tie platoon on my own. I was sitting in a *lugga*, stark bollock naked, up to my navel in running water, when these chaps appeared over the horizon and insisted on surrendering."

The Italian army in East Africa was famed for its caution and not noted for its aggressiveness.

At precisely eight o'clock Hector finished the last drop of his last glass and called, *"Chakula tyari?"* (Is food ready?)

"Ndio, bwana," replied the cook in the affirmative.

We moved from the comfort of our canvas and wood chairs to two others, identical, but placed on either side of a wooden table set with a white tablecloth. Soon after a delicious supper of steak and baked potatoes we moved off to our tents. As is usually the case in Africa, we did not sit up late. Sleep followed easily.

My next conscious action was to open the tent flap and take the tea from a tray presented by the cook's assistant after his friendly, *"Chai, bwana."* (Tea, sir.)

"Look sir," he said, pointing to the ground. I stood and gazed in fascination at the huge footprints of a bull elephant that had passed between Hector's tent and mine. As our guy ropes intersected, the animal had had to step extremely carefully. Neither of us had heard a thing.

Without hurry we moved off down to the *lugga* and prepared to get our breakfast. Nothing had prepared me for what was to come. Within 15 minutes I had shot as many grouse as I cared to. As Hector had been banging away as well I was sure that we had enough to eat. For the next 45 minutes I sat and marveled at the sight. Wave after wave of birds came in from every corner of the compass. In the distance they appeared like little swarms of insects. These soon got close enough to be distinguished as groups of ten to 30 birds, and every now and then a small number of birds, two or four, would join a band. Occasionally the bands would coalesce. There might be as many as three or four layers of flocks flying above in different directions, like jetliners stacked above an airport. The twittering sound continued throughout. They would soon descend to the water's edge. Then there would be a general splashing and bathing. After a few minutes the entire band would rise, as if at a signal, and head off across the desert.

Breakfast that morning, for the entire camp staff, was a delicious dish of creamed sand-grouse breast, although the cream, in this environment, was actually sweetened condensed milk. Coffee never tasted better.

The sale itself was something of an anticlimax for me. Hector sat still, surrounded by his staff, and watched the proceedings. It was my job to ensure that nothing obviously sick was entered into the ring, and I had to check the mouths and feet of each animal as it entered through the crush.

As Hector began paying cash for the cattle that he had bought, I realized that he had, all along, been carrying a large sum of money.

"Don't you ever worry, carrying so much cash?" I asked later.

"It is a helluva lot," he agreed, "but I've never even been threatened. One time I had a pretty close call. I was on my own in the middle of the night, lying on the open ground, and a band of *shifta* moved into camp. The only thing to do was to pretend to be asleep. After a while I heard one of them say, 'We will leave him alone. He brings plenty of money into this area.' I waited for a while to be sure that they had left and then broke out into a muck sweat. It's nice when even thieves know not to kill the goose that lays the golden egg."

The duties as DVO Isiolo involved other less exciting activities, such as the monthly administrative meetings with the District Commissioner. Sometimes these were frustrating, even downright maddening. On one occasion when Tony was present, my tendency to call a spade a spade created a minor stir. The DC had asked me about the cattle dipping program in the area.

"We have had some complaints about the number of ticks on the people's cows. I arranged for the dip fluid to be tested and the results have just come in."

He handed me a report sheet which indicated that the dip was so far under strength as to be almost useless, then said, "I do not have any money in my budget for dip replacement. Would you advise the herdsmen to bring their cattle more often, say twice a week, in order to overcome the problem?"

"No," I replied. "You might as well dip the cattle in fresh water as use this solution. It is simply a waste of time to continue until you have the dip at the right strength."

I'm not sure he was used to such direct responses. I never heard if any action was taken. Tony commented as we headed back to his home for lunch, "That was refreshing; I'm not sure he appreciated the candour though."

Two weeks later, the DC called a special meeting to deal with another problem. The attendance included local missionaries of one denomination, several of another group who had come up from Nairobi, and one or two senior government administrative officers.

The problem boiled down to the inability of two rival Christian sects to agree on almost anything. One of them had a zealous young doctor ready and willing to work in the Northern Frontier District. They also had a Land Rover modified as a fully equipped mobile clinic, complete with a sliding operating table that fitted in the middle of the back section. The problem, said a senior member of this delegation, was, "We do not have any accommodation in Isiolo for our doctor."

He turned to the DC. "Can you help? Do you know of any empty housing that we might use?" The DC looked at the senior cleric of the local mission. "I know that you have two empty houses on your compound. Can we use one of those?"

The answer was a flat no. Even after a couple of hours of circular negotiation, the answer did not change. In the end, the Nairobi delegation returned home, and the Land Rover never appeared in Isiolo. The same kind of "tribalism" which is widely condemned in both the local and international media, and which holds back co-operation between Africans, was evidently a force among the people carrying subtly different versions of the "word" of "their" god, or is that God?

CHAPTER 16

SAMSON KABWITHIA'S
SIMPLE IDEA

A team from the Meru office, including men from four different Kenyan tribes, gets into the field and carries out a widespread rabies control program. I nearly become a meal for safari ants. The rabies control campaign is soon followed by a campaign to contain an outbreak of foot-and-mouth disease.

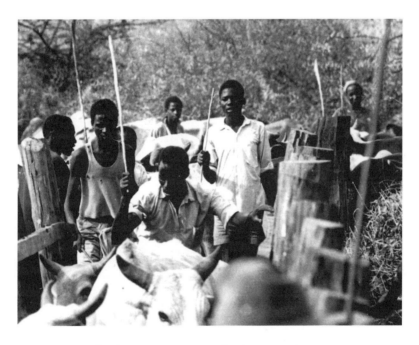

Cattle management; vaccination campaign.
Karimbene crush, getting cattle ready for vaccination.

"I HEAR THERE'S BEEN AN INCREASE IN rabies in several areas recently," I told Vitalis and Mr. Muhoma, the livestock officer, who had just come into the Meru laboratory. "Only last month there was a report in *The Standard* of an American volunteer dying of it in Machakos district. I think we must take some action."

My work in Isiolo was still going on, but in the meantime I still had to attend to my duties in Meru. An annual task was the rabies vaccination campaign for dogs in the district. Vitalis had been showing me the ledger, which revealed that we had fallen well below the annual figures for the last two years, and that our recent safari had had a very poor response.

We would routinely vaccinate dogs brought to the office, but in outlying areas we had to take a more active role, and also ensure that licence fees were paid. A traveling team would vaccinate cattle against anthrax, and herders were required to present all unlicensed and untagged dogs at the vaccination sites. The team would also go into the villages and issue licences. Dogs had to be vaccinated every three years, but the licence fee of five shillings was due annually to the County Council. Treated and licensed dogs wore a collar with a current tag. A County Council bylaw stated that "the Veterinary Officer may destroy by any means at his discretion" any dog that was not suitably identified. To send out the vaccination team again would probably be a waste of effort. It was time to find out what official policy existed at headquarters for the destruction of untreated dogs.

The deputy director in Kabete, Dr. Marcus Durand, told me, "For years we have used strychnine. It's supplied under strict security here at Kabete. The technique involves taking a small parcel of meat, about an inch square and half an inch thick, and making it into a sachet. Just slice it half way through to make a slim purse and insert a small amount of the poison. Don't put in too much, or a dog will vomit it up and you will lose the effect and expose other animals to risk."

I decided to go to the veterinary laboratories store myself, as it seemed unwise to trust such a deadly substance to the bus service.

The information for strychnine use was quite detailed. "The purses of meat should be impaled on small sharpened sticks around a selected village late at night." So read the instructions on a rather heavily used piece of paper. The paper, held around the bottle with a rubber band, had been folded many times, and the print had worn rather thin.

A team of us set out to test the poison: myself, Kipsiele, Vitalis, who relished the chance to get out of the office for a few days, and Austin Ciaji, a senior animal health technician with both smarts and enthusiasm for his work. Austin was a Luo, tall, patrician, very dark-skinned, with a smile like a halogen lamp. He had an infectious good humour and his involvement was always a pleasure. He was also an excellent animal man. I had once shown him how to stop a cow kicking by squeezing in the middle of its back. I had also shown him how to pull a cow to the ground, in order to carry out foot trimming or other treatments, with strategically placed ropes around its belly. He was so strong that he was able to combine the two methods: by squeezing over the withers he could make a cow lie down, which was an impressive sight.

Once we left the office on our mini-safari I told them about the methods and risks, as it was essential that no careless mistakes be made.

"We must purchase some meat from Maitima, the butcher, and keep it in a thermos flask." I described the "purses" and continued, "We have to make sure that we don't poison anything except unlicensed animals. We must warn the villagers, both to ensure that no people take any meat, and that licensed dogs are kept in so that they do not eat the poisoned bait. We must collect the sticks before dawn and the number of baits remaining must be recorded. I've brought along some rubber gloves, and I suggest that I be the only one of us to handle the poison." They seemed to need no coercion on this last idea.

After the first night I realized that while this method may have accounted for a few dogs, it could equally well have taken small predators such as jackals and members of the cat and weasel family. I also realized that there were two marked disadvantages. First, a single animal might eat several baits, thus invalidating any attempt to estimate the number of animals poisoned, and second, people would simply lock up their unlicensed dogs at night and so avoid both the penalty and the fee.

In order to overcome both of these problems at once I decided to use the lethal poison purses under controlled conditions in daylight. Kipsiele, Austin, and I drove to Giaki, a village where only two dogs had been licensed or vaccinated a month before — which seemed an unlikely figure in a community with over 50 buildings, including several shops, and a busy market. After driving down the increasingly rutted and very dusty road, we picked up the local animal health technician, Simon Marangu. He was short, almost as short as Kipsiele, but slimmer and not nearly as dark skinned. With him as a guide we moved to an area near the local slaughterhouse, where we had a good chance of finding stray dogs.

Simon asked why we were carrying out the program. "Rabies is a very dangerous disease," I explained. "We can control it, at least in dogs, which have more contact with people than do wild animals. The only way we can do that is to enforce licensing, even though the cost of issuing the license and the vaccine is more than the price of the tag."

"I see. So how will we test the poison?"

"We will find a dog without a tag, and try and see if anyone owns it. If not, we will throw it a small piece of meat with the poison inside and see what happens."

We sat in the Land Rover and waited to check for dogs that had no tag. There were about 15 of them roaming in a loose pack around the marketplace. The first two to approach the Land Rover were each thrown a piece of treated meat, and we then watched them carefully.

Quite soon after eating the bait the dogs started a frenzied run and then fell over. They recovered briefly and continued running and falling for several minutes, yelping in pain. Finally they stayed down.

"Why don't they die sooner?" asked Simon.

I explained, "The poison has to dissolve in the stomach and then enter the body. The muscles are stimulated, until finally they're unable to relax, and then the animal suffocates as it can no longer work the breathing muscles. There is a poison called cyanide that works right away, when it gets into the animal's mouth or even when the animal smells it, but this is much too dangerous for us to handle."

Until we started this program I had not realized what a gruesome poison we were dealing with. The convulsions and struggles that these poor dogs underwent were horrible to see. Although there was no doubt that we must keep the much more horrible scourge of rabies at bay, I decided that as long as I could find another way of killing these dogs, strychnine was not going to be used again while I was veterinary officer. The next morning I placed a call to Kabete.

"Dr. Durand, yesterday I witnessed two dogs dying under strychnine poison. It's pretty nasty, and I have a gun of my own. Am I allowed to use it for rabies control?"

"I don't think that there's any problem, but you'll have to be very careful around villages," he replied.

"Oh, of course. But I don't think it's any more dangerous than the strychnine. At least with a gun I won't be leaving poison around for anything to eat, and I won't be killing indiscriminately."

"You can pick up some ammunition from the stores here at HQ. Good luck. Let me know how you get on."

The next task was to organize a team to go round the district and bring the rabies situation back under control. We kept the team small. I took my shotgun and a supply of number four cartridges, and we set off in a southward direction among the villages at higher altitude along the mountain slopes. The news spread along the heavily traveled road much faster than our safari. After the first couple of days, we were met in several villages by groups of dogs and handlers waiting for vaccination. The gun could be kept in its case.

By five each evening we called it quits. This gave us time not only to set up camp but to get in a little R & R. For me this was simple. Several glacier and spring-fed rivers tumble off the heights of Mount Kenya towards the plain below. I was glad of the opportunity to dip a line into a few of them. In one pool in the Igoji River, aided by a large Mrs. Simpson streamer fly that I had carefully cast with an upstream roll, I landed two fine brown trout, one of them over three pounds. Austin, a Luo from the shores of Lake Victoria, was more than pleased to help in eating them, and Kipsiele showed no hesitation either. Vitalis was not so sure; as a Meru he had no tradition of fish-eating behind him, but his hesitation soon broke down after he had tried a morsel. Our store of butter dwindled quite quickly as all of us relished a supper of trout cooked in a large government-issue frying pan until their skins turned a crispy brown.

The following evening, after visiting half a dozen more local villages, I succumbed to temptation and returned to the Igoji River, trying a few casts just below the spot that had yielded last night's supper. As I watched the white wings of my Royal Coachman drift down the fast water, and begin to swing out of the current into the belly of the pool, I suddenly felt an excruciating pain in my groin. My left testicle and the tip of my penis felt as if someone had pierced them with a red hot needle. Naturally, I looked down the front of my shorts and was horrified to see about 20 *siafu* (safari ants) on my upper thighs and the nearby family jewels. Most of the ants were of the small variety, but a few, including the ones clamped to my most tender parts, were the large and vicious soldiers. A further look showed me that while intent upon my fishing, the lie of the pool, and the action of my fly, I had managed to step right into an ant's nest. Another hundred or so of the creatures were swarming up my legs. I had antagonized the creatures, and they had *ant-agonized* me. I did not stop to get an accurate count, despite my scientific training.

There was only one thing to do. Abandoning my rod over my shoulder with a flick of the wrist, I jumped into the river. It took about ten minutes to rid myself of the unwelcome pests. I'm not sure if the immersion had any direct effect upon the *siafu*, but the water certainly acted as an anesthetic, and considerably reduced the area of skin for the beasts to attack as my cremaster muscles went into a rapid reflex contraction, reacting to the change in temperature from the balmy equatorial evening to the glacier-fed stream. My fishing trip was a bit of an *ant*-iclimax.

I related the scene to the team as we sat over supper; there was a sort of pregnant pause and I guessed that they were unsure whether to laugh or not, considering that I was not only the boss, but also a *mzungu*. Eventually Austin cracked a smile, and then there was a round of good raucous laughter, in which I joined. Once we had settled down, there was a general discussion about the fact that the large soldier ants are used as sutures by some traditional medicine practitioners. The ants are held to a cut, and allowed to clamp on to either side of it. Then their bodies are broken off behind the head so that the mouthparts are left closed on the wound.

We carried on down the tortuous road to Chuka, vaccinating as we went, and from there dropped down towards the arid plains of Tharaka. This region was more isolated than the communities along the hairpin contours above, and news of our activities had not yet filtered through. It took no time for the message to spread once a shot or two had been fired.

Supper changed from fish to guinea-fowl or yellow-neck — I had slipped a box of my own number six bird-shot into my gear. None of the rest of the team had ever tried yellow-neck before.

"This is very good," said Austin, wiping some fat off his chin as he tucked into a piece of leg.

"Yes, almost like a good chicken, but more flavour," chimed in Vitalis.

"I like going on safari with the doctor," said Kipsiele. "This yellow-neck is better than the guinea-fowl we had last night."

"Oh, I think the guinea-fowl was better, but neither was as good as the trout at Igoji," was Austin's contribution. As a Luo he tended to be a bit biased toward fish.

After our rabies campaign had covered the southern half of the district, we stopped for the weekend and passed through Meru to pick up more vaccine and receipts. It gave us all a chance to relax and get a decent wash. Jo was happy to chat as we sat on the verandah and enjoyed a couple of ripe avocado pears from the two small trees in the garden. From home base the vaccination team ventured north and made another circular trip, this time through the Northern Grazing Area, past Kangeta and Lare, the little market town of Maua where there was a small mission hospital, and even to the borders of the Meru National Park.

County Council revenues were strong that year because so many people were inspired to pay their license fees.

Before I even had time to write up the campaign in the monthly report, the success of our efforts had surprising and far-reaching consequences.

The party line phone pealed its one short and two long rings. This meant that the call was for us and not others on the line.

"Hello, Dr. Haigh here, district veterinary office."

"Good morning Jerry, this is Marcus Durand in Kabete."

"Good morning, Dr. Durand. What's up?"

I assumed he was calling to enquire about the use of the gun on the rabies outing, but I was wrong.

"Jerry, we have a problem. South Africa Type II foot-and-mouth disease has broken out up at Moyale and is moving south with the herders. We need to take action. Can you please arrange a meeting with the DC for Thursday or Friday? Geoff Smith and I will try to be there early." Dr. Smith was my immediate superior in the provincial office.

Type SAT II foot-and-mouth, one of only seven known types worldwide, had never before been reported north of the Zambesi river, some 1,400 miles south of us on the border of Zimbabwe and Zambia. How it had made such a huge jump was a mystery. The problem was that the entire cattle population of Kenya was at risk: none of them had ever been exposed to this strain of the virus. The major problem with foot-and-mouth disease virus is that the blisters it produces cause severe pain in the mouth and feet, and prevents cloven-hoofed animals from eating and walking. The high fever that results from infection can also lead to abortions. Some cattle may die, especially if they have never been affected before, or some other virulent agent takes the opportunity to set up shop in the already compromised animal. Some types of the disease had been around in the country for years. Many cattle had been exposed to one or other of the local strains, and so did not suffer so severely when a fresh outbreak occurred. This new threat was quite another matter, and it could potentially cause devastation at several levels.

I called the District Commissioner and asked him to request the attendance of his District Officers, and as many of the chiefs from the northern part of the district as possible, at a Thursday morning meeting.

Drs. Durand and Smith arrived in plenty of time. At the Pig and Whistle, over a breakfast of scrambled eggs and bacon, large quantities of slightly damp toast, and lashings of marmalade, Dr. Durand explained the planned strategy.

"Meru lies between the semi-arid deserts of the NFD and the heavily populated agricultural land of the highlands, with its millions of valuable dairy and beef cattle, as well as places like Marania and Kisima with their thousands of sheep. So we want to create a *cordon sanitaire* across the Northern Grazing Area of Meru, and at the same time extend it into the adjacent Nanyuki district. Peter Gamble will lead the campaign in Laikipia, so that we have a belt across from Lare, at your northern limit, all the way across beyond Rumuruti. Do you think you can manage to get something organized?"

"It will depend upon convincing the DC, as well as making sure we get all the cattle in the Northern Grazing Area, the NGA," I replied. "The tricky part will be to ensure compliance, and also to recognize those cattle that haven't been treated, so that we can prosecute those who do not bring their beasts forward."

The NGA was a strip about 20 miles wide and 75 miles long that was leased to the people of the area under county council jurisdiction. Fortunately, as it turned out, the entire zone was under the direct control of one very energetic chief named Festus Kiautha, whose location headquarters was at a place called Liliaba.

At the meeting that morning, the District Commissioner called for maximum co-operation from all of his staff and asked for suggestions on how to ensure compliance.

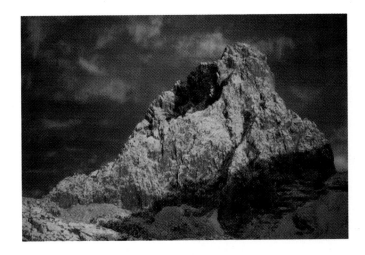

Nelion at dawn, 17,022 feet (5,188 metres), Mount Kenya's second highest peak.

Mount Kenya's peaks from the north at about 13,000 feet.

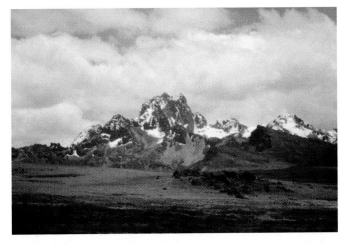

The author looking east into the dawn light from near Point Lenana, Mount Kenya's third highest peak at 16,356 feet (4,985 metres).

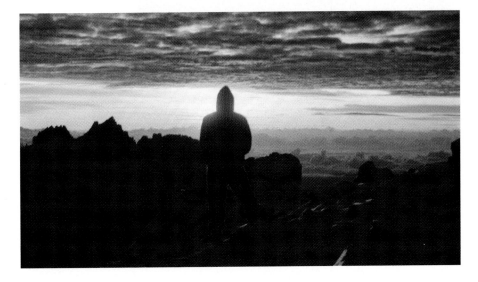

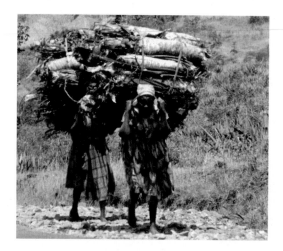

Two heavy loads of firewood being carried by Kikuyu women. The weight is borne by tump lines across the forehead. In the late 1960s many older women could be seen with permanent furrows in their foreheads after many years of carrying such loads.

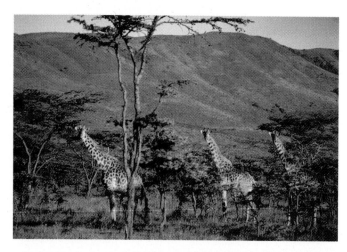

Masai giraffe among the thorn trees below the Ngong hills.

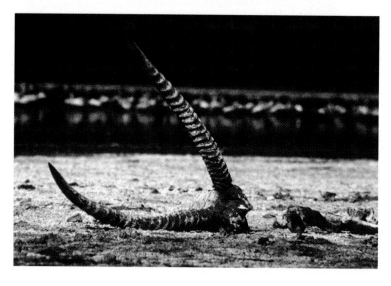

The circle of life. All that remains of a waterbuck on the shores of Lake Nakuru.

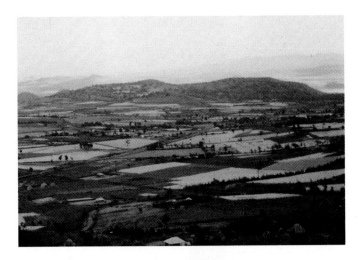

From the road above Kirua village the small farms look like a patchwork quilt as the wheat ripens.

From the road below Marania looking out over Isiolo and the Northern Frontier District. On a clear day one can see Marsabit Mountain.

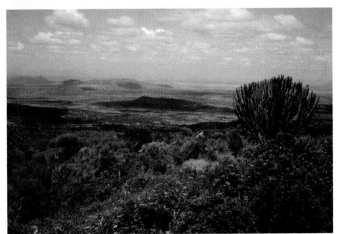

Homesteads near Tigania.

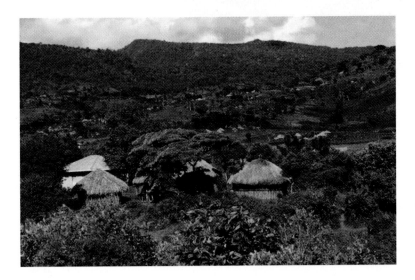

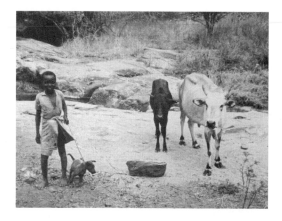

A boy, his dog, and the family cattle. Near Ciokarige, Tharaka.

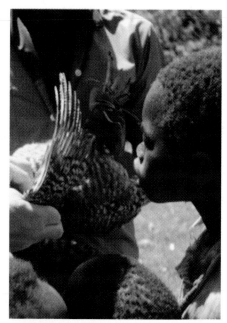

Curious eyes to see what vaccinating a chicken is all about.

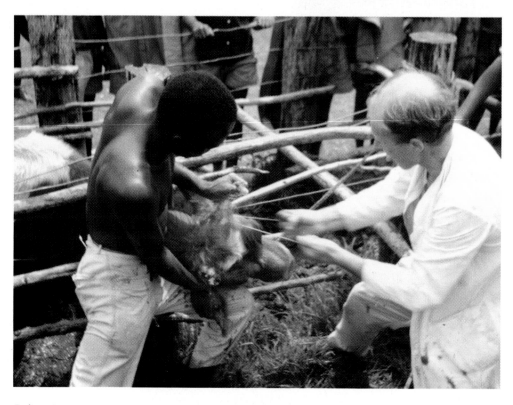

Dehorning a Guernsey cow near Maua. Austin Ciaji holds her head.

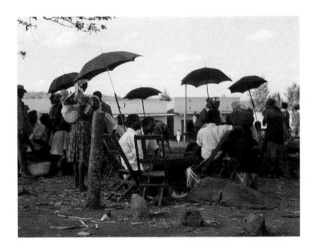

Come rain or come shine. Umbrellas are a standard feature on market days.

Sunning themselves. A group of youngsters from the paediatric ward. Meru District Hospital, 1968.

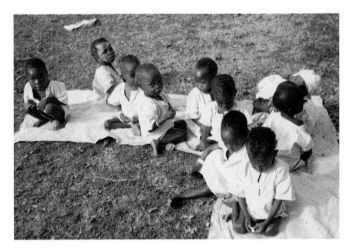

Driving hazard. A tire change for the Marania Land Rover.

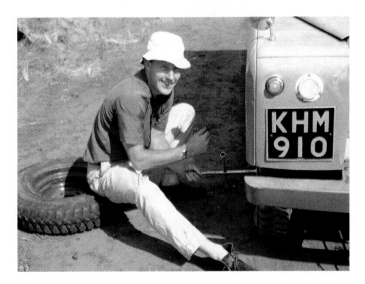

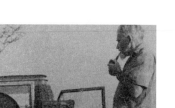

Jonny Baxendale, George Adamson, and Boy at Mugwhango.

Joy Adamson and Pippa the cheetah.

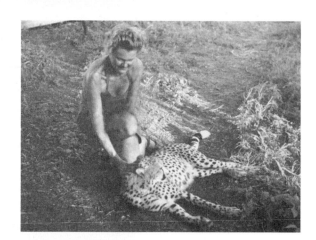

A young male lion checks us out from a tree fork at Mugwhango.

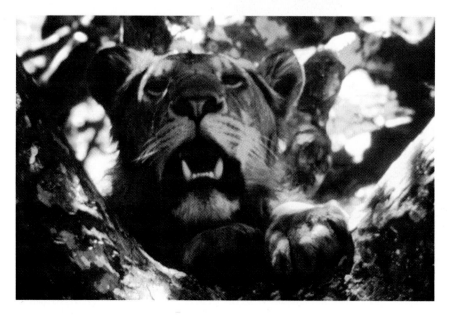

Leaving the cathedral of the Highlands. December 22nd, 1939. Margery and Paddy Haigh. Also seen are Mr. & Mrs. J.C. Mundy — Mr. Mundy gave the bride away. He was the Commissioner for Inland Revenue! The best man (on right) was also in the KAR, and was Captain the Hon. Roderick Ward (brother of the Earl of Dudley).

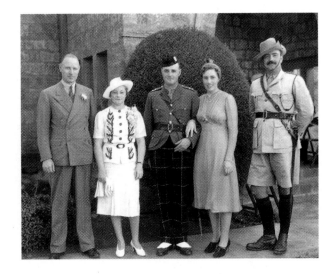

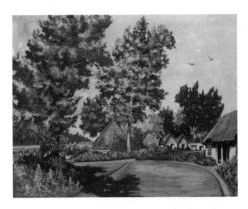

The painting by R. Snoaden done in 1944. The scene was almost unchanged in 1969. The drinks at our wedding were kept in the building at right, and the cake cutting took place about where the artist's easel must have been standing.

On the lawn at the Nanyuki Sports Club. From l to r, Lorna O'Callaghan, Mrs. Haigh senior, Tim Roberts (best man), the newlyweds, and Judi Gamble, who made the cake.

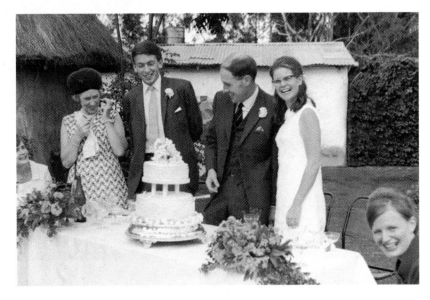

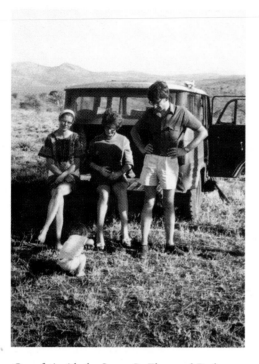

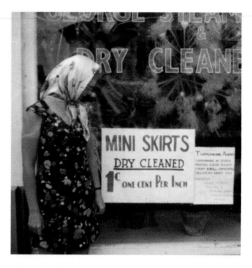

Knysna, South Africa, 1969.

On safari with the Sayers. Jo, Elma, and Paul,
with Nicola checking out the dirt.

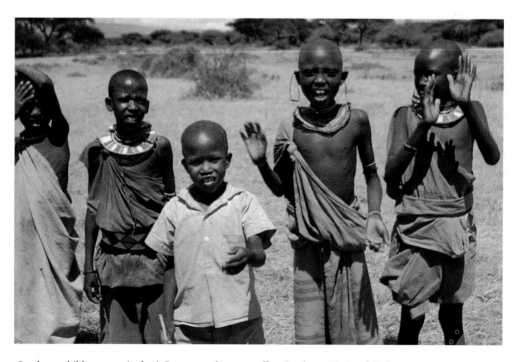

Samburu children near Archer's Post, near the turn-off to Samburu National Park.

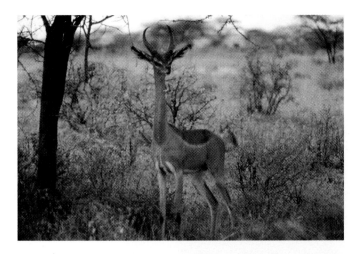

A male gerenuk checks us out. Samburu Park.

On that same safari we sat and watched an elephant group as they came to the Uaso Nyiro River, all to drink, the young to play.

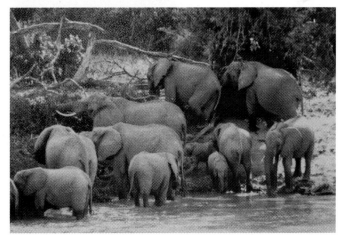

A young male elephant flexes his teenage muscles and tries to scatter a herd of buffalo, just for the devilment. This was his fourth try in ten minutes and the buffalo have become blasé.

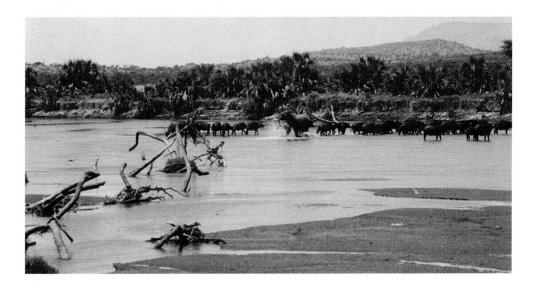

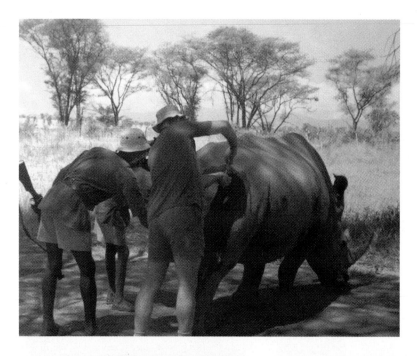

A big injection
of antibiotics
into an awkward
patient while
two *askaris*
keep her happy.

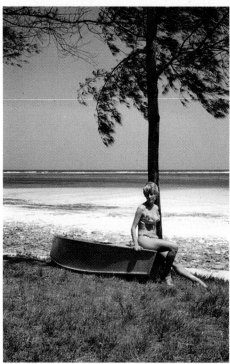

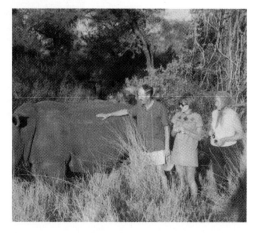

The Haigh family, on holiday, are not quite sure
about this ex-patient.

A break from dealing blackjack at the London
Playboy club. Brigid on a visit to the Ocean
Sports Hotel at Watamu.

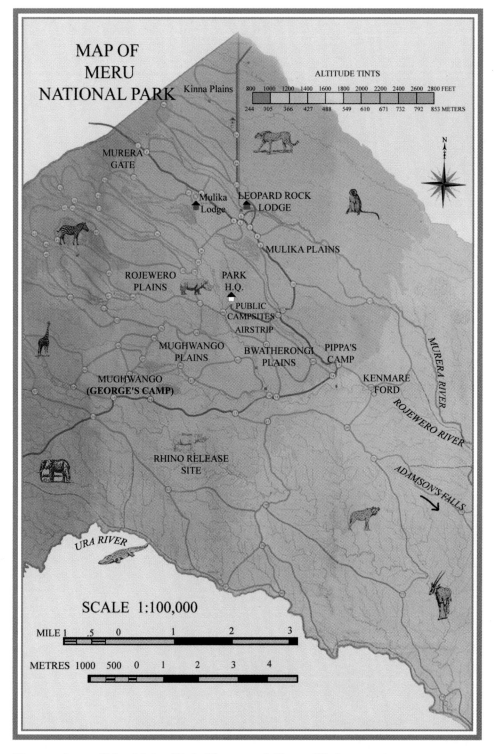

MAP OF
MERU
NATIONAL PARK

Kinna Plains

ALTITUDE TINTS

800	1000	1200	1400	1600	1800	2000	2200	2400	2600	2800 FEET
244	305	366	427	488	549	610	671	732	792	853 METERS

MURERA
GATE

Mulika
Lodge

LEOPARD ROCK
LODGE

MULIKA PLAINS

ROJEWERO
PLAINS

PARK
H.Q.

PUBLIC
CAMPSITES

AIRSTRIP

MUGHWANGO
PLAINS

BWATHERONGI
PLAINS

PIPPA'S
CAMP

MURERA RIVER

KENMARE
FORD

MUGHWANGO
(GEORGE'S CAMP)

ROJEWERO RIVER

RHINO RELEASE
SITE

ADAMSON'S FALLS

URA RIVER

SCALE 1:100,000

MILE 1   .5   0   1   2   3

METRES 1000 500 0   1   2   3   4

The central part of Meru National Park. The eastern half was off limits to tourists.

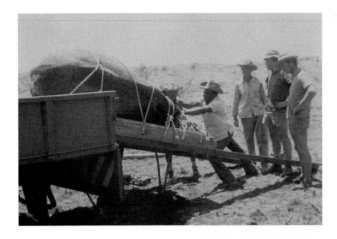

Despite appearances, Alexander is not doing all the work. Two men are cranking a winch that is dragging the sled up the ramp and into the lorry.

Back at camp, Mutua collects ticks before the rhino is unloaded.

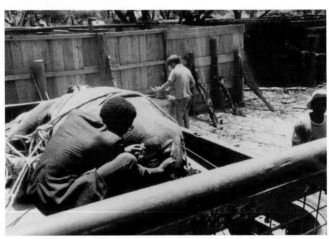

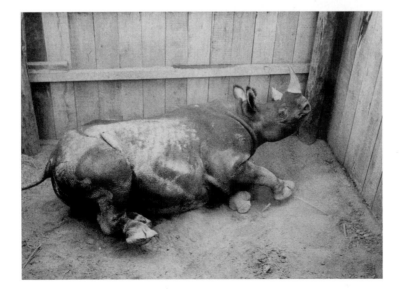

A newly caught rhino wakes up in strange surroundings within seconds of being given an antidote to his capture cocktail.

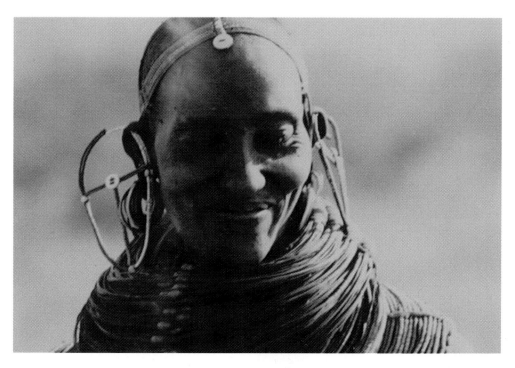

A Samburu woman near Wamba.

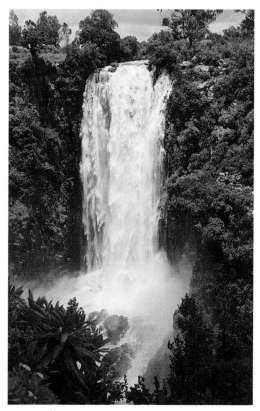

Thomson's Falls.

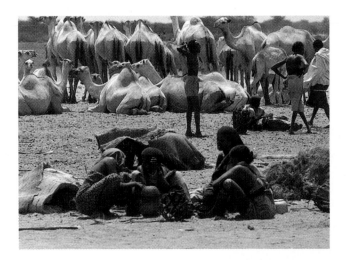

Just relaxing. A group of Boran people at Wajir.

We are not amused.

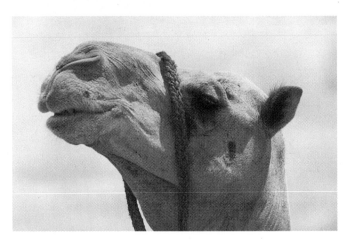

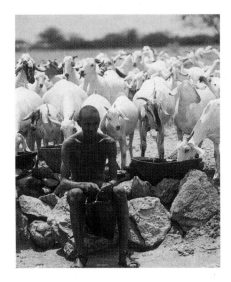

At the well. Goat herder and his herd at Wajir.

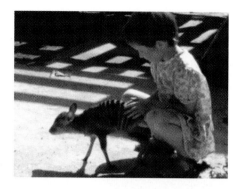

Karen and a tiny zebra duiker at
the Mombasa Quarantine station.

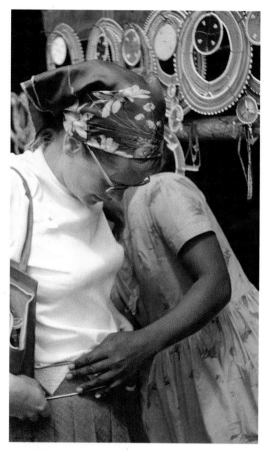

Jo being fitted for a belt at
the Masai trading booth.
Namanga, on the Kenya–
Tanzania border.

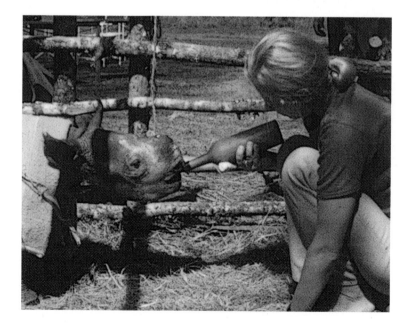

Iris offers break-
fast to a warmly
dressed young
rhino after a
sleepless night.

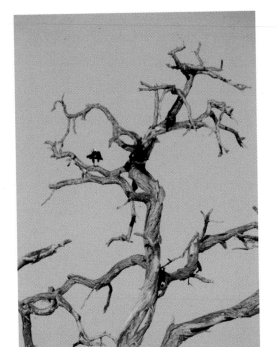

African fish eagles.

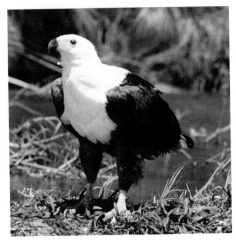

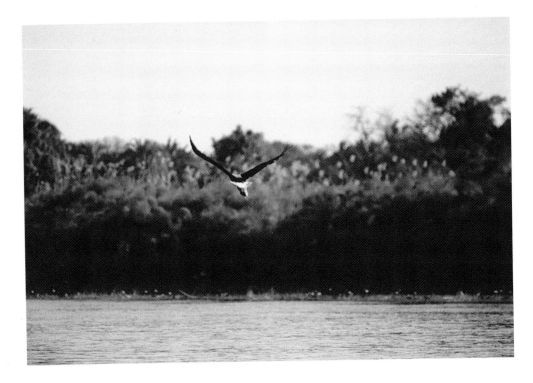

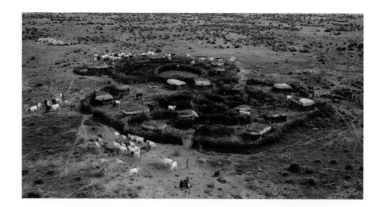

Samburu manayatta
near Maralal.

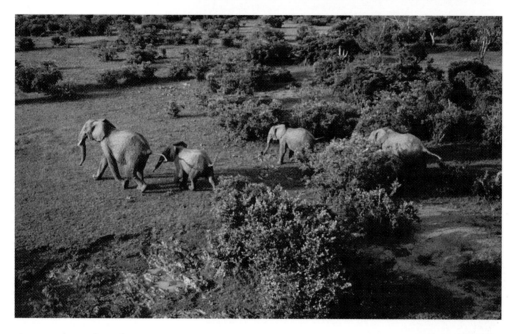

A group moves through
the bush near Maralal.

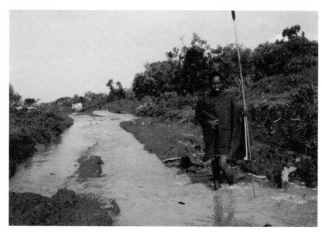

Driving during the rains can
be difficult. Near Maralal.

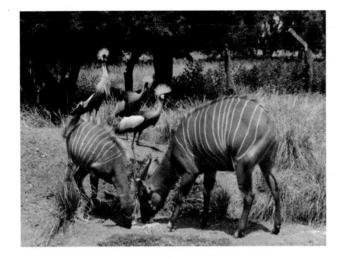

Bongo and crowned
cranes at the Mount
Kenya Game Ranch.

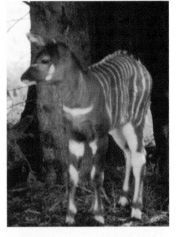

Born on the ranch; a young bongo
gets the benefit of some shade.

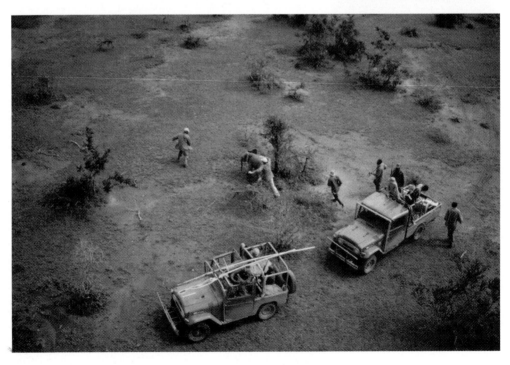

The ground crew moves in as the young elephant, trunk relaxed under
the influence of drugs, comes to a halt. Don Hunt is first there.

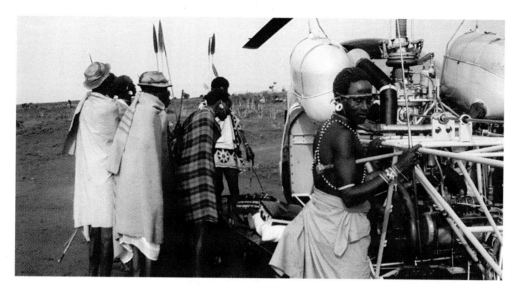

A clash of two cultures.
Samburu men gather
round the Hughes 300.

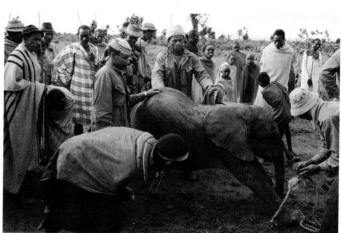

Boy or Girl? Near Maralal.

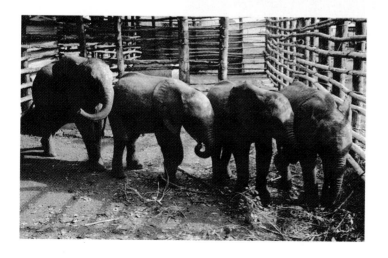

In quarantine, getting
ready for a trip to
Nigeria.

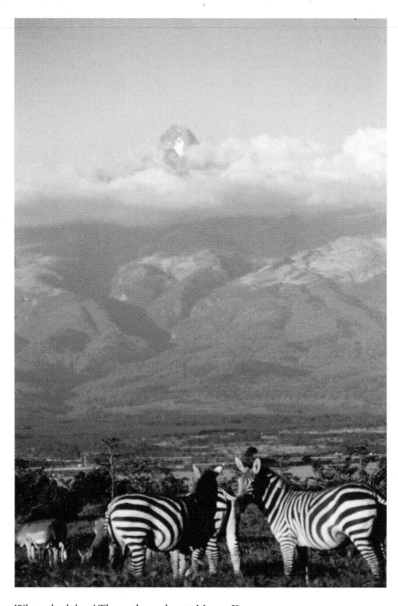

What a backdrop! The peaks peek out. Mount Kenya.

"We can prosecute any owners who fail to bring their cattle," said Dr. Durand, "but it is more important to make sure that the cattle are brought than to worry about charges. This is a really urgent matter. Any unvaccinated cattle will be at risk and can spread the disease."

I explained that it was not long since the cattle owners had had to bring in their animals for the annual anthrax campaign. The memories surrounding the rinderpest problem of a few years previous had diminished. Would the herders be fed up with so much interference with their cattle?

It was Festus who came up with the solution. He reminded us all of what had happened in our recent rabies safari. Then he asked me to attend a *barazza* to which he would call all the graziers who paid annual fees to the county council.

The morning of the *barazza*, Kipsiele, Austin, and I left the office early and motored up the dusty road past Tigania to the lookout point just short of Kangeta at the northwestern point of the Nyambenis. In the clear morning air we could see a prodigious distance. Shaba, and the smaller Shaba Dogo, seemed to be almost within a stone's throw, although we knew them to be at least 20 miles away. The intervening rounded hills of varying sizes, partly shrouded in early morning mist on their lower slopes, resembled nothing more than the mud bubbles in a hot spring, ready to burst and re-form. A thousand feet below us were a group of two or three *manyattas* (groups of family dwellings) around a cattle crush. Festus had designated this as the meeting point. We descended gingerly over the heavily rutted track and eventually parked GK 881 under a convenient thorn tree.

Many people were already gathered, including some of the subchiefs whom I already knew. I recognized and greeted a couple of the elders from *manyattas* where we had recently caused such consternation with our dog campaign. They did not appear to be in any way upset, but perhaps they were either showing inherent good manners or were superb actors. We sat around drinking the sweet milky tea that was brought to us in glasses and waited for Festus to call the meeting to order.

Timothy Mutiga, an animal health technician whom we had picked up in Kianjai because Austin spoke only a smattering of Kimeru, acted as translator for me. Festus went through the rituals of greeting and introduction, and then he described the problem and its solution. Turning towards me at the correct moment, he paused for dramatic effect.

"Remember what this *mzungu* daktari did to your dogs last month when they were not vaccinated? Think," he said, "what the veterinary officer will do to your cattle if you do not bring them when he tells you to."

This statement came as a complete surprise to me and, no doubt, to the assembled crowd. It would have been more than my life was worth to even appear to threaten shooting cattle. I just played stupid and hoped that we would get away safely after the meeting.

Festus's threat had startling consequences.

The first organizational challenge was to decide how best to cover all the cattle in the NGA. Second, we had to estimate how many animals would turn up at the vaccination stations, and how to be sure both that we treated them all, and that we did not treat any of them twice. Eventually we decided to have three teams of six people each. Mr. Sigilai, a junior livestock officer and fellow tribesman of Kipsiele's, would lead one, Austin another, and I would take on the third. Each team also had a driver and a technician. The latter would ensure that sterile needles were available, fill syringes, keep the vaccine cool in refrigerated boxes, and stoke the branding fire. The other four men would vaccinate and brand the cattle.

Through messages to the chiefs, passed on to assistant chiefs, the herders were told to bring their animals to one of two cattle crushes, well known to all of them, where the anthrax vaccinations were normally carried out. One site would be at Liliaba, where we had held our *barazza*, the other at Karimbene, much closer to town, and down a less hazardous track than the one from Kangeta. Each owner was also told to bring a supply of firewood. My third team was to act as a rover and be available to go to whichever of the crushes had the greater number of animals to deal with.

The brand with which we would mark vaccinated cattle had to be chosen carefully. During our planning session, I explained, "We must not let any cattlemen know what the brand will be. We'd rather not spend money on a new brand, and there is no need to give the animals a permanent brand that will actually burn the skin. Something that will last a month or so will be enough."

After some discussion, it was Samson Kabwithia, the oldest man in the group, who came up with the answer. Enjoying the chance to be heard among his colleagues, he tilted his head slightly to one side, as we had all seen him do when acting as a cattle auctioneer, which he did in the deliberate African style. His resonant voice and slow pace riveted one's attention.

"Perhaps we can use the 'N' brand that is given to every animal as a life mark to show that it has been vaccinated for rinderpest, but we can turn it on its side to make a 'Z.'" He turned his wrist to demonstrate. "We can also place it on the hind leg, instead of on the hump."

This simple solution needed no further discussion.

The campaign started on a Monday morning. Taking the rover team with me I visited the first of the two crushes, at Liliaba, and things seemed to be going well. Each owner, with assistance from several young children, and the staff of the veterinary department, was waiting his turn to run his cattle into a long crush constructed of local logs. Once they were ready they were vaccinated, branded with our "new" hair brand, and let go. Work was proceeding at a steady pace, and a check with the technician indicated that there would be enough vaccine to last the day. After a couple of hours, we moved off to see how Austin and the others were doing.

We could see clouds of dust hanging in the still air as we drove down the slope to Karimbene crush. It seemed as if all the cattle in the district had gathered. The bellowing and shouting could be heard from a couple of miles away. The leaves and thorns of the flat-topped acacias seemed to emerge from the dust cloud fully formed without any sign of a trunk.

Here, our men in the vaccination team were spending most of their time pushing, shoving, and generally cajoling reluctant animals into the corrals and chute, rather than actually vaccinating anything. Two men would go down a line of cattle, one with a multi-dose syringe in his hand, and the other with the branding iron, and do every beast in about ten minutes. Then it would take another half hour or so to get the next lot of animals ready.

It was evident that we would never get the job done if we continued to use the crush, as the problem was the rate at which cattle could be persuaded to enter it. With the team in my Land Rover we had double the available staff, but this would not increase the rate at which the cattle were actually treated.

One of the most remarkable things about pastoral herders in Africa, at least to those unfamiliar with cattle, is the extent to which the herders, be they small boys or old men, know and can control their charges. Within an area less than half a mile across there were probably 10,000 animals. Each herd was tightly packed together. Any straying would be promptly dealt with by a shout, or, in extreme need, a thrown stick. The herder knew each animal by name, and although he may not have known the exact number of head, he certainly knew if any were missing, or alternatively if any stranger had joined the mob. Small boys controlled their animals at the water hole nearby with a real sense of order and decorum. Herds would stand 20 or 30 yards off, and wait while a particular group finished drinking. The next group in line, and I could not determine how this was decided in the absence of a line, would then come forward, and even the individual cattle would drink in turns, as directed by the boy.

Naturally, most of the staff members knew about this control as they themselves had carried out similar tasks in their own youths. I let the discussion flow, and soon Vitalis, Kabwithia, David, Austin, and the others had come up with the solution to our problem. As Austin, the senior among them, summed it up: "We should organize into two groups of six men. We can then go through and process each herd in a few minutes. Two men can vaccinate, two men can mark the cattle, and two more can do the brands. Geoffrey will mind the fire and help Vitalis with filling the syringes of vaccine." Geoffrey Kanyuru and M'Ichoro Iraku were quiet during the discussion. They usually worked as cleaners and general messengers around the office, but I'd had to enlist every possible staff member into the campaign. The office could go unswept for a few days. Geoffrey was relishing every moment. M'Ichoro, older and more experienced, had seen it all before, well before my time.

The first two men walked quietly among the cattle, an automatic syringe in each hand, and injected animals in the loose skin behind the shoulder or over the neck. Two more walked immediately behind the needle holders, and as an animal was vaccinated they would pick up a handful of the manure that was by this time spread just about everywhere, and daub it along the spine. When every animal had been decorated in this fashion, the third pair of men would move in with their brands. Naturally, as the animals turned, some of them would be double branded, one on each side, but that hardly seemed to matter.

The swirling dust, the lowing of the cattle, the smell of burning hair, the crackling of the fire, and the shouts of the herdsmen combined to make an unforgettable scene. We broke for meals in relays. The kettle was on the go the whole time. I joined in as a spare hand whenever someone needed a break, filling syringes, wielding a branding iron, stoking the fire. It was all grist to the mill. We continued into the growing dark, the headlights of the two Land Rovers turned towards the spot where each herdsman waited his turn. At nine o'clock I called a halt.

When we realized that we did not have enough vaccine with us to keep up the furious pace, the fact that we had an extra driver really paid off. Kipsiele was able to run a shuttle, and also to carry messages and replenish vaccine supplies from the office. By lunch time on Wednesday we had passed the original estimate derived from our annual census, and were running out of vaccine again; Kipsiele was dispatched directly to Nairobi to collect more, as the bus service would not get supplies to us in time. He was back that same evening, and now we did not have to worry about running out.

By Friday the pace was slowing. Both sites had been using the "new and improved" method of herd vaccination, and we had treated an enormous number of animals. In retrospect it seems likely that two or three things combined to bring this about. First of course was Festus' warning. I am sure too that the appearance of the deputy director at the DC's meeting, and the fact that we had called a meeting over so routine a matter as a vaccination campaign, made an impression on the cattle owners. And the fact that we issued dire warnings about the threat of a new disease from the north probably played a role. "Bush telegraph," or "coffee row news," is one of the fastest means of communication in any rural community, be it in Africa, Saskatchewan, or the English countryside, although this method of news dissemination has lost ground where television has invaded our lives. The threat probably brought cattle out of the woodwork from areas well outside our target. It seems quite likely that animals came in from neighbouring Isiolo district, as well as from more distant parts of Meru. It was fortunate that we had enough vaccine available to accommodate them all.

The eventual tally, estimated from the amount of vaccine used, was just short of 100,000 head in six days! Soon after we finished the campaign the short rains began. What effect our six-day madness had upon the spread of the foot-and-mouth disease is difficult to estimate. Certainly the problem never appeared in Meru, and the threat to the dairy cattle in the lush high country did not materialize, so perhaps we did some good. Alternatively, the change in the weather may have been the key. I suppose we'll never know, but we did establish a precedent for quick, widespread emergency reactive programs, which could be used again in similar situations.

Another change: Geoffrey applied for the new Animal Health Technician position. His experiences had whetted his appetite, and in any case the pay was twice as good as that of an office cleaner.

CHAPTER 17

WRESTLING WITH RHINOS

*Following a series of teething problems, I catch my first wild
black rhino. Soon others follow. I meet a Turkana camel herder
who has scant regard for rhinos.*

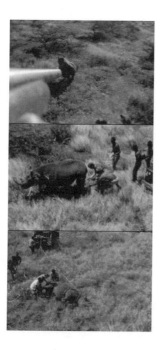
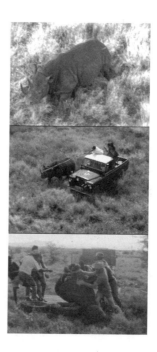

Rhino capture, taken from Super-8 movie clips.
1–6. Lining up the target, drugs taking effect, the animal either comes to a
complete stop against a small object, falls over on its own, or is pulled over
after a loop is placed over its neck. It is then hobbled, rolled over, and
flipped on to a sledge before being transported back to base.

THE ANNUAL TENNIS TOURNAMENT, which drew mixed–doubles teams from clubs around the country, was in full swing at Makuyu. Between matches that Saturday, Tony Parkinson and I sat at the bar in companionable silence. He was there representing Kabete's Vet Lab Sports Club; I had been asked to come across from Meru and play with the Nanyuki side. We had played together on the winning Vet Lab team in 1966.

As we sipped our pints of chilled gin and bitter lemon, topped up with lemonade, Tony suddenly looked up. "Jerry," he said, "John and I have been catching rhino for years using trucks, ropes, and chases. We're thinking of changing to the new drugging methods that are being developed. Would you be interested in getting involved?"

"How do you mean?"

"Well, I have a dart gun, but we need a vet to administer the capture drugs, work out doses, and make sure that we get into no trouble. Would you be free for a few days at the end of next month?"

About five seconds later my career took a 90-degree turn, as I replied that I would be more than willing. It's funny how little things can create big changes.

Tony had been involved in conservation for almost 20 years, and had worked with his godfather, John Seago, since his teenage years. John, the brother of East Anglian landscape artist Edward Seago, had served in motor torpedo boats during the Second World War. He had contracted TB and had been advised to move to a better climate, so once the war ended he'd moved to Kenya, and had never been back to England.

The two of them had a reputation as a very efficient team who knew a tremendous amount about the capture and translocation of a wide variety of Kenya's wildlife. There were two basic ways in which the crew earned their keep: the capture of animals for zoos and the translocation of animals within the country. As the human population increased, so the land hunger of the new generation of young people grew ever more urgent. The only solution was to open up new tracts of undeveloped land, and of course this led to displacement of the wildlife that lived there. They had recently been involved in a well-publicized translocation of the scarce roan antelope from an area near Embu that was destined for settlement. Pictures of Tony riding herd on a group of roan as they entered a huge trap, several acres in size, surrounded by piled thorn bush, had appeared in a local wildlife magazine.

Schemes of this sort had been tried many times before, seldom with success. Noel Simon records in his book *Between the Sunlight and the Thunder* that J.A. Hunter shot 1,088 rhino in one area in order to clear it for settlement. The current desperate plight of the rhino becomes even more poignant when viewed in the light of such history.

In the late 1960s and '70s there were still large numbers of rhinoceros in many parts of the country. Rhino are highly territorial, a fact which has made them an easy target for the unbridled poaching that has devastated their populations throughout the continent. It is easy to find out where a rhino is living, simply by identifying manure heaps, which accumulate at the boundaries of his home range as he patrols.

A large and stubborn animal such as a rhino would be an impossible tenant on a small farm. Not only would the beast be obstreperous, but it would also be highly likely to lay waste to any attempt at crop agriculture. Building a heavy thorn *boma* around a planted crop might well prevent gazelles or zebras from eating maize or tomatoes, but it would be a complete waste of time as a rhino deterrent. Their thick hide and wedged shape mean that rhino can go through thorn bushes like a hot knife through butter.

Tony and John and their team had captured many species of large animal by using heavy vehicles to chase their quarry through the bush until they were close enough to drop a noose over the neck. The noose was pre-set with a bulky knot so that it would never tighten sufficiently to throttle the subject. In turn, the rope and noose were loosely attached with woolen threads to a long bamboo pole, and as soon as the noose had been dropped over the animal's head the threads would break, releasing the pole. The animal would thereby be attached to the vehicle. This method had disadvantages for both the animal and the personnel involved, and it also took a fierce toll on the vehicles. A running rhino can reach speeds of almost 30 miles an hour, and turn at right angles even when going all out. At such speeds, charging through, rather than around, small thorn scrub and across a seemingly unending field of rock-strewn bush, or in a sea of tall grass, one could never tell when the vehicle might hit an ant hill or drop into an unseen hole and come to an abrupt halt. The chase vehicle was a converted wartime Ford 4 x 4 with a very high clearance, which it certainly needed. Tony's unerring eye for terrain was just as important. The new dart gun, if it worked, would certainly make the whole process much easier and safer.

I had treated only a couple of white rhino in Meru National Park at this time, and had no experience working with free-ranging black rhino at all, having not even seen film of the old method of capture. I decided to load my darts with the drug cocktail that I had used successfully on the white rhino, but much trickier was the question of needles. Rhinos have about the thickest hide of any land animal. The ordinary thin needle that most folks see at the doctor's office, or even the one used by a vet to treat cows, was simply not going to do the job. Even the commercially made darting needles available at the time were not robust enough for this task.

I took the problem to my friend Buster Cook, who had a farm called Endarasha near Nanyuki. Buster was a keen amateur engineer, and had his own metal shop as well as an abiding interest in fresh challenges.

"Buster, I wonder if you could give me a hand with these?" I said, showing him the needle that I had obtained, as well as the dart barrel and other bits and pieces.

"I need a needle that is stout, has a small barb to stop it jumping out, will go through thick hide without cutting out a plug and getting blocked, and most awkward of all, will fit into the thread of the barrel, which seems to be an odd size. I have tried several bolts, just to see what fits, and I am stumped."

"Let's have a look," he said, leaning forward and looking over his half-moon glasses. He took out a micrometre gauge from the top pocket of his overalls, just like others might pull out a pen. He adjusted the glasses on the end of his nose, and began to measure things in silence.

"Hm. This is a special thread; we will have to manufacture the thread to fit it ourselves. Let's walk over to the workshop and see what we have."

Before long he was lost in a neat collection of bits and pieces of equipment. A metal lathe, drills, automatic saws, welding gear, and a host of other paraphernalia filled the shop. Buster soon had a brass rod, metal tubing, and small tools lined up on the bench.

He turned his head. "Leave this with me for a couple of days, and I'll give you a ring when I think I've got something."

As good as his word, Buster had half a dozen needles ready for me two days later. They were beautifully crafted. The three-inch tubing was set into a brass base. A short piece of spring wire had been soldered on about an inch from the base as a barb, and to solve the problem of the needle cutting a plug out of the skin Buster had soldered a small drop of alloy into the tip and drilled holes in the side of the tubing just below the sharp point.

Tony had given me clear instructions on how to find his camp. It was situated beyond Isiolo on the road to Marsabit. It was well hidden from the main road, set in a large grove of flat-topped acacia, and far enough back not to be enveloped in a cloud of the fine white dust that rose from the surface every time a vehicle went past.

I parked the car in the shade and was greeted by Tony and John, whom I had met once or twice at his Kabete home, where I had encountered the lame giraffe. John, at only about five foot seven, with a stoop that emphasized his size, was slim, almost to the point of skinny — perhaps a legacy of his TB.

Tony introduced his solidly built foreman Alexander and his head catcher Mwaniki. We wandered over towards the mess area, where several folding canvas chairs were set around a table, beneath the canopy of two large overlapping trees, which provided deep shade. Tall woven papyrus mats erected on three sides acted as wind breaks.

"Jerry, before it gets dark, take a wander around the camp, and then come and have a cup of tea. That's your accommodation over there," said Tony, pointing to one of the several Karen tents that had been set up, each under a separate tree, in such a way that no sun beat on them after about ten in the morning.

I took him at his word. Not far away was a cooking area, and back beyond the tents were a shower and a lavatory shelter. Each of these was surrounded by papyrus mats.

After getting out my gear and organizing my tent, I wandered back over to the mess area to find it deserted.

"Where are the others?" I asked the cook.

"*Bwana chai* has gone to the *bomas*. There was some dispute over there," he responded.

"*Bwana chai?* Who's *Bwana chai?*"

"*Bwana* Seago. He likes tea a lot, so we call him *Bwana chai.*"

That evening, as we sat around the mess area, John explained, "We have an arrangement with the government that we will remove as many rhino as possible from this area, as it has been scheduled for settlement. We're working on a 'one for one' basis. We have to catch one animal for movement to a national park, and we get another one for ourselves. Most of the latter will go to American zoos, after we have held them here and acclimatized them for about a month."

"Where do you take the ones that the government gets?" I asked.

"Several will go to Parfet's place at Solio, and the rest will go to Meru National Park. It'll depend upon how many we get," replied John.

"How many do you think we'll get? How far away will we be working?"

"The estimates are that there may be as many as 50 between here and the Nyambenis, and that will be our main area of operation, as it's the settlement area, but we will also take as many as we can this side of the Garba Tulla road, as they have a huge home range. Some will undoubtedly be found as far away as Shaba."

As we chatted the evening drew in and we switched from tea to beer. We sat around the campfire and enjoyed the night sounds. Cicadas chirped in the trees, there was the occasional manic, eerie moaning and chuckling of a hyena in the distance, and much closer the high, clear, *hjuuh, hjuuh* call of a Scops owl. The muffled tinkling of a wooden camel bell indicated that a herdsman had corralled his animals nearby.

Every now and again the cook's helper announced that yet another batch of hot water had been prepared. I was invited to take a shower, and discovered that it consisted of a large canvas bucket with a sprinkler nozzle, controlled by a chain, underneath. The whole was suspended from a stout thorn-tree branch and a wooden pallet had been placed on the ground for something to stand on. Leaving the papyrus cubicle, clean and dust-free, wearing only my *kikoi* and sandals, my eyes now accustomed to the night, I was plunged into true dark under a star-spangled African sky quite unpolluted with industrial waste or any extraneous city light. It was magic.

In the morning, as we ate a leisurely breakfast, the plan for the day unfolded.

"Meru and Maina went out at first light and are trying to find a rhino. We've been checking out an area where there are known to be some, and when an animal lies down to sleep they will pinpoint it and come and fetch us. Then we'll go with the vehicles and see if we can catch it," said Tony.

"I'll wait until we hear something before I load up syringes, then," I responded.

"Certainly. We might not get anything, or we may have only a juvenile. Who knows?"

The trackers returned and we piled into the big Ford, an ancient Land Rover, and an International three-ton truck loaded with gear. Near a small rocky hill we transferred an initial capture team to the Ford. Meru, John, and two other team members stood in the back with me. Meru guided Tony towards a patch of thorn bush, and suddenly a rhino exploded from it and charged us. As it turned away I prepared to fire when Meru, who had been standing next to me, inadvertently moved into my line of fire. At that time we knew little of the dangers to humans of the very potent immobilizing drugs being used, but in hindsight it was a blessing that I did not shoot. My father's early lessons in firearms safety came to the fore and prevented a disaster.

There was a general kerfuffle as we sorted ourselves out, and after some discussion we set off after the same animal. It had not gone far. I stood directly behind Tony and he drove straight through everything in sight as we got near our target. I discovered that shooting at a moving target from a wildly bucking truck is not easy. We got within five yards and I fired. The dart emerged from the gun, powered by a pair of carbon dioxide cylinders, struck the rhino square in the backside and bounced off into the grass without ever even penetrating his hide.

There was no point in continuing. Tony headed for Nairobi to track down a better dart gun and I returned to Meru and a couple of days of more mundane tasks. We agreed to continue on Thursday.

Two days later, armed with a new gun, which propelled darts with enough force to penetrate the target's hide, we set out again. We were still having teething problems; we came close to two rhino and put darts into both of them but, for some reason that I never did fathom, neither worked. At last, five days after this second start, we made our first capture. After all the struggles it was a huge relief, rather than a big high. I watched from the back of the Ford as Tony, Mwaniki, Meru, and Alexander piled out in a mass, like a swarm of angry bees, and soon had ropes around the bull's feet, effectively hobbling him.

Here I was, confronted close up by my first downed black rhino, and not really knowing what to expect. He was a very different proposition from the half-tame white rhino in Meru Park. Would the drugs kill him? Would he wake up and create havoc? What would I be able to learn?

It was back to basics. Heart rate, temperature, breathing. The last of these was almost impossible to gauge with a stethoscope through the thick crinkled hide, so I simply put my hand in front of his upper nostril and began to count.

"How's he doing, Jerry?" asked Tony, looking over at me from where he stood directing the approaching three-ton lorry.

"Seems fine. Breathing at 16 breaths per minute. Heart rate of 60. He's covered in ticks. I'll try to collect some," I said with more confidence than I felt.

The next step was to take the rhino sled off the truck, roll the trussed animal on to the sled, and then winch the whole thing up special ramps after we had secured him even more thoroughly. We also laid his head on an old tire and covered his open upper eye with a bit of sacking, after I had instilled some drops into it to protect it from sunlight, insects, dust, and possibly even fright. We did not really know if an immobilized animal could still be aware of his surroundings, although the modern drugs we were using probably overcame consciousness; they were related to morphine, but much more potent. Perhaps 6,000 times as potent.

The next two hours were spent doing a sort of slow-motion bull riding exercise in the back of the truck, as Mwaniki drove us back across country.

We dragged the sled off the truck bed and into the newly constructed pens. All the ropes were removed, and I gave an antidote into the vein in the ear.

"Is everybody out of the way? Watch out!"

One moment there was a recumbent animal, seemingly unaware of its surroundings — then, in a flash, it was up and showing its considerable displeasure with the new situation.

I stood on the top wall of the pen and gawked at my new patient. A success!

Several times during the evening I walked over to see how our newest guest was doing. At least that's the excuse that I gave myself. I'm sure that I was also going over simply to marvel. A couple of times Tony came over as well. After all, it was a first for him, the first rhino with drugs. On one trip I even found John, who had climbed the ladder set against the side of the pen, gazing over the wall with quiet interest.

The camp was only four miles north of Isiolo, and the eight *bomas*, set under a group of shady trees, were something of a draw for local people. Within a few days of that first capture we had a visitor.

At least he was almost a visitor. We could hear the sonorous clapping of wooden bells before we could see anything. About 50 yards from the perimeter of the camp a group of dun-coloured camels wandered slowly along. A tall, scantily-dressed old man accompanied them. He was immediately identifiable by his coiffure and the oddly-shaped neck stool that he carried in one hand. The coiffure, a grey packing of mud at the back of his head, is used only by the Turkana people, whose home lies mainly to the north and west of what was then known as Lake Rudolph, but has since been re-named for the tribe itself. The Turkana are renowned for their indifference to outside influences and the seemingly bizarre activities of other people. This old man was no doubt curious about the heavy wooden structures, but he was not going to show it by coming too close. I am sure that he viewed our activities as another example of the craziness of *wazungu*.

I wandered over, and we chatted for a while about his camels. His Swahili was somewhat rudimentary, but at least he spoke it, unlike some of his people who had never traveled outside their homelands. He made a small income from the sale of camel's milk in Isiolo, hence his need for the *lingua franca*. I told him that we were catching and translocating rhino.

"Rhino!" he said with obvious contempt, turning his head and spitting vigorously. "They are bad news. They run through my animals and frighten them. I've had to kill two of them when they came too close." He brandished his long spear and demonstrated a thrusting motion.

The next few days brought us a couple more successes, but it was slow going, and on many days we saw nothing. One day, upon arriving in the camp, I was surprised to see a little red-and-white helicopter parked nearby. The painted sign on its side said "AutAir Helicopters."

Tony greeted me as I walked over from the old Toyota to the ring of canvas chairs set around the dining table.

"Jerry, we've decided to try using a helicopter for searching and darting. I'd like you to meet Andy Neal. He's our pilot. That's his machine over there." Andy, round-faced and solidly built, half stood and shook my hand, as I moved towards a seat and the usual, very welcome, cup of tea.

The next morning, Tony and Andy headed off in the helicopter on a spotting expedition. They took off and sloped away to the east. I stood with the crew, waiting for their return. Within half an hour, we heard the characteristic whop-whop of the blades before we saw the aircraft. It landed, the mechanic poured some fuel into the tanks, and Andy led me through the essential safety procedures.

"Never, ever, go behind the cab or try to cross under the tail boom of a helicopter. There have been some nasty accidents that way. When you get into or out of a chopper, always bend low until you are well beyond the arc of the prop. Never, ever, get out of a chopper on the uphill side and try to walk away from it. The prop may be circling just a few feet from the ground."

He didn't need to expand. The image of chopped carcass in my mind's eye was vivid enough. I climbed in and sat on the floor, the passenger seat having been removed, and securely strapped myself in with a jury-rigged harness. I taped my spare darts into the cab, and before I knew where I was, we were airborne.

Speeding above the overgrown terrain was certainly easier than trying to walk or drive through it. At ground level, there were many obstacles. For instance, there is a bush known widely throughout sub-Saharan Africa as the "wait-a-bit" thorn. Anyone unlucky enough to be caught in its grip will indeed wait a bit. The reverse curved thorns, all set in a slightly different direction from one another, can wreak havoc with one's clothing, not to mention one's skin.

"We found a bull across by that hill, about half way to the Nyambenis," said Andy through the intercom.

By now I had learned that a darted rhino may take several minutes to fall asleep, depending on the placement of the dart and the dosage used. [Many television shows inaccurately give the impression that the immobilization is almost instantaneous, I suppose because watching an animal gradually fall asleep can hardly be considered good drama.] We were still testing to find the best drug combination.

We saw an animal almost at once.

"He has moved about 50 yards since Tony and I saw him," said Andy. "Wait a moment and I'll try and manoeuvre him away from that hill and those rough rocks. Then I should be able to get you in for a shot."

I aimed for the animal's left rump and took my shot, but something caused the machine to veer, and the dart sped across the rhino's backside and buried itself in the ground just beyond him. As quickly as possible I grabbed another dart and, as Andy turned round and climbed, I inserted it into the gun. Within about 40 seconds we had managed a good shot and Andy climbed away so as not to further disturb our patient.

"Tony, Tony. This is Andy. Do you read? Over."

"Andy. This is Tony. Reading you loud and clear. Any luck? Over."

"We've got an animal darted. A male. I'll make a wide circle around him and we'll keep an eye on him. Can you see us yet?"

Six minutes later Tony's old Ford crept rather slowly out of a grove of flat-topped thorn trees. On the back were half a dozen members of the capture crew.

"How's he doing, Andy?" asked Tony, forgetting about radio protocol in the excitement of the moment.

"He's looking a bit dazed. He's walking strangely, sort of trotting.

Jerry's drugs must be working."

On a patch of clearer ground, less strewn with large rocks, the Ford was able to speed up. As they came around a clump of bush we could see that someone on the back — I could not make out who — had spotted the rhino and was leaning over the side of the vehicle and frantically waving to Tony. The truck turned and before I knew it Mwaniki was holding out a long bamboo pole with a large noose attached. Tony quickly drove up alongside the animal, which showed no signs of running, or even recognizing the thing as something foreign, and Mwaniki dropped the noose over its head. At once Tony turned away and, as the rope tightened, the rhino fell onto his side. Quick as a flash Tony was out of the cab, running towards the rhino. He had a couple of lengths of rope in his hands. Meru, Alexander, and Mwaniki were not far behind. Alexander was a trifle stout, but the stimulus of a catch seemed to spur him forward. Between them they tied ropes around the animal's legs and pulled him over. As Andy and I came to rest about 50 yards away I could see Tony gesturing towards the vehicle, but I couldn't hear what he was saying, as the helicopter engine was still cooling down.

As I ran over, the rhino gave a convulsive heave, seeming to want to get up again. By this time I could hear Tony telling Meru to get behind his back and pull on the ropes that joined the feet. I could immediately see what he was driving at. The barrel-like shape of a rhino made it simple to lift the hobble ropes and so roll the animal back onto his side, or part-way on to his back, if he got too far over towards his feet.

The team began to clear bush and get things ready for the heavier trucks, which we could hear grinding away over the rocks.

By the fifth day we had another bull and a cow and calf in camp. When I shot at the calf, I had the misfortune to send the dart right through the middle of its tail. The hub of the dart was on one side, the three-inch needle showing about two inches on the other. Luckily the calf stayed with its mother. Tony caught it with a noose, then I moved in and gave it a sedative. We were very lucky with its tail. I got the needle out without causing too much damage, and gave it a generous dose of antibiotics. It made a full recovery.

That evening we sat around the fire and reviewed our progress. John and Tony seemed well pleased, and I was having a great time. I was learning fast, working out of doors, and being paid for it! I mused on how my early boyhood wishes of becoming a zookeeper seemed to have been partially fulfilled. As I sipped an after-dinner cup of coffee I turned to John.

"John, I don't know if Tony told you, but Jo and I are off on leave next month. Then we're coming back to Nanyuki, where we're going to try and start up in private practice. Will you be doing any more rhino before then?"

"I don't know. How long will you be gone?"

"About six weeks. We should be starting again in mid-April."

"No, I doubt we'll do any more before then."

"What happens to these animals?" I asked.

"We're taking these ones to Meru park for release, once we have them settled," said Tony.

The rhino were held in a stout *boma* for about a month while they were acclimatized to captivity and trained to enter a crate without harming themselves. Truck loads of thorn bush were cut every day and brought in as feed. The pens were cleaned daily. Usually within three days the animals would settle down, and some would even take hay from one's hand. Within a week or two they would be sleeping in the crate, because it offered shade and security. They were eventually loaded on to another truck and taken to Meru National Park.

CHAPTER 18

FAREWELL TO MERU

A move to Nanyuki is put into the works. A farewell party in Meru has a memorable menu, and Kipsiele, among others, is promoted. Years later we greet him as a long-lost friend and meet his grown family.

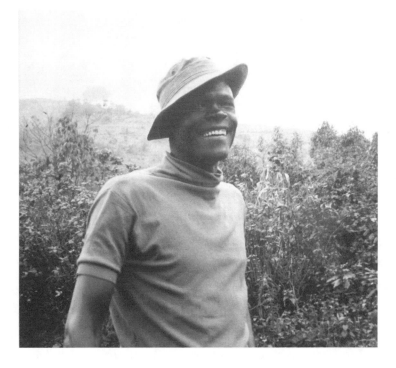

Austin Ciaji

Y SECOND CONTRACT AS AN employee of the government of
Kenya, sponsored through the British Ministry of Overseas
Development, was coming to an end. We had no wish to
leave Kenya, and every desire to stay in the Mount Kenya area. Had the
spirit of the mountain captivated us?

I visited several of the large-scale farmers in the Timau area and put out
the idea of some sort of contractual agreement to allow me to start up in
private practice, based in Nanyuki. It was a risk for me, and also for them.
George and Irralie Murray and Bob Wilson gave me every support, and so
we made the decision to move. We planned to make the jump after our leave
as we wanted to take Karen to Europe and let her meet her relatives, particularly her great-grandmothers. Being only five months old, she wouldn't
remember anything of the trip, but it would be fun for the old ladies.

Before we left we were invited to supper by Lily, one of Jo's former
midwife colleagues at the government hospital.

"Dr. Riet," she said, when they met outside Kens and Sons, the hardware and general goods store in town. "You must bring your husband to our house for some supper. Can you come next Friday?"

"That would be lovely. Can we bring anything?"

"No, no. I want to give you some typical Meru traditional food. Maize — *ugali* — cabbage and some other things."

Over a delicious meal we all fell to a discussion of local problems, including the highly addictive *mira'a*. "Lily, we saw one of those *mira'a* vehicles near Kaaga, as we came here. He nearly ran us off the road. What is it about *mira'a* that makes everyone so dangerous?" Jo asked.

"Those traders are crazy. Also dangerous. They never save anything. They live in hotels and are completely irresponsible. They often take a new wife. They are like the Luo by Lake Victoria. With fish always present in lake, there is no need to cultivate. They may not harvest anything even if it does grow."

"I understood that desert people take it because it reduces appetite and gives great endurance. Don't they even stay awake for huge lengths of time?" I asked.

"It also makes men impotent. Perhaps that is why they keep taking new wives."

Lily's sense of the absurd and her cheerful giggle were irrepressible. However, her view of the effects of *mira'a* may have been a bit one-sided, as she no doubt saw some of its worst effects in her medical capacity at the hospital. I had seen men chewing it on every visit I had ever made to Isiolo, and it was on sale in many of the little shops there. At any cattle sale in the Northern Frontier, many men would be openly chewing on a thin stick of the stuff. I had tried it, but only once, and only for about six jaw movements, as I found it incredibly bitter.

We later learned that the active ingredient of *mira'a* is an amphetamine-like chemical, a sort of natural "speed." No wonder it is so addictive.

"The various types of beer are another local thing that used to give me all kinds of problems," said Jo.

"How do you mean?" I asked.

"I used to get a lot of patients — mostly men — who were alcoholics. At first I couldn't figure it out. They would come into the out-patients complaining of stomach pains. Daudi, Stanley, or Erastus would send them on to me, and it would often turn out to be a stomach or duodenal ulcer. I would ask them if they drank beer, but always they would say "No." As I got more experience I could ask them directly, without having to use one of the fellows to translate, and I would say *pombe* for beer. It took quite some time for me to figure out that there were lots of different kinds of beer, and these men would avoid answering unless I named the actual drink with its Kimeru name."

"Oh, they make beer from many things," said Lily. "There's sugar cane, maize, millet, doum palm, and then there's *katheroko*. That can be deadly stuff. In pure form it's just straight alcohol, but some of the worst people add all sorts of things to give it more kick. They may add meths, formalin, and other bits of goodness-knows-what."

"That's what those fellows drank the other day, the ones that were reported by *The Standard* as having gone blind," I remarked. "I would imagine that it must have contained a load of meths. That's certainly a deadly poison, and often it causes blindness."

We finished our superb meal and headed down the hill. Our destination was the Mulika Coffee Hotel, where Tim had first lived when he came to Meru over four years ago. About once a month a movie was shown in the main hall. This month it was to be a Bollywood potboiler, with subtitles for the non-Hindi speakers. We sat and watched the show and gradually began to feel uncomfortable. I surreptitiously undid the waistband on my trousers. A couple of minutes later Jo did the same to her skirt. We looked at each other and by mutual, unspoken signals we stood and headed out of the door.

"We shouldn't have had those second helpings," said Jo. "I feel so full. Let's go for a walk."

This was the only solution. We headed across the road and walked behinds the veterinary office and so up across the fairways of the third, fourth, fifth, and six holes of the golf-course. The Sports Club house was in darkness. Our time as Meru residents was coming to an end. A break, and then a new life in Nanyuki beckoned.

Our last social function in Meru was the farewell party thrown by the veterinary department staff. At three o'clock that afternoon, GK 881, now looking somewhat worn, rolled through the gap in the hedge onto the lawn. Kipsiele stepped out and watched as Geoffrey and M'Ichoro removed a variety of bits and pieces from the back. First came two halves of a 44-gallon drum, each with metal angle iron welded to them as legs, and then a motley assortment of chairs. The drums were set on the ground next to each other, and sacks of charcoal were poured into each. The charcoal was lit, and then grills were placed on top of them. The chairs were placed in a semi-circle around the braziers. The men stood and waited chatting in a rather self-conscious way. Half an hour later about 30 members of staff walked up the drive. Some had come in from nearby posts and I recognized each of them.

Daniel seemed to take charge of the cooking. The meal was strictly for carnivores. *Nyama choma*, definitely *nyama* (meat) and very definitely *choma* (burnt). Rare would not be an adequate description, but raw would not be quite right either. This time it was goat's meat. There was plenty of beer, luckily Tusker, rather than anything local and more potent. A few bottles of Fanta orange for the teetotalers, Jo ranking among them as she did not like beer.

Short speeches were made. Daudi reminded Jo how she had removed something from his eye and had told him to stay away from work for a day. One or two of the speeches became somewhat incoherent, especially as the afternoon sun dipped towards the slopes of the mountain and time passed by. I received several ceremonial gifts. A fly whisk, symbol of strength, and an ornate walking stick, symbol of respect. Kipsiele's wife

Pauline had made an elaborately decorated belt for me and a woven bag for Jo. Kipsiele himself had found a traditional Kipsigis knife and had made a sheath of red-stained leather for it.

Before wrapping up my final report after four years and a few months of service, I had made several proposals for promotions. Chief among them was for my friend Kipsiele, for whom I made a strong recommendation for promotion to Driver Grade 1. The thoughtful Kabwithia had brought many thousands of shillings into County Council coffers with his masterly conduct of cattle auctions, so his name too had gone forward. Austin's potential had already been spotted and he had made the move to Kabete and the Animal Health and Industry Training Institute several months previously. Two or three others were due promotions for long and reliable service, and Geoffrey Kanyuru, the youngster who had started his working life as an office cleaner, was confirmed as an AHT.

Twenty-eight years later we were able to track down Kipsiele on his farm in Bomet. He was an old man by now, but we had a wonderful visit. Several of his sons were there, and we were offered an excellent spread of curried chicken. We reminisced about our times in Meru, and he was more than happy to tell us of his adventures since leaving the district. He had been duly promoted and had ended up as the senior driver in the provincial headquarters at Nakuru. He had eventually been given his own vehicle, a stripped down British mini car called a mini-moke, in order to make the rounds of the several government department garages and check on standards of care. He was much more interested in recounting his successes at home. The initial loan that he had repaid so assiduously had remitted serious dividends. He was living on the seven-acre farm that he had purchased with that first seed money. It was a thriving tea-growing operation, but he had added a flour-mill and a small general store at one corner. He had two other farms; one was a 40-acre plot — almost a spread by local standards — where his hired hand farmed maize and ran a few beef cattle. The other was also a tea farm. He greeted

Jo as a long-lost friend and recounted how she had dealt with him right in my office when he had complained of feeling sick. Rolling back his sleeve he said, "Doctor, don't you remember? You told me to put out my arm, and you took a blood sample from me right there."

We went for a slow walk on the farm. He showed us his few cattle and reminded me of my prediction that the fancy AI schemes of our Meru days could not last. The first thing to go had been the maintenance of communal cattle dips for tick control. This had inevitably been followed by disease and death among the cattle. Combined with a lack of funds to keep the fleet of inseminator's vehicles on the road the scheme had fallen on hard times.

Kipsiele had just sold an in-calf heifer to pay for school fees for his youngest daughter, who was away at boarding school in Narok, taking her last year before trying to go on to university. Of his seven children, two were university graduates, two were teachers, one an accountant, one had been an army sergeant, and he had high hopes for the last-born girl.

Less than three months after we returned to Canada, in March of 1998, Richard, his eldest son, sent us an e-mail telling us of the passing of our friend. We had found him just in time.

CHAPTER 19

THE COTTAGE
ON LUNATIC LANE

*We set up house, and vet clinic, in a fishing cottage on Nanyuki's
Lunatic Lane. Fixing a defunct X-ray machine proves relatively easy,
but finding a good cook presents a problem.*

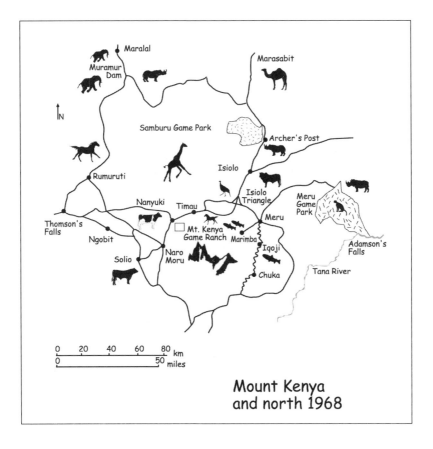

Mount Kenya
and north 1968

AFTER MY CONTRACT WITH the Veterinary Department had expired, and we had taken Karen to Europe to meet her relatives in Holland, Scotland, and England, we returned to Kenya and a change of venue. We had decided to give private practice a go, with Nanyuki as our base. We had many friends in the area, having been involved in the rugby scene for several years, and their promised support, in the form of forward contracts, helped us get started.

There would be big changes for both of us. Meru was a market town of about three thousand people, with only small numbers of Asians and Europeans, about 40 of each. My caseload was built around dairy practice, with a large beef herd that needed little attention outside the routine government work. I probably saw no more than one pet a month.

Nanyuki was the economic centre of numerous large-scale farms. The first European farmer in the district had arrived in 1910, with 13 chickens and four dogs, but from that meagre start the area had become a thriving agricultural community. There were many high-quality beef animals, with famous breeds such as Aberdeen Angus, Hereford, Galloway, South Devon, Charolais, Boran, and even Simmental. The dairy mix was also varied, with Channel Island breeds, Ayrshire, and Friesian. To round out the cattle mix there were dual-purpose breeds such as Brown Swiss and Sahiwal. There were several flocks of sheep numbering in the thousands, and of course more than enough accompanying horses and household pets to keep a veterinary practice on the go. Many more of Jo's patients would be of European extraction, and she could expect a steady caseload at her new office in the Cottage Hospital.

Before leaving Meru we had searched in Nanyuki for a house to rent. As we sat in the Sports Club at lunch time, having had a fruitless morning, Anne Allen, an acquaintance from rugby days, overheard our conversation. She came over and greeted us, then said, "I hear you're looking for somewhere to rent. There's a place down Lunatic Lane, right opposite me. It belongs to a Nairobi couple. I have a key to get in. Why don't you come down after lunch and have a look?"

We readily agreed, and after lunch we headed down this oddly named murram road. I was intrigued.

"Anne, why Lunatic Lane? Is there a dark story behind it?"

"There are several stories, but the one that I hear most often stems from the early days. The entire road was developed in the mid-thirties because it lies on the ridge between the Nanyuki and Liki rivers. The land was divided into ten-acre plots and used for weekend fishing cottages or for retired people. An old couple bought one of the plots and moved in. Pretty soon, drama developed. About twice a week the wife used to appear at the club and start screaming, 'Get that lunatic away from me! Help me! Help me!' Invariably she would very soon be followed by her husband, usually brandishing a kitchen knife or an axe."

It was not long before the word got out that we had arrived. As we sat around the cottage on the two boxes that did not have anything else stacked on them, gathering our wits after the moving lorry had departed, and trying to remember which crate held our sheets and blankets, the first of our new neighbours arrived at the door. She was a tiny, elderly lady, slightly stooped with osteoporosis, holding an old-fashioned hearing aid box in front of her, with its twisted cord snaking up under her hair, accompanied by a pack of what seemed at first to be about 15 miniature Yorkshire terriers.

Muffin, our miniature long-haired dachshund, after his initial frantic barking as the visitors arrived, showed that he was more than pleased to meet a set of individuals not only of his own species, but of his own size. The pack turned into a group of no more than six, most of them with little ribbons on their top knots to keep the hair out of their eyes. Tail, ears, and head erect, Muffin checked out his new acquaintances, and let them know that they were on his turf now.

"Good evening, my dears," she boomed loudly, in the manner of the very deaf. "I'm Enid Pipe, from just up the road. (Down, Bertie.) I thought it must be you. I had heard from Anne Allen that you were coming, and when I saw the lorry I thought I'd come down and say hello. (Oh don't mind Jenny, she's just inquisitive.) Anyway, you must come round and have a drink and some supper. What about tomorrow night? I do hope you've got some distemper vaccine, as these characters need their injections."

I shook my head and pointed at the shambles around us.

"No vaccine? Oh well, I'm sure you'll get some in, dear. Let me know right away when you do. I'll let you get on with the unpacking. Tomorrow night at seven. Good night. Come on, dogs. Bertie! Jenny! Freddie!" She marched off with a determined stride and disappeared round the corner of the house.

Jo soon got her practice going at the Nanyuki Cottage Hospital. At that time it had ten private rooms, a six-bed maternity ward, a surgical suite, a broken-down X-ray machine that looked as if it had been discarded by someone soon after Noah had landed, and not much else except a fabulous view of Mount Kenya through the podo trees that lined the river bank. The matron explained that the local government hospital had a good laboratory, but there was no X-ray unit in town.

Late one afternoon, Jo said to me, "Can you come up and look at the X-ray unit with me after supper?"

"Of course, we'll go and take a look. Speaking of supper, I think I'll go see how Njoroge is getting on with it."

Njoroge was a Kikuyu from Karatina who had arrived at the door the morning after we had moved into the cottage. He had said that he was looking for work, and bore a testimonial from some former employer that stated:

"To whom it may concern. This is to certify that Njoroge Kamau was employed by me as a cook cum house servant during the period February 1966 to January 1968. His employment ceased when I left the country."

It was signed with a completely indecipherable scribble, and underneath was printed "Jason Oblenski. Volunteer. Karatina Secondary School."

Needing a cook, and seeing no other candidates, we took him on. He did a good job keeping the house clean, but his knowledge of cooking lay somewhere between the rudimentary and the non-existent. At least his knowledge of cooking the types of meals that we liked. Perhaps he was a whiz at maize meal, cabbage, and boiled eggs, but we did not intend to find out. His biggest failing, at least in my books, was his inexperience at cooked breakfasts. His porridge was OK, but his eggs were a disaster. Neither Jo nor I knew much of cooking beyond the simplest things, and we owned not a single recipe book, so something had to be done. Perhaps we could teach him ourselves, step by step. For this evening we had set Njoroge to making mashed potatoes, peas, and fillet steak. Surely that would not be too difficult.

Jo set off to see one more patient, while I had a look in the kitchen. Seeing that the potatoes were on the boil, and the peas shelled, I decided that nothing much could go wrong for an hour or so, and decided to head for the river. My rod was already set up and hanging on hooks in the passageway. With net in hand and rod over my shoulder, I stepped out through the gate at the bottom of the garden and set off down the path. Muffin and Njugu, the Staffordshire bull terrier whom we had inherited from departing residents, decided they wanted to come along. Both immediately disappeared into the bushes beside the path.

The fish were not biting, but that didn't matter as the rushing water, the shade cast by the big podo trees with their spiky waxed leaves and rough bark, and the cooing of the doves made for as relaxing a scene as one could want. Muffin, his hair now a mass of burrs, and the plume of his tail a complete tangle, came to the water's edge but decided that he would go no further. Njugu, whom we had been warned was not overly intelligent, simply stood and barked at the little waterfall at the head of the pool. *Njugu* is the Swahili for nut. She seemed appropriately named.

It was time to check the progress of supper. We all arrived together. Ester walked round the side of the house, Karen looking at me from over Ester's shoulder where she nestled in the traditional back sling used throughout Africa. Jo drove in through the gate, and the dogs rushed up the path, Muffin jumping up in greeting, as if he had not seen her for days.

The potatoes and peas were fine. I cooked the steaks myself on the old wood stove.

"Look, Njoroge," I said in Swahili, as he had no English, "you must get the frying pan very hot, with just a little butter in it. Then put in the steak, leave it for a short time to lock in the blood, and turn it over. *Memsahib* likes her steak done for four minutes on each side, so that it has no blood when she cuts it. I like mine done for a shorter time. About three minutes each side. Do you understand?"

"Yes, sir."

"Right. Tomorrow, when you cook our boiled eggs, remember that I like mine done for three and half minutes, while *memsahib* likes hers hard, at least five minutes boiling." He seemed to understand.

After supper, once Karen had been put to bed and Ester had been detailed as babysitter, we set off up the road. The X-ray machine was ancient, but the reason that it was not working seemed to be rather simple, as it had no plug, just loose wires. Five minutes later I announced to Jo that we seemed to have power. "The warning light comes on when I plug it in and we may be able to do something," I called into the cubbyhole where she was checking the developing tanks, which were quite filthy. Searching in the drawers we found several yellow-faced cassettes of differing sizes that seemed to be in reasonable condition.

"We can get some new chemicals from Mr. Minja's chemist's shop, but let's try the thing first," she said.

For the next few days, we puzzled over what to do for a test. There was no way we could use the thing on human patients until we knew what settings to dial in. The biggest danger would lie in too high an exposure, but too little would be a waste of time and money, as films were expensive.

Then luck intervened. One of Jo's early patients was Sue Sewell, whose husband Bob was an undermanager at a large ranch, Ol Pejeta, about 20 miles out of town across the Laikipia plateau. Sue told Jo that she had been a radiology technician before moving with Bob to the Nanyuki area, and also that she had a good guide book containing lots of information about focal lengths, time for exposure, development techniques, and the like.

"Could you come and help me set up this machine?" asked Jo. "I'd really like to get it going."

"Of course," said Sue enthusiastically. "I'll send the book in with the driver tomorrow so that you can be sure of getting everything you need and have some idea how to start. Let me know if you need more help."

"Wonderful! We'll order some films and new chemicals, and hopefully we'll have a service to offer."

Two days later the films arrived from Nairobi, and by this time I had figured out what to do about the test run. We would use Njugu as our test specimen, as she was a spayed bitch, so anything we did in the way of X-rays was not going to damage her reproductive potential. She seemed the obvious candidate for the furthering of science.

With a long-acting anesthetic in her system, it was easy to manipulate her on the table and make a series of exposures based upon the advice in Sue's book. There was only one lead apron in the hospital, so I banned Jo from the area and carefully donned both the apron and the lead gloves before going any further. I could probably make several exposures without creating any danger for the dog. Each time, I recorded the voltage, the milliamps, the number of seconds shown on the spring-loaded dial, and the thickness and kind of tissue that I was shooting through, as bones need quite different settings than stomachs. Using the chemicals in the darkroom was simply a matter of following the excellent directions in the book. After two hours and a dozen X-rays, I had some ideas transferred to paper and we could make up a chart that might work for humans, or even horses.

Njoroge made little, if any, progress. The morning after the steak lesson, I found him boiling two pans of water on the stove.

"What are those for?" I asked.

"One is for your egg, the other for the *memsahib's*." I suppose it seemed logical to him.

We determined to persevere. As his previous efforts with fried eggs had produced a leathery concoction of greasy yellow stuff resembling a chamois cloth fit for cleaning windows, Jo suggested that I show him how I liked them done. Saturday seemed to be a good day.

"Put in a little butter, and make sure that it does not go brown, but that it is bubbling. Then break the egg directly into the pan. Make sure that the heart is not damaged, so that it stays as a yellow hill in the middle. When the clear part turns all white, but before the yellow is hard, the egg is ready." I hoped it sounded simple and logical.

I demonstrated as I spoke, and fortunately did not break the yolk. At that moment I noticed something out of the corner of my eye. It was a cat groggily staggering out of the open front door of the cottage. Fearing the worst, I left the kitchen and tried to catch it, but my sudden movement startled it and it ran for the flower bed. Realizing that it could only be a patient that had come in for surgery the previous afternoon, and that I absolutely must catch it, I shot back into the house and grabbed my fishing net. As I passed the spare bedroom I checked the cages and confirmed that somehow the door of the crucial one was not bolted.

Half an hour later, after quite some drama crawling about flower beds and thorn bushes, I had succeeded. The cat was safely back in her kennel, seemingly none the worse for wear. Returning to the kitchen after relating the drama of the cat to a still sleepy Jo, I checked on the breakfast situation with Njoroge.

"Here is your egg, *bwana*, just as you said you like it." He presented me with the same egg, now lying in a congealed mass of cold grease. At least he had had the presence of mind to take the pan off the heat.

When Njoroge finally parted company with us, neither he nor we were particularly unhappy about it. He returned to Karatina, and we put out the word for a new cook.

After one dud, who proved to be "light-fingered", but not in the culinary sense, we took on Abuyekah, a slim, slightly balding Abeluhya from Kenya's Western Province. He had cooked for Frank Douglas at Marania for a number of years, and Frank warned us to keep an eye on his habit of making home brew for commercial purposes, a problem that we never experienced. Abuyekah proved to be a talented chef with a fine sense of humour. He was able, with virtually no notice, to produce a hot breakfast — scrambled eggs, sausages, toast, coffee, the whole bit — for as many as eight or ten of the Mt. Kenya rugby team, whom he would find dossed down all over the cottage on a Sunday morning after a game. When I appeared one evening with some doves, he instructed me to go and buy cream and some spices so that he could make a "doves braised in cream sauce" dinner the following evening. It was simply sublime.

After we left he rejoined Frank. We saw him again some years later, when his daughter, whom we had helped put through high school, had children of her own.

CHAPTER 20

A GNOTHER GNU

*The horses and birds at the Safari Club become regular patients,
and I meet Don and Iris Hunt. It takes longer than
expected to capture a few wildebeest.*

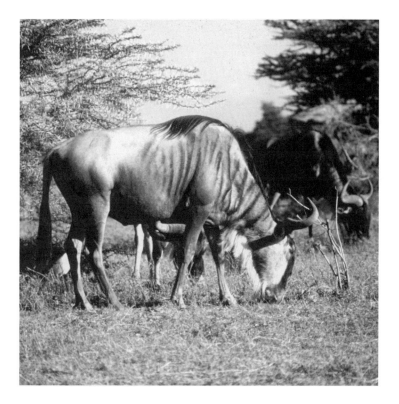

Wildebeest (gnu) — smarter than they appear.

MY FIRST CALL TO DEAL WITH horses came from the Safari Club, where we had had the unusual experience with the little dachshund on the first morning of our marriage.

Since the earliest days of the club's development there had been a string of horses available for guests to use, either for trips around the superb grounds, or further afield on small safaris into the forest towards the peaks of Mount Kenya. Even the earliest owners, "Bongo" Smith and his wife, had been keen horse people. Later the Prud'hommes, who had had possession from 1938 until 1947, had developed the site to an incredible extent, adding a menagerie of exotic birds, and numerous ponds full of fish, creating an aura of opulence second to none.

After their divorce and Gabriel Prud'homme's death the property was purchased at auction by the well-known Kenya hotelier Jack Block, and turned into the Mawingo Hotel. Mawingo is an accidental corruption of the Swahili word *mawingu*, meaning cloud, and a better name could hardly have been used for this beautiful setting on the equator at 7,000 feet, right under the peaks of Mt. Kenya.

The Blocks passed the hotel on to the three men who were its owners when Jo and I were there. They were Ray Ryan, a Texas oil millionaire, Carl Hirschman, a Swiss banker, and the film star William Holden, who was at the peak of his fame. They had re-named the place The Mount Kenya Safari Club and had developed it further as a retreat for the rich and famous. Lucinda de Laroque, in her book *Paradise Found*, has documented much of its history, and provided a long list of celebrities from many walks of life who visited and became members.

Just before we took Karen to visit her relatives, we had paid a visit to the club to see the Burrows. Jenny knew that we would return to Nanyuki and private practice, and she had asked me to take on the regular care of the riding string. While we were still settling in at Lunatic Lane, and before I had even had time to build any kennels, the phone rang out with its characteristic *rrrrrrrrr . . . rr . . . rr*. A long and two shorts, our own code on the seven-subscriber party line. It took me a moment or two to recognize the pattern, as my office line in Meru had had just the opposite set of rings, but I picked up the old black hand set and gave my name.

"Good morning, Jerry. This is Brian Burrows from the Safari Club. The *syce* reports that one of the horses has a nasty cut. Can you please come up and take a look?"

"Do you know when it happened? Is it still bleeding?"

"Hold on, I'll check." A muffled conversation in Swahili with someone, presumably the *syce*, followed, and Brian came back on the line.

"He found it cut this morning when he went into the stable. There was blood on the floor, and on the horse's leg, but it has stopped now."

"Right ho! Brian, I'll sterilize some instruments and be up in about half an hour. Please tell the *syce* I'll meet him at the stables. Ask him to have a couple of buckets of warm water available." I put down the receiver and gave the handle a generous double turn to signal that the line was again free.

I called Mutua, who had started with me as a trainee technician, and asked him to get the instrument bowl boiling. Mutua, whose full name is Bilasio Mutua wa Mugambi, the *wa* meaning "son of," was a young man from Meru who had been the only applicant to arrive on time when I had interviewed potential candidates for the position before I left Meru. His punctuality outweighed his lack of experience, as it indicated responsibility and enthusiasm.

"*Jambo, mzee. Habari gani?*" I asked as we pulled up beside the stables.

"*Jambo, daktari. Mzuri tu. Habari yako?*"

"*Muga muthee,*" said Mutua, somehow recognizing the *syce* as a fellow tribesman, and greeting him in their own tongue. "*Muga muno,*" replied the *syce*.

We got our gear from the station wagon, and I warned Mutua about horses. This was the first time that he had ever been near one.

"Never walk behind a horse that you do not know, and even if he does know you, never frighten him or make sudden noises. They are large and powerful. Unlike cows, which you have seen on your father's farm, horses will kick straight back. Also, watch out near the head. A horse can bite very hard." Mutua kept his distance throughout.

The bay gelding was the only horse in the stables, and I talked to him as I went up on his left-hand side. "Woo boy, good fella, steady now, steady now." The words probably did not matter at all, but the soothing tone and confident approach were crucial.

There was a substantial amount of dried blood caked on the outside rear face of his left front leg, starting about ten inches off the ground, and contrasting plainly with the white hairs of his sock. I stroked his leg, and he didn't flinch. Gently smoothing the hair above the site I asked the *syce* for some tepid water, and taking a cloth from my kit, I cleaned things up as best I could. The wound was small, only about an inch long, but deep into the skin.

"This is not a fresh wound. When did he get hurt?" I asked the old man.

"Last night, just after I brought him into the stable, I noticed the blood," he replied.

Rather than remonstrating with him about his failure to act sooner, I decided to get on with doing something about it. The blood had already clotted over the wound, and it was too late to do anything about stitches.

"Put a handful of Epsom salts — the white powder in that plastic bag — into that bucket and fill it half full with warm water," I told Mutua. "We'll wash the area thoroughly."

The *syce* did not know if any of the horses had ever had injections for anything, as he was a new employee. "I am going to give him two injections," I told him. Turning to Mutua I said, "Bring me the white bottle marked 'penicillin,' and also the thermos flask that we put the small bottles in at the house. Those bottles that I took from the fridge. Also bring me the small, round bottle of blue powder called Negasunt. It is in the large wooden box."

The flask contained anti-tetanus vials, and of the two injections this was perhaps the most important.

"The blue powder contains a sulfa powder as well as a *dawa* to keep flies away, and the injections are to keep him from getting sick," I told Mutua.

I turned to the *syce*. "I will return tomorrow and see the horse. Make sure he is here, and do not let him go out for exercise until I say so. Keep him nearby in that small field for today, and at four o'clock bring him in and wash his leg again with this *dawa*, using warm water, just as I did now. Not too hot or you will hurt him." I handed him the bag of Epsom salts.

After we had cleaned up, I left Mutua and the *syce* to check around the stable and yard to see if there were any nails or other sharp objects that might have caused the injury. While they were doing this I went up to the club house to see Brian and tell him about the horse. He and Jenny were both in the office, and they invited me to join them for a cup of coffee. We sat looking out over the immaculately manicured lawns to the kidney-shaped swimming pool. The colourful birds that we had seen on our honeymoon stay were still wandering about looking for scraps.

Suddenly a large, brown, flightless bird, with a crest on its head and blue wattles hanging down on each side of its neck, appeared from behind the swimming pool.

"Good heavens! You've still got that cassowary. We saw it when we were here on honeymoon. I wonder how it got here in the first place."

"Oh, it was here when we arrived," said Brian. "It was probably brought in by Mr. Ryan, but it may even have been here before that."

"As far as I know the cassowary is one of the few birds that will attack humans on sight. They are reputed to be exceedingly dangerous, leaping into the air and using those deadly looking toes to disembowel their adversaries. I hope it never attacks anyone here," I said.

I never pursued the matter any further, but a few weeks later the cassowary seemed to have disappeared.

We returned to the subject of the horses, and Brian asked me to make regular visits and get the string in shape. As far as he could make out there were no records of any vaccinations, although Jenny recalled that they had been done for African Horse Sickness on several occasions. There also seemed to be no record of any treatments for worms.

The next day, with no other cases on the books, we returned armed with equipment for working on horses' teeth and a generous supply of de-worming medicine. I checked the progress of our first patient, whose wound was now healing nicely. Then I carefully examined all the horses, and found that several had sharp edges to their teeth. These would interfere with proper digestion, as the food would not be adequately ground during chewing. They needed a good go with a rasp.

Those who have done it know that rasping a horse's teeth is demanding work, and one has to be fit to do it properly. This seemed as good a time as any to let Mutua get some hands-on experience.

I turned to the *syce*. "Hold the horse firmly by his head collar. I am going to use this file to remove the sharp edges off his teeth. Mutua, you hold him on the other side, and watch carefully what I'm doing."

The rasps were small blades, no more than six inches long, held in place on a long handle with a set screw, so that they could be replaced when dull.

"You put the file into the mouth, feel for the sharp outside edge of the teeth, and then push and pull it back and forward." I began the motion, applying upward pressure as I went. Pretty soon I could hear and feel the characteristic sound of a rasp doing its job. I pulled it out and showed it to the two men.

"See, the sharp points on the teeth have been worn flat, here is the powder on the file. Now we will do the other side, and then I will do the lower jaws with the straight handle. This one has a bend so that I can work on the upper jaws properly."

Eight horses later I had had enough. We dispensed the worming doses, and I told the *syce* that we would have to return as there was one horse that needed a special treatment for his teeth.

Sweating, tired, and feeling that I would not need to go on my daily rugby training run that evening, I went up to the club to see Brian. With him was a solidly built open-faced stranger, whom he introduced.

"Jerry, meet Don Hunt. He owns the Mount Kenya Game Ranch. The zebras and things that you saw on your way into the club belong to him. Don, this is Jerry Haigh. He has just moved here with his doctor wife, Jo."

"How'd you do, Jerry. It's nice to meet you," said Don, leaning forward and putting out his hand. "I've heard about you from Brian, and I know that you've been doing a bit of rhino work with Tony Parkinson and John Seago down at Isiolo. I'd like to talk to you about that. When can we get together?"

We arranged to meet at his house the following morning, after I had dealt with the horses again. The house was situated some 500 yards below the Safari Club, itself on the grounds of the ranch. It consisted of two rondavels joined by a large central rectangle, which made up the living area. There were numerous interesting masks from many areas of Africa, and several unusual paintings decorating the walls. Over coffee on the verandah, which faced the mountain, Don told me something of his operation.

"We have a small animal orphanage, which I'll take you to in a minute, and out in the park we have a variety of hoofed stock. We've been building the ranch up slowly since we started in 1967. Like Parkinson and Seago, we're involved in capture and translocation, and we could use your services with rhino and elephant. I even plan to try to capture some reticulated giraffe in the near future, and I could use your help with those."

"Who are the 'we'?" I asked.

"Oh, there's Julian McKeand, who is the professional hunter at the Club, Deane Johnson, a lawyer from the States, and William Holden, who also has a share in the Club."

"And how did you get involved?"

"I used to do a wild animal TV show, back in the dark ages in Detroit. It was called 'Bwana Don.' We were doing a documentary for the show out here and I fell in love with the place. Before we knew where we were, we were negotiating for purchase and I had obtained a permit to change the land use from agricultural to conservation."

At that point a car pulled up outside and an attractive blond woman emerged. As she came over to the verandah, Don introduced us.

"Jerry, I'd like you to meet Iris. Iris, this is Jerry Haigh, the vet I was telling you about. His wife is the new doctor at the cottage hospital."

As I stood to greet her she said, "Hello, Jerry. Nice to meet you. I've just met Jo at the clinic."

"Jerry and I were just discussing the ranch, and I was about to tell him that from time to time we need to have some of the park animals captured, as the herd grows and they become surplus." Turning to me, Don said, "Would you be able to capture some wildebeest for me fairly soon? I need three females and a bull."

I nodded, not sure what this would involve, and Don said, "Let's take the Land Cruiser and go have a look at the orphanage. We can go via some of the tracks on the ranch, and I'll show you the lay of the land. That may give you some ideas about how to catch hoofstock when we need them."

"How often do you need to catch stuff, and what are the main species?"

"It varies. When there get to be too many I like to pull a few out. From time to time we need to fill an order for a shipment to the States, and then we have to get a load ready to go to the Mombasa quarantine station. We like to hold them for acclimatization in the *bomas* behind the orphanage before we move them, so you can catch the wildebeest as soon as you like, and we also need half a dozen impala females, as well as a ram. Other than those we have zebras, some eland, half a dozen oryx, and a few giraffe."

At the orphanage Don and Iris showed me their pet chimpanzee, Jon Jon, who had been rescued from poachers. He was already nearly full grown, and becoming a very powerful animal. Because of the threat he posed to visitors, he was restrained with about 15 yards of strong chain attached to a collar round his neck. This was anchored to a huge flat-topped acacia. A low wooden rail marked the limit for visitors to approach, and a sign warned people not to go any closer.

There were a few other species grazing on the lawns. A pair of cranes had come over from the Club, and three pet eland were nosing around. Two men, one tall, one short, were standing by an office building looking at something and chatting.

"There are John and James. Fellows, I'd like you to meet Dr. Haigh. Jerry, this is John Kariuki and James Mutuoto."

"Good morning, John, James," I said, shaking hands.

"Dr. Haigh will be coming up to the ranch from time to time to help us catch animals and look after things in the orphanage, as well as Iris's cheetahs and the lemurs down at the house. He'll let you know if he needs any help, and if Iris and I are away you can call him."

The reference to cheetahs and lemurs was news to me, but I let it go for now.

As I would be coming up to tend to the injured horse again next day, it seemed pointless to dally. I arranged on the spot to have a go at catching a wildebeest early in the morning, before any tourists might be up and about. I included my capture kit in the boot of the car. Don had left his dart gun at the orphanage, and so I picked it up and worked out a plan with John Kariuki, the taller of the two men that I had met yesterday and, as it turned out, the foreman of the orphanage crew. We got into his Land Rover and drove to the edge of the field, where we had seen a group of wildebeest (gnus) grazing as we drove in.

There was one problem. What dose was I going to use? I had, by now, become quite familiar with the dart gun, and had a good supply of needles of various sizes, but the only animals that I had captured were rhino, and this was a very different situation. I could find nothing written about dosage for the drugs I had, only some older information about drugs that I could not obtain. I would simply have to trust to luck. I calculated something based on the animals' size relative to rhinos, and loaded up the dart.

The first animal was deceptively easy. John simply drove up and stopped about 30 yards from the herd. The animals were thoroughly used to seeing ogling tourists and took no notice of us. The tiny *crack!* of the .22 blank was followed by the thump of the dart in a rump; almost at the same time came the muffled crack of the charge inside the dart emptying the syringe. Within a fraction of a second there was a mad scramble of alarmed animals. Tails flapping madly, heads bobbing as they charged off across the field, they quickly disappeared from sight. John started up his engine and began to chase them, but I signaled for him to wait. I did not want to disturb them further.

After a couple of minutes we went around behind the spot where they had disappeared to see what was happening. We saw our patient, dart sticking out of her backside, wandering aimlessly on her own. Before we had gone more than 50 yards further, she stumbled once and then went down.

This outcome seemed to surprise John, but I pretended to take it in stride, as if I had expected nothing less, and I asked him to go back to the orphanage and get a couple of guys to help while Mutua and I kept an eye on the wildebeest.

By the time John returned, riding with two others in the trailer behind the ranch tractor, Mutua and I had treated the animal with antibiotics and removed the dart. We soon loaded her on the trailer and moved her to the holding pens behind the orphanage. Within 30 seconds of a dose of antidote into her jugular vein she was standing, checking out the 30-by-30 foot pen in which she suddenly found herself.

"Right, let's go and get another one. Don wants three females and a young bull," I said.

But I quickly gained an insight into the wildebeest mind. There was no way any member of the herd was going to let any vehicle, particularly a green Land Rover, anywhere near it that day. If we even slowed down at a hundred yards, they were off. We soon gave up and went to look after the horses.

Jo and I began to use the Safari Club as a place to go for a treat. A favourite time was at about four o'clock on a Sunday afternoon, which of course is tea-time in any part of the world where the English have made their stamp. Tea-time was also a good time to observe the large and varied bird collection.

Usually we would take a walk, and stop to watch the rookery in a much-used tree that overhung one of the sculptured ponds below the main club building. It seemed to be a constant hive of activity. Grey herons, sacred ibis, and marabou storks all jostled for nesting space, and there was a constant to-ing and fro-ing as adult birds flew in and out.

Then as we sat and drank our tea, accompanied by cake and biscuits, we watched the birds as they gathered on the sloping lawn in front of the large bay windows in anticipation of their afternoon feast. The manicured grass sloped down towards the open-air swimming pool. Smartly dressed sacred ibis, in their black-and-white garb, helmeted guinea-fowl, wild starlings free-booting on the goodies, and at least two dozen Egyptian geese crowded on to the stage. Five marabou storks, with their red heads and baggy throat pouches, appeared among the group, seeming incongruous and ugly compared to the others. Four stately sarus cranes, dressed in smart pale grey, except for their white collars and red heads, towered above everything else, almost as tall as the man dispensing the feed. The geese, with their raucous calls, tried their best to lord it over everything else, but they could not keep up with the scurrying guinea-fowl, which rushed about in a seemingly aimless fashion, heads bobbing as they feasted on the treats. A single pelican waddled up from behind the pool, and Jo could not resist quoting her favourite nonsense limerick:

A wonderful bird is the pelican
His beak can hold more than his bellican
He can take in his beak
Food enough for a week
But I'm damned if I see how the helican.

[We both believed this to be an Ogden Nash classic; it was not till years later that Nadia Halim, while editing this book, discovered that the true author was Dixon Lanier Merritt.]

As if to prove this right, the keeper dipped into a bucket and flipped two or three dead fish into the gaping maw. In the background, low clouds obscured the view of the mountain and even most of the forest above the manicured gardens.

■

It took over four weeks to get the rest of the wildebeest. We used several techniques. These included ambush, me lying in a clump of grass or under a bush; stalking, at which I had only one success; and a variety of different vehicles, as I joined a tourist group as a "Judas" viewer on one occasion — much to the delight of the American tourists, who must have dined out often on the experience afterwards, especially back home. As a time-and-motion exercise it was rather unproductive. However, I learned some new things about animal behaviour and gained a great deal of respect for the sagacity of the wildebeest, which had always seemed to me to be a rather stupid creature, inclined to panic at the slightest provocation, and having an almost clown-like gait as it bobbed along. When I listen to the gnu song in which Flanders and Swann use the phrase 'a gnother gnu' my attempts to catch the second and subsequent shaggy-bearded wildebeast spring to mind.

CHAPTER 21

THE TWO FACES
OF LADY LUCK

*A lucky case in front of a crowd gets my practice off to a good start,
but then a mistake in judgement keeps me on an even keel. A Jack
Russell terrier survives being run over and a toy hammer plays a role.*

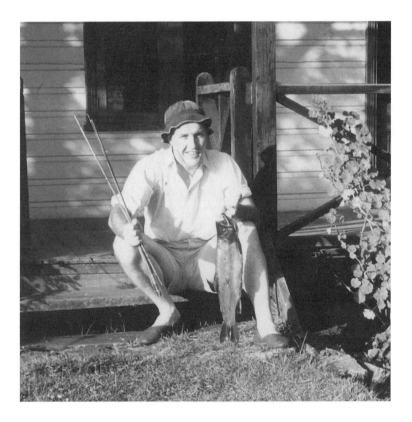

Supper for two, with some leftovers to come.
Almost four pounds of rainbow trout.

WE SOON BEGAN TO GET TO know some of our neighbours. Anne Allen lived just about opposite, and we would see her from time to time, especially if I had a yen to fish the Nanyuki River. She'd issued me a standing invitation to walk through her garden to get there. With the Liki River only 45 yards from our back gate, and with plenty of hungry rainbow trout in its pools, it might seem strange that I'd make the longer walk to another stream, but it was hardly a burden. The Nanyuki River, tumbling through a series of enticing pools, was no more than 125 yards away. The fish here were brown trout, but seemed no less hungry. What a strain, to have two good fishing rivers within a three-minute walk of our front door!

In Meru I had started out with a case that had provided all a new vet could ask for: a simple diagnosis, an easy remedy, and a huge slice of luck. Nanyuki did not give me quite such an easy start. The lucky case occurred a few days before an unlucky one.

Three weekends after we arrived, while I was still finding my feet, I

240

was asked to act as honorary vet at a polo tournament. A limited number of people from around the country played the game, which required a string of several ponies, an athletic bent, and a pocket book deep enough to be able to maintain the animals and the *syces* to look after them. Two hotbeds of polo were in my practice area, one at Timau, up at about 8,000 feet on the north slopes on the mountain, and another right in Nanyuki, at the Sports Club. The polo ground was right next to the rugby pitch, in the middle of the old racetrack.

I sat in my station wagon, the rear compartment packed with as many things as I could think of that might be needed, my stethoscope on the passenger seat beside me, and watched the game unfold. Horses shook the ground as they raced up and down, clubs flew over the head of the riders as they swung in a full arc, and there were audible *thwacks!* as the white ball was struck and flew down the ground.

Suddenly everything came to a halt. Horses and riders moved back from a melee in the middle of the pitch. One rider was standing next to his horse, which was lying on its side. A referee signaled to me, and as I started up the car and drove onto the pitch I could feel the weight of dozens of pairs of eyes on me.

The bay gelding was lying on his left side, puffing hard, and seemingly resting. I pulled out my stethoscope and put it on his chest. The heart sounded fine, but was a little difficult to hear through the heavy breathing. There didn't seem to be anything wrong with his legs, and the owner told me that he had just fallen over.

"I just managed to throw myself clear," he said, as he dusted himself off. "I think he's just exhausted. I'm short one pony, and he had to play a second *chukka*."

I went over the pony as carefully as I could, and noticed that his breathing seemed to slow a little.

"I'll give him a couple of injections," I said, opening the rear door of the car. I got out a dose of cortisone, and a multivitamin shot used for shock patients, and gave both injections into the muscles of the horse. One in his rear end, the other in the chest muscles between his forelegs. At least they would do no harm.

As I put my empty syringes back into the car and chatted to the owner, the pony rolled part way up, back down again in a rocking motion, and then, almost in a single movement, got to his feet.

I knew, as I drove back to the sidelines, that sheer luck had been at my elbow. A couple of minutes more and the horse would have stood without any help from anyone. The treatments had played no role. To have done so they would have had to go directly into the bloodstream with an intravenous injection. But it could do no harm for this incident to have been seen by a large segment of the local population, and many members of the horse-owning community, who might pass on their impressions to friends and neighbours. There was no way I was going to enlighten them.

The next morning my huge luck took a reverse. I had been called out to visit a bull with a broken leg. Full of bravado after my stroke of fortune, I made a silly mistake. The break was high up, above the hock, in mid-tibia. The bull was a less-than-gentle Boran, a breed not known for ease of handling.

Instead of remembering my lessons, I decided to foray an attempt at a cast. An hour later we had built a metal brace that fitted the leg, with a loop around the thigh, and I had applied my entire stock of plaster of Paris to the limb. First on the broken area with slabs, then a series of wraps, finally wraps that incorporated the brace. The bull was still deeply asleep from his anesthetic when I left for the next call, about 15 miles up the rough gravel road to give some horse sickness vaccinations.

As I was about to leave from this call the owner came running back out of the house waving. "Jerry, there's a call for you. It's Mickey."

The news was bad. "That bull got up, walked a couple of paces, looked round at his leg and started to kick. He shook the thing off, and his leg is dangling." I was stuck, I had no more plaster, and there was nothing I could do. The bull had to be put down.

In retrospect I would have been much wiser to accept the inevitable and suggest immediately that the bull be put down. A leg broken so high up in an intractable patient would have been hard enough to repair in a fully equipped veterinary hospital 30 years later. What I had attempted was virtually impossible. Worse, the drugs that the animal now had on board would render his meat unsafe to eat.

Back in town, my efforts with the X-ray machine paid off and helped restore some of my self-faith.

Nigel and Muffet Trent arrived from Lolomarik soon after I got back for a late lunch. Nigel was about my size, but had a full head of hair, a ruddy complexion, and a face that seemed ever ready to break into a happy smile. He also had one distinguishing mannerism. When making a decision he would say "Right," raise his right thumb and point with his forefinger, but not in any particular direction. Muffet, his wife, was a keen horsewoman and gardener, as well as a good organizer.

Nigel had a Jack Russell terrier in his arms. "This little fellow got himself in trouble this afternoon," he said. "Can you have a look at him please and see what you can do?"

"Good afternoon, Nigel, Muffet, poor little fellow. Isn't this Ranter? What happened?"

"We had Tim and Carol to lunch, and as they went to leave Ranter moved out from under their car wheel, where he had been hiding from the sun, when Tim started the engine. Then we got chatting about something or other and the dog got bored and went back again. Tim started off and went right over his hind end. Then Muffet and I called out and in the confusion Tim at once backed up, driving over him again. Poor little chap."

I led the way into the spare-room-cum-clinic and Nigel put the little dog up on the table. I popped a cotton bandage around his muzzle, although he was not in the least aggressive, as I did not want him to bite either of us if I inadvertently hurt him while checking things out. His heart and lungs sounded fine, his gums were the healthy pink hue that they ought to be.

"Nigel, please hold him by the scruff of his neck, and put your hand under his chest. I'm going to examine his rear end and see if anything is broken. Hopefully it won't be his pelvis, as he seems to be supporting himself on his right leg without much trouble."

I felt up and down his spine. There seemed to be nothing amiss. Pressure over his hip bones produced no response. Then I picked up his rear end and compared his legs. The left one looked about an inch shorter than the right. Pressing the two legs together, the difference became obvious. The shortening was evident both at his toes and his hock joints.

"I want to examine this leg more closely. I hope it isn't broken. Let's lie him over on his side. If you put your forearm across his neck and hold his bottom leg, the right one, with your hand, he won't be able to do much. Then I can have a good feel."

The next step was to check the bones in his leg. They seemed fine, no palpable breaks.

"From the feel of things this is either a dislocation of the hip, or possibly a fracture of the neck of the femur. We've now got the X-ray unit at the Cottage Hospital working, so let's take him up there and see what's what."

"Right you are," said Nigel. "Let's go in our car."

"You know what's amazing about this thing?" I asked rhetorically as we drove up the lane. "By rights he ought to have been squashed flat. He could easily have been killed. He is a very fit, muscular little dog, and that, with a good dose of luck that the wheel didn't cross his back four inches further forward, has saved him."

"Well, he and Bluey, Nigel's lab, come riding with me every day, so they are very fit," said Muffet.

Half an hour later I was showing Nigel and Muffet the results of our efforts, using the window as a light source, in the absence of a proper viewing box.

"There doesn't seem to be any sort of break. That's a relief. If there was I'd have to send you down to Paul Sayer in Nairobi, as I'm not equipped to deal with that sort of thing just yet. However, you can see the dislocation here. That I can probably deal with."

Back at the house I gave the little dog a dose of anesthetic. This allowed me to lift his leg high up in the air and pull the bone back over and down so that the ball and socket slipped together.

"Normally the ball is held in by a strong little ligament. When a dislocation occurs the ligament ruptures. Now we have to rely on the heavy thigh muscles to hold it in, and I'm going to give them a little help for a day or two."

What I needed was a small hammer. The only one I could think of weighed about 12 ounces, and was much too big. Then came inspiration. Many years ago I had been given one of those toy tool kits. Square saw, plastic ruler, compasses, pencil, screwdriver, and a tiny claw hammer. The hammer was made of cast iron, and was more or less useless for anything larger than thumb tacks. The claws had long since broken off, but the head was just what I needed, and I knew that the thing was stored — logically of course — with the shoe-cleaning gear.

Nigel recounted the scene to friend and boss George Murray about a month later.

"Before we knew what was happening, Jerry had stepped out of the room, leaving me to hold the sleeping dog, and returned with miniature hammer. Holding the leg firmly in place, he proceeded to pound the hip area around the joint. We could hardly believe our eyes. 'This should create some bruising and swelling in the muscles, which should hold everything in place for a few days,' he said. And Ranter has never looked back. He was hardly lame at all, but those little Jack Russells often run around on three legs just because they feel like it. Now you'd never know he'd even been hurt. I must say, it was news to me that a hammer could be considered a veterinary instrument."

CHAPTER 22

THE STOLEN WATCH

*I find a strategically located new office in town. A fine old horse
is put to sleep. During a visit to examine some cattle
my wedding-present watch is stolen. Too late, I remember
my father's account of a similar theft 30 years before.
One of Jo's patients self-medicates with leftover dog pills.*

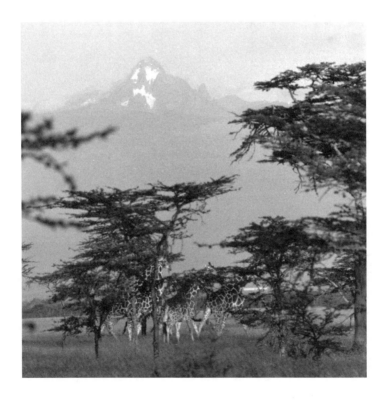

A
S BUSINESS IMPROVED, AND the limitations of our little cottage as a clinic became more obvious, I searched for a spot in town where I could set up shop. Lady Luck was with me again, as the first site I examined was the old office of the East African Power and Lighting Company and had just about everything one could ask for. It was located on the main street, was roomy, and had a back yard, a lockable room with a wall safe for dangerous drugs, a large sink, and a frosted glass divider that allowed me to set up a surgical suite out of sight of public scrutiny. Better still, it was only three doors from Mr. Minja's chemist's shop.

It took little time to find some old furniture: armchairs, a low table, several cupboards, and we were all set. My own old copies of weekly newsmagazines supplied the usual reading material, and I augmented these with several copies of *The Shooting Times* and a little cheaply produced magazine called *The Fly Tiers Guide*.

In order to ensure continuous service to clients, even when I was out on calls, I took on as an office assistant a young Meru man named Njeru

Nyaga, who had been sent over for interview by Vitalis, the laboratory technician from my Meru days. Mutua had found accommodation just down the road from our home, and the owners had another room for Njeru. Each morning the young men would walk the half mile or so to our cottage and at about eight o'clock we would set off up the road to the office.

If there were no calls we would knock off at about five o'clock and head home. I'd usually walk though Anne's garden — always a pleasure, mainly for the anticipation of standing at the river, rod in hand, but also for the beauty of the property itself. Set in 20 acres, the house was one of the many that had been built in the mid-1930s as a home for a retired couple. The land also contained two fishing cottages. The 20-acre plot was full of a marvelous variety of trees, some indigenous, like the podos and cedars, others planted, like the rough-barked eucalyptus or grey ironbark, an Australian transplant distinguished by its spiky leaves and fluffy flowers. As I walked through the back gate towards the river, I was brought to a sudden stop by the litter of yellow leaves about my feet. A deciduous tree in Kenya. Not a common sight. This was the pappea, and like the larger cape chestnut, which produces a shower of delicate pink blooms on an irregular basis, it would occasionally shed some leaves.

In the background I could hear an unfamiliar steady thumping, which got louder as I went along. Right at the river's edge, I discovered the source of the sound. A ram pump, driven by water pressure from a furrow that ran alongside the river, presumably arising upstream, was pulsing with a rhythm somewhat like a heartbeat. Not quite like the classic *lub-dup, lub-dup*, that we had been taught as students, but close to it. The pump was connected to a pipe that headed back up to the house. Anne later told me that it supplied water to her household tank.

As the evening gathered in, and three raucous Hadada ibis flew in to roost I wound my way back towards the house. Anne met me as I stepped out of the trees on to the drive. She looked as if she had been waiting for me.

"Jerry, I'm afraid the time has come for poor old Nicky. He's 36 years old, and has been fine until just lately, but he's going downhill fast, and I think it's only kind to put him to sleep before he suffers too much."

"I'm sorry to hear about this. He's a grand old horse."

"When can you come?"

"I can call in and do it before I go to the office. Say about eight o'clock tomorrow. Would that suit?"

"That'll do well. I'll see you then."

"I'll bring my shotgun. It's very quick that way. They're usually gone before they hit the ground."

"Oh no!" she said in horror. "I've shot off his back. He knows what a gun is. Can't you give him an injection?"

"I'm sorry. Yes of course I can. He shouldn't feel a thing."

At supper Jo and I discussed the situation. For her there was no such option if her patients reached a point of no return.

"I was having tea with Christopher and Alfreda Hazard yesterday afternoon," she told me, "and he let out one of his dry witticisms. 'We'll call you if we get sick, and if you can't help us then we can always call Jerry to put us to sleep.'"

We both sometimes wondered how much this sort of sentiment was really in jest.

In the morning I went over to Anne's, taking the car instead of walking in order to lend a professional air, but leaving Mutua at the house to be picked up when I had finished.

Anne had the old horse on a halter, and as she stood by biting her lip I did what was necessary. He reared up as the drug took effect, and then dropped stone dead.

Anne was badly shaken, and I walked back to the house with her after she instructed her gardener and *syce* to bury him in the hole that she had already arranged to be dug.

Trying, and largely failing, to hold back her tears, she recalled, "He was a remarkable horse. I bred him and after that we really did nothing with him until he was five. We didn't even castrate him until then. Six months after breaking him my brother introduced him to polo, but straight into fast games. Six weeks later he played in the most senior tournament in Kenya, and, you know, I controlled him throughout with just a rein from his noseband. The following weekend I rode him to second place in a three furlong race at Njoro, and then later he placed second in a hunter trial at an agricultural show. He was a natural on the polo field, one of those that watches everything, and he could follow the ball as it flew around the field. When he was 26 I played polo on him again, and he was still keen, still first on the ball, at least during the first *chukka*. My son Marcus learned to play polo on him."

Knowing that grieving often has to be a private thing, I let her continue until she seemed to have run out of steam, and then made my excuses. It took her a long time to get over it, but she had grand memories of a fine animal.

I picked up Mutua and Njeru on the road, halfway to the office. They had decided to go and open up in case any early clients came round seeking vaccines, de-wormers, or other medications. We chatted as we drove along the bumpy road and I avoided a donkey cart laden with firewood.

"We have to go to Burguret this morning, then in the afternoon we have to spay those kittens for Mrs. Clarke," I said.

Mutua and I set off on the 15-minute drive to Burguret, where we would be doing one of our routine monthly visits centred on the breeding program. Burguret, 10,000 acres in size, was predominantly a dairy farm, owned by Sir Alfred Beit, a wealthy South African who had also been a minister in one of the Tory governments in Britain, and managed by Mike Littlewood. Mike's father had managed the place from 1951 until his death in 1968, then Mike had stepped into his shoes. He and his mother lived in the large house, which the owner would occasionally visit.

We pulled into the top dairy and started to get to work.

"Morning Jerry. Bit late aren't you?" said Mike in his gruff manner.

"Morning Mike. *Ajamage"* — this to arap Ruto, the tall, very dark Nandi headman. *"Hamjambo"* — this last to the dairymen and other members of Mike's staff. "Yes, Mike, sorry about that. We had to deal with some problems, but I didn't think we'd be more than 20 minutes late. Didn't they ring from the office?"

"Perhaps they did. I've been up here, so I wouldn't know."

One of the mainstays, in fact the bread and butter, of the practice was the routine work on cattle breeding programs throughout the district. Mike and I had established a system for the monthly checking of all his Friesian cattle. Some checks would confirm that the animals were pregnant, others would see why they were not. It was a team effort that required the keeping of excellent records on Mike's part, and the donning of plastic sleeves and thin rubber gloves on my part. I would examine each cow by feeling her uterus and the rest of her reproductive tract.

There was no point in spoiling good clothes. The first job was to take off my watch and shirt, which I put on the table as usual, and don a protective apron. I then applied some gel to the sleeve and started down the line.

"Pregnant about 16 weeks." I moved on to the next one, a heifer.

"Open. No palpable structures on the right ovary, which is tiny, the left ovary is about the same. How old is she, Mike?"

"Twenty-one months. There are four or five in here of about the same age. I'm worried about them, the herdsman says that they aren't bulling, and those that do don't seem to be catching. Even some of the milk cows seem to have the same problem. I'll get you to look at them tomorrow, if you're free."

We went down the line together. There did indeed seem to be a problem. Of the 17 animals, eight of them that had never been pregnant, only five were in calf, and none of these were heifers.

"What sort of feed have you had them on?" I asked. "It's been very dry, and since the failure of the rains in November I've seen similar problems elsewhere. Up at Timau there are even a couple of fellows who have not put out their bulls, because they've had no grazing to speak of for quite a while."

"We aren't as badly off as Timau, but it's not pretty. I've had the milking cows on lucerne for a while, but we haven't got enough to cover everything. Can you suggest anything?"

"Well, there's no substitute for good green grass, but everyone's in the same boat at the moment. One or two of the fellows are using monthly injections of vitamins A, D, and E, which are certainly important in breeding. You could try that, but I'm not entirely sure about the evidence that it actually does anything to bring animals that have ceased to cycle back into heat."

As we chatted I cleaned off, discarded my glove and sleeve, and reached for my shirt. My watch was not there.

"Mutua, did I give you my watch?" I said, hoping that memory was playing me tricks.

"No sir. You put it on the table under your shirt."

I did all the obvious things. I checked in my trouser pockets, I checked my medical kit. I looked under the table, behind the dusty plastic bottles of disinfectant and partly used de-wormer on the shelf above it. Nobody in the barn moved a muscle. Somebody was doing a good job of concealing their feelings. My watch had "walked." Somebody had decided that they needed it more than I did.

To lose a watch was bad enough. To lose this watch was particularly bad. A good quality Omega, it had been a wedding present from Jo.

There seemed to be only one thing for it.

"Mike, can I use your phone? If you could ask arap Ruto to make sure that no one leaves this barn until the police arrive, I'll go and call them."

The police acted as swiftly as anyone could ask. They arrived within half an hour, took statements from all of us, generally looked around and did their best to help, but with no success.

Realizing that I would almost certainly never see the thing again, I set off for home. Halfway home, ignoring the sight of several zebras under the cloud-encircled peaks of the mountain, I slapped the steering wheel and uttered a series of curses: "Damn! Damn! DAMN!" thinking, "I must be daft! I wish I'd remembered my father's story." Mutua kept his own counsel.

Over lunch, which we tried to share as often as possible, as long as neither of us had calls, I related my tale of woe to Jo. Then I voiced my thoughts.

"You know, I must have had a mental lapse. I remember Dad telling me about something similar that happened to him before the war. I wish I'd remembered the story."

"What story is that?"

"Someone stole his gold watch and racecourse winnings, about 200 shillings, which was a fair sum in 1939, from a drawer in his house. This was before Mum came out to join him. He called a witch doctor who lined up the five men who looked after Dad and the other bachelor with whom he shared the house. A cook and an orderly for each man, and a gardener. He remembered the names, tribal roots, and serial numbers of each of them. The witch doctor produced some revolting-looking dough and prayed over it. He then announced that all the men would in turn eat a dough ball, and the guilty man would choke on it."

The third man in line refused to have anything to do with it, and of course the witch doctor simply said, "There's your guilty man." To cut a long story short, the man ran off. He returned later and tried to replace the watch and money, but the other staff had lain in ambush for him, and he was duly court-martialed and sent home."

"Fascinating, psychology I suppose," said Jo.

"S'pose so, but I wish I'd remembered it this morning. Dad gave himself a mental kick in the rear end for having been stupid enough to leave his valuables in the way of temptation. I know that in a camp like Burguret, where they have 80 staff, never mind all the families and hangers on, there is bound to be a witch doctor. Some farmers won't use them, but at Kisima they do, although I've no idea how successfully. Blast. I don't suppose I shall ever see that watch again. Anyway, enough of that. Have you had a good morning?"

"Well, I had a pretty funny, but annoying, thing happen. One of my ladies came in asking for a prescription. I don't give them out just like that, and so I asked her what it was for.

"'Well,' she replied, 'I have just had a bout of cystitis. It got better after I treated it with some Bactrim for a couple of days, and I want to be sure and have some on hand for the next time.'

"I told her that two days was definitely not enough for a proper course and asked her where she had got the Bactrim.

"'Oh, I had some left over from when Jerry treated our Labrador for cystitis a couple of months ago. She got better after three days, so I stopped the course.'"

All one could do with a story like that was grin and bear it.

"I lectured her about the risks of stopping a course of antibiotic before its prescribed time, and even more about the switch-over from veterinary to medical treatment, but I don't think she took any notice. She's one of those know-alls."

This description confirmed in my mind the name of the client cum patient. There were quite a few like her in the district, but only one whose Labrador had had cystitis two months previously.

CHAPTER 23

THE HORN OF THE RHINO

*Jo receives an alarming telephone call. To get the full story
she first has to find me, 50 miles from home.*

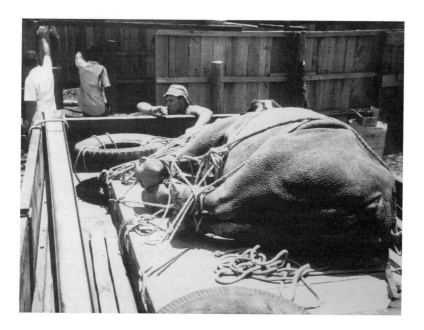

Everything OK? Checking the breathing near the rhino pens
back at the Isiolo camp.

THE CALL CAME IN OVER A crackling line via the operator. He had been unable to maintain the contact between Meru and Nanyuki, but the gist of the message for Jo was, "Your husband is in hospital in Meru because he has been horned by a rhino." No doubt at least one of the other seven subscribers on our party line had also heard the call, as the "bush telegraph" soon had the news around Nanyuki.

The message was so garbled that it was difficult to make out the truth. The first thing to try was a call to the government hospital in Meru.

"Hello, this is Dr. Haigh. Is my husband in your hospital?"

"Who is calling please?"

"Dr. Haigh."

"Who please?"

"Dr. Haigh from Nanyuki. I used to be Dr. Riet."

"Ah, Dr. Riet. How are you? How do you like Nanyuki?"

In Africa the formalities must always be attended to. Greetings are ritualized, even in a dire emergency.

THE HORN OF THE RHINO

Eventually Jo was able to make herself understood, and it turned out that there was no white man in the government hospital. Nor had they seen anyone who had been injured by a rhino. Jo set out for Meru, almost 50 miles away.

I had been doing rhino capture with Tony Parkinson and John Seago about once a month, except during the rainy season. I had begun to refine my techniques, and to pass on my experience to Mutua, who had now become an integral part of the team. As we sometimes caught two animals in a single helicopter run (usually a female and her calf), I could happily let him ride on the truck with one animal, while I traveled with the other.

On the day of the accident, a Japanese television crew were with our team in the field, shooting a documentary. They had lots of action to film as the crew made their way through a dense thicket of wait-a-bit thorn, attacking the bushes while trying to stay out of the grasp of the curved thorns.

One truck and the ancient open Land Rover made it to the site of capture, and we successfully rolled the rhino onto the sled. The beast was partially tied down, we had splashed it generously with the water that we carried in jerry cans, and I was taking a series of measurements to check how it was doing. I had also collected a blood sample from the vein in the ear. As the needle puncture was still bleeding a little, I used a swab to apply some pressure to the site.

Events after this are somewhat confused in my mind. This is what I think happened.

As I leaned over the animal, it started to thrash its head. I lost my balance, slipped on the wet wood of the sled, and managed to fall directly on to the tip of the rhino's horn just as it made a violent thrust. As it was lying on its side I was flipped about ten yards away, turning at least one somersault in the air. I could feel a terrible pain in my side, but I had no idea how serious it was. Like all good cameramen, the film crew kept the film rolling all the way through, offering no help, and not pausing to check how things were. I have never seen the footage. If it has not been consigned to a trash heap by now, almost 30 years later, I suppose it is gathering dust in a vault. If any of the crew are reading this, would they please let me know, as I would love to see the film and check if my memory is accurate.

Two or three capture crew members rushed to help, and quickly determined that I had better be taken for help as soon as possible. Mwaniki and Alexander checked my abdomen and saw that it had been punctured. They gave me a cloth to staunch the wound and helped me into the only small vehicle that we had present. The helicopter had returned to camp, we had no radio with us, so the old Land Rover was the only solution. By the time that we reached the tarred road the combination of thorn bushes and sharp rocks had led to three holes in the tires. There was no option but to keep going, as far as the team were concerned, and I wonder to this day how the rims stood up to the insult. To ensure that we got a ride quickly, Alexander and Mwaniki stood out in the middle of the road, giving the approaching vehicles virtually no choice but to stop. We were lucky; the first one was a local Peugeot taxi, and I was soon in Meru.

Things were not as bad as they had at first seemed. By the time the taxi driver arrived in town I had somewhat recovered my wits, and had asked him to take me to the clinic of an old friend, Dinka Bhatt. I had treated his family dogs for a variety of ailments over the years, and we had played many a game of snooker in the Meru club. Dinka quickly determined that the injury was not as serious as had at first appeared. The skin was broken and even the muscles were torn, but by good fortune the abdominal cavity had not been punctured. There was of course a good deal of bruising, but nothing more serious. After cleaning things up and dressing the wound, he started me on an antibiotic course and moved me to a friend's house, and it was here that Jo found me a couple of hours later.

I had to re-tell the story to her, and we gabbed more or less inces-santly, using the noise to mentally drown out the much deeper concern of what might have been.

Within a month I was back to full strength, and was able to drop into the rhino camp on my way to another job. I was happy to hear that the rhino which had clobbered me was doing well, and had just been translo-cated to Meru National Park and the care of Peter Jenkins.

CHAPTER 24

THE RHINO BABY

Mutua and I head for Don Hunt's luxurious camp at the Muramur dam, just outside Maralal, where we begin to remove rhino that are under severe threat of poaching. I fly with the world's only one-handed helicopter pilot, and I sit up all night nursing a baby rhino.

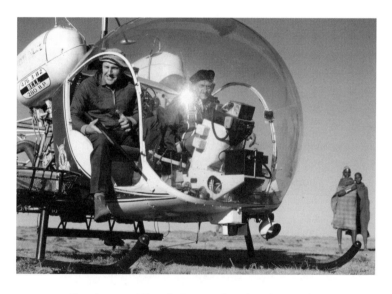

Ready to go! Punch Bearcroft and author in the
Hughes 300 at Maralal.

ONE AFTERNOON, SOON AFTER my belly blow from the rhino, Don Hunt dropped by the office to see if I had recovered and was still interested in helping with captures. He explained that the rhino in the Maralal area were under severe threat of poaching, and he had a licence to capture a number for transport to zoos in the U.S.A. We were soon discussing details.

"Bring a change of clothes, including something warm for the evenings, and your drug kit," he told me. "We'll look after everything else."

"I'll bring Mutua as well, if that's not a problem. He has plenty of experience and can help with downed animals."

"Fine, then. We'll see you both at camp."

It was about a two-and-a-half-hour drive to the camp, near Maralal. Across Laikipia to Rumuruti, the murram road, washboard hard in places, was fine as long as one kept up speed to ride the crests of the little waves.

The plume of dust stretching behind the car hardly moved in the still air. We left the fenced areas and the region of large cattle ranches, and drove along the edge of the Lerogi Plateau. Scattered herds of Grevy's zebra stood eyeing us with suspicion, and small antelope lifted their heads briefly as we sped by.

We arrived at the camp, where Don and Iris greeted me and showed me around. Even in such a "bush" environment, Iris managed to look as elegant as ever. Clad in khaki trousers, a white shirt and a smart waistcoat, she looked as if she had just come from a salon. Her blond hair had no strand out of place.

This camp was more luxurious than the one at Isiolo. There were seven spacious, well-shaded Manyara tents. The mess tent, a large, open-sided affair with mosquito-proof walls, boasted a table that would seat 12, and a well-stocked kerosene refrigerator. A series of robust animal pens lay nearby, located under the densest of the thorn trees to ensure maximum protection from the sun.

Over lunch we discussed the plans. "Punch Bearcroft will be flying in in the police helicopter later today. He has only six days, so we'll be done by next Thursday. We'll get going in the morning," said Don.

"How early?" I asked.

"Well, I'd like us to be flying right at first light. As soon as Punch says it's all right. Iris will be staying in camp and I'll be up to the north-west here —" he pointed over his shoulder "— with the Toyota and the fellows in the lorry. We'll probably leave about five o'clock."

"Are we just after rhino?"

"We know that there are supposed to be at least 56 rhino in this area, and they're already being poached. I'd like to concentrate on them, but if you see some small elephant, no more than about 52 inches, we can also take them as I have a couple of orders to fill."

"Will there be some breakfast before we go? I need a good start, especially if we're out for a long day," I said.

"What sort of breakfast do you like, Jerry?" asked Iris. "Cereal? Toast? Eggs? Coffee or tea?"

We established that a full English breakfast would be most welcome, even at five in the morning.

The Hughes 300, with its blue Kenya Police Airwing colours prominent, circled the camp once, the rotors creating a crescendo of sound as it dipped over the dam, signaling the arrival of the last and crucial member of the team. I moved down to camp and met up with Don and Iris as they walked over to the clearing a hundred yards beyond.

The pilot, his right hand behind his back, stepped out from behind the machine, where he had been going through his closing-down procedures, and walked towards us. He stood about five feet nine, walked with slightly bowed legs, and had grizzled hair and the general appearance of someone who had lots of experiences under his belt. It seemed odd when Don made no effort to shake his hand but merely greeted him with a cheery, "Hello, Punch. It's good to see you again. Hope you had a good flight. I'd like you to meet Jerry Haigh. He's our vet for the next few days. Jerry, this is Punch Bearcroft."

Punch still had his hand behind his back and did not bring it forward as I tentatively reached out in the normal way so we simply exchanged verbal greetings.

The reason for his reluctance was soon apparent. He had no right hand. From time to time he would fold his sleeve over the stump of his wrist, but he made no reference to his condition. He seemed calm and relaxed over a beer as he and Don exchanged stories about mutual acquaintances whom I did not know. At supper he kept his forearm out of sight below the table, and had no trouble dealing with the delicious steak that Iris had organized for our opening supper.

After breakfast, we set off. Iris had thoughtfully provided a good pile of sandwiches and a thermos flask of tea. As the lorry carried two drums of helicopter fuel, we would be independent of camp for most of the day, especially if we had no luck in finding animals.

The dawn mist was still clinging to the lower yellow-green branches of the trees, and the doves were heralding the day as Punch began his pre-flight checks. I could still not fathom how a pilot with only one hand would be able to fly a helicopter, so I watched with particular interest as he pulled a two-inch wide section of car inner tube from under his seat and passed it over his wrist six inches or so up his forearm. He then laid the stub of his arm against the joystick, passed the inner tube around the rubberized handle, using the indentations intended for fingers as slots to prevent it from slipping, and brought the loop back over the end of his wrist. He was now firmly attached to the controls.

I put on my headset and strapped myself into the safety harness. The right-hand side door had been taken off and I was sitting on the floor, my legs on the skids. I made a few practice movements with Don's new dart gun in my hands, as I had not flown in a Hughes 300 before. Leaning over, Punch tapped me on the shoulder with his left hand.

"We'll try and keep radio contact to a minimum," he said. This did not make much sense until I remembered that in order to speak to me he would have had to press the transmit button on the joystick with his right thumb.

We peeled off and began a search, meandering westward. The searching was quite different than the work that I had done with Tony and John in the Isiolo area. Here we were working over thick forest, the ground completely obscured at times, the gaps between the trees and bushes seldom more than ten or 15 yards across. After a while we turned north, and then further west. Finally we turned south and then Punch, after locking the collector lever, reached across and, using his left hand, called up Don on the radio. I got a brief glimpse of a moving grey object beneath us, and turned towards the pilot. He was way ahead of me.

"Don, we have spotted a rhino. I'll get back to you." None of the "Over, over" stuff for him, at least not up here in the bush when talking to the ground crew.

We circled and picked up the lone bull. This looked as if it was going to be a very difficult proposition. However, we got lucky. We could see a reasonable opening about 400 yards away on a ridge, and Punch held back and began to manoeuver the animal towards it. Knowing that chatting was more or less useless I depressed my radio switch and said, "I won't fire until you can get the chopper moving at the same speed as he is, so the dart won't overshoot. Let's drop in when we get to the edge over there. A shot at about 40 feet gives me the best chance."

Skillfully Punch moved the machine behind and to the side of the rhino, as we tried to get a good look at him through the trees. As he approached the clearing we lost height and it only took a moment to get the dart away. I could almost feel the smack as it hit the beast square in the left rump. The whole thing, from spotting him to hitting him, had taken less than a minute.

Punch got back on the radio. "Don, we have an animal darted." As he gave directions on our direction and location, the animal headed away from the forested areas. After about six minutes, he began to stagger. We watched as he fell over, struggled a bit, then lay still.

Punch put down, the skids only just touching as I piled out with my drug box and gun, and took off again to guide the team to the rhino.

By now I had done enough rhino work to have established a routine. Check the breathing; check the heart; cover the upward eye. Check breathing and heart again. Insert a thermometer into the rear end. Once I knew that all was well I could relax a little. Before I forgot the rates, I wrote them down on my clipboard. The temperature read 102.2 degrees Fahrenheit. There were no centigrade thermometers available, so one had to be bilingual in this area as well. All this information would be crucial in judging how the animal was doing. Then it was time to remove the dart and inject the dart wound with an antibiotic.

Before long, Punch returned, setting the helicopter down about 50 yards away. The truck came grinding up the slope, moving slowly over the boulders. The Toyotas appeared like a couple of dodge-em cars, weaving among the rocks, searching for the best route.

As always, Mutua assisted with the next part of the routine. Body measurements; calculate the weight; figure out drug doses; collect sample of manure and ticks; check the vital signs again, every few minutes. Record everything.

The team soon had ropes on the animal and began loading him on to the sled and then the truck. I sent Mutua with the animal, arming him with a bottle of antidote in case the patient got too deep and needed resuscitation. I also gave him the record sheet so that he could write down information on breathing. We had found that trying to listen to a heart while on the back of a moving truck bouncing across country was a fruitless exercise.

Punch and I climbed back into the helicopter, flew back to base, and sat with Iris telling her of our good news. After an hour the ground crew arrived bearing the cargo.

Now came the tricky task of unloading the rhino. Just over two hours had elapsed since I put the dart in his backside. Mutua told me that his breathing rate had increased and that his temperature had gone up to 104 degrees. After the lorry had been backed up to one of the pens, and even before we rolled the sled off the vehicle, the first thing was to undo the head rope and see how he reacted. He promptly thrashed his head, which told me that he had made quite a recovery and that a small top-up dose was needed. I injected it into his muscles. By the time the sled had come down off the lorry and been manoeuvred into the pen, the animal had settled down. We got the ropes off with ease and after his antidote injection, he soon came to.

After a lunch of tea and sandwiches, we were soon airborne again. The place seemed to be teeming with rhino, and by early afternoon we had another animal in camp, this time a sub-adult female. We set out in the chopper yet again, and after about an hour we spotted a single animal, sporting a broken front horn, among the trees. At least it seemed to be a singleton. Pretty soon it was quite evident that it was in fact a cow, with a small calf. As it began to get dark, I worried that we might not be able to get the job done in sufficient time to ensure safety for ourselves or the animal. Then luck played a hand. The animals ran within about 30 yards of the trucks, and quick as wink Don had his team on the move. The calf was captured using the old roping technique, and we broke off the aerial chase as the mother had moved into impossibly thick stuff and we could hardly see her.

There was no need to tie the little guy to a sled, and Don brought him back to camp in the Toyota. There was plenty of powdered milk on hand for just such an event, and now Iris took over. Rhino calves spend most of their time closely attached to their mothers, frequently taking a drink. So the milk is diluted, but they need lots of it. For the human sur-rogate mother this translates into numerous bottles and a disturbed sleep pattern, which was nothing new for Iris, an experienced animal person.

The dense thickets of mixed woodland made chasing rhino difficult, but the numbers of rhino meant that we continued to have good luck finding them. I felt sure that Punch's seemingly haphazard search method played a role. Either that or he was the luckiest pilot imaginable.

Early on the morning of the fifth day, we caught a cow rhino. There was no doubt that she was the mother of the little calf in camp, as her torn ear and broken front horn were so distinctive.

"Look," I said to Mutua and Don, who were standing close by, "you can see by the rub marks along her spine that she has been breeding.

Often, if an animal is nursing a calf, the reproductive cycle is shut down as the stimulus of sucking prevents ovarian function. As soon as the milking stimulus stops the ovaries can start to function again."

When we returned her to base and put her in a pen on her own, Mutua asked, "Why can't we put the calf in with her? It would be better if it had its mother's milk."

I replied, "It's been tried before, and even if the mother and calf are caught at the same time, the bigger animal almost always turns on the little one and kills it. I think it's probably the stress of captivity and unfamiliar surroundings that causes the behaviour."

By the end of the fifth day we had seven rhino in camp, including the calf. I had been doing the rounds every time we came back, and there was always a pile of fresh-cut brush near the pens. The old branches, thoroughly chewed off, were piled like a giant bonfire behind the *bomas*. The calf had been drinking well and was already getting into mischief, squeaking when called. He would throw up his head, the faint beginnings of a horn just showing as a bumpy ring at the end of his nose, and butt the bottle as Iris held it out to him.

As we sat enjoying a sundowner in the mess tent Iris said, "Jerry, I'd like you to take a look at 'Junior' after supper. He hardly drank anything at his last feed, and he seems to have a runny nose."

"We could look now if you like, while there's still some light. I'll get my bits and pieces."

We walked over to the shelter that had been rigged for the calf. He had rapidly settled into his new life, as black rhino do, and there was no robust fence, just a canvas wall about three feet high to act more as a draft screen than a real barrier. The rhino was lying on his side, seemingly asleep, but his breathing did not sound quite right, even from a yard away. When I touched him his body seemed a bit cold, and he was slow to respond when I scratched his ear and talked to him.

"How much fluid has he had in the last 12 hours?"

Iris checked her records. "About five and a half pints, but this last time he hardly drank anything."

The youngster was about the same size as a five-month-old pig, 150 pounds at a guess. I did a bit of quick mental arithmetic.

"At his weight he should be getting around 15 pints a day, seven or eight in 12 hours. He's probably a bit shy on that, even if I have overestimated his weight. Iris, please can you hold his head while I examine him?"

While my thermometer did its thing at his rear end I put the stethoscope to my ears, knelt down in the straw, and concentrated. There were faint scratching noises that should not have been there, but none of the nasty fluid sounds that would mean that he had breathed in some of his milk. If that had happened he would have been in serious trouble, but as it was he needed help.

"Iris, I think that his main problem is hypoglycemia, but he may be starting a bit of pneumonia. I don't have any record of what a normal baby rhino temperature should be, but if he was a foal, 98.2 would be a bit low. It's very cold at night and despite the shelter he may have caught a chill. I want to start him on some penicillin, but I also think we must get some fluids into him."

"Fine, Jerry," she responded. "Don, what can we do about the cold?"

Don, who was naturally standing nearby, a very interested spectator, responded, "I do have that old quilted jacket that you wanted to throw out. I brought it along as a spare. Why don't you use that?"

I went off to get some bottles of saline and dextrose, with their attendant drip sets and needles, and Iris got out a sewing kit and got busy.

I could see no handy veins that would suit for the drip. The ear vessels, into which I normally put antidote in rhino, were too small for the purpose. The only solution was to run the emergency fluids directly into his abdomen, where his system would absorb them almost as quickly as if I had put them directly into the bloodstream. Relying on my knowledge of pig and horse anatomy, I inserted the needle just behind and slightly to one side of his belly button and fixed up the drip. The fact that he lay there and hardly reacted when the needle went in told me that he was far from well. Iris draped his new coat over him and we sat up in the gathering dusk.

We ate our supper on our laps, Don sending over generous helpings from the mess tent, and drowsily watched our charge and chatted.

I changed the empty drip bottle and curled up in the corner of the pen. As the air chilled to only a few degrees above freezing, at the elevation of well over 6,000 feet, I walked over to my tent and grabbed a couple of blankets. We sat up the entire night, dropping off into a doze every now and again, and once disconnecting the drip as our patient grew restless. Iris tried him on some milk formula at about 2:00 a.m., but he did not show much interest. As the pink dawn light began to creep into the sky I suggested that we try to feed him again. He suddenly rolled over and pulled out the needle. He would not stand still enough for another one to be put into him for more drips. I gave him a second dose of penicillin and even this he objected to. He definitely seemed much more frisky, although not completely back to his mischievous self. He drank a full wine bottle of milk and after Iris tickled his rear end with a damp cloth he even passed a small amount of dung.

"He seems to have turned the corner," I said. "I'm heading for some shut-eye. Why don't we let him sleep now?"

"Can you just give me a hand with his coat," said Iris, "and then we'll leave him."

Now that he was standing, we could dress him properly. The fit was perfect. Iris had made some ties which she knotted under his belly and chin, and then we left him to it.

As is often the case with young animals, he made a quick recovery.

By the afternoon feed he was back to full strength, guzzling his milk at a furious rate and inspecting anything that looked interesting in his pen. He tried his best to eat the hoses on my stethoscope as I checked him over.

After a well-deserved morning's rest, during which Don and the crew went out eastwards onto the plateau and managed to find a couple of Grevy's zebra with which to fulfill one of his orders, we took off for one more try in the forests.

This time we got really lucky. We managed to dart two rhino in the space of about 45 seconds. A mother and large juvenile had been running together, and even after we dropped down with the chopper to shoot the mother, the youngster did not break away. As we were flying into the breeze, Punch was able to maintain a straight flight, although we had to stay high up to avoid upsetting the animals. I was able to quickly insert the single spare dart that had once again been taped to the firewall behind me. There was no back-up dart, but Punch and I had by now worked out most of the bugs, and he knew that I would not fire unless everything was right. The darts in both animals were exactly centred in the heavy muscles alongside the tail. Even handier, both animals went down in the open, not more than 30 yards apart.

We had exceeded all expectations. An exuberant Don was obviously delighted as we sat and sipped our evening beers.

"Fellows, we have a problem. We have filled our licence, and anyways we have no more pens here for rhino. I think we'll call it off and try again at the end of next month. I'll get in touch with you to see when you are free."

Some problem.

Next morning, after a more leisurely and certainly later breakfast than usual, Mutua and I headed for home. It would be great to see Jo and Karen again.

Looking back with the 20:20 vision of almost 30 years, the notion of collecting animals from the wild for zoos seems unacceptable. However, the
massive destruction of rhinos in the last 25 years of the 20th century,
which was merely the culmination of over a century of unbridled killing,
changes the perspective somewhat. The most authoritative text on rhino-
human relations is *Run Rhino Run*, authored by the husband and wife
team of Esmond and Chryssee Bradley Martin. Quoting various authors,
including Richard Burton and Frederick Selous, they relate that early in
the 19th century the white rhinoceros were present "in almost incredible
numbers" and "the black rhinoceros . . . [was] as common as the elephant." This situation did not last long. Commercial hunting took place
on a huge and organized scale. By 1870, the white rhinoceros in South
Africa had dwindled to something less than a hundred animals. Between
about 1900 and 1931, hunting of black rhino was especially intense.
Hundreds of horns were exported annually from Somali ports around
1900, and between 1927 and 1931 huge gangs of up to 50 hunters were
employed by French hunters to kill as many rhinos as possible in French
Equatorial Africa. "There must have been well over 10,000 white rhinos
shot" in this brief period.

While the bulk of these early hunts were for commercial purposes,
some were conducted by "sportsmen." Earlier European visitors, the first
of a long line of sportsmen that would later include Count "Windy-
Scratch" and his Hungarian museum pieces, had hunted rhino for no
more than the bragging rights. An Indian army captain and two friends
on safari had killed 66 just on the eastern slopes of Mt. Kilimanjaro, and
Count Teliki had fallen one short of the cricketing goal of "a ton" by
managing only 99.

Although most rhino destruction was for commercial purposes, and
some for sport, one remarkable cull occurred under government aus-
pices. J.A. Hunter probably holds the record for killing more rhino than

any other single person, and it was all done in order to clear the area of Makueni, south-east of Nairobi, for settlement. Hunter is variously reported to have killed either 1,088 or 996 rhinos between 1944 and 1946, as well as various other animals. The numbers are mind-boggling, and he himself queried the killing in his autobiography.

In Kenya alone there were possibly as many as 20,000 rhinos left in 1969, but by 1982, the year that the Bradley-Martins' book was published, there were probably no more than 1,500. The collapse of rhino populations was underway well before African independence. As Jonathan Kingdon has shown, rhino were present in varying numbers throughout almost all of East Africa in 1925, but had vanished from over half their range by 1950. In the last 180 years over 95% of Africa's rhinos have been shot, and in the decade following 1970, the numbers were halved.

The Bradley-Martins also address the obvious question: Why? In a wide-ranging investigation in many countries, they found some answers. Rhino parts, particularly the horn, have had a cash value in Eastern countries for a long time. The markets for rhino horn are very considerable. The stuff has been used for centuries in Asia for medicinal purposes (mainly as an anti-fever agent), and despite what the Western media would have one believe, its use as an aphrodisiac has been limited to a small region in the state of Gujarat in India. The Bradley-Martins also point out the extensive use of whole rhino horns in Yemen. There they are used to make dagger handles, and ownership of such a dagger is a definite status symbol. The development of the oil-based economy in the Middle East, and the increased number of men with disposable incomes from work in the oil fields, served to exacerbate the pressure on an already fragile world rhino population.

■

There are some sad postscripts to all the work that we did capturing rhino near Maralal and translocating them out of the Isiolo area.

The first is that, for the local people and most of the rhino, the whole exercise was a complete waste of time. We had moved rhino near Isiolo to make way for settlement, which completely failed. How could farmers hope to make a living off five or ten acres in an area where, in an average year, it takes about 20 or 30 acres to support one small native *zebu* cow? With rainfall no more than ten inches or so a year, and temperatures often above 30 degrees, maize crops would often wither before they reached a couple of feet in height, long before any cobs appeared on the stalks.

All the rhino that the Seago/Parkinson team moved to Meru Game Park were dead by the mid-eighties. Peter Jenkins must have had quite a scare when he came across a gang of 22 poachers in the park. They were all armed with Russian and Chinese automatic weapons and, not surprisingly, they cleaned out many areas of rhino and elephant. The small group of semi-tame white rhino, several of them my ex-patients, which had been guarded for years, were taken in a single night. The antiquated Lee-Enfield rifles of the rangers were not much of a match for modern automatic weapons, and pay scales for guards may not have been enough to motivate them to risk their lives against well-armed gangs. All our efforts there were in vain.

There are two small glimmers of a more cheerful nature. While it is estimated that the Maralal rhino population had completely disappeared by 1980, some of the 25 or so that we captured and moved survived and may have bred, albeit in zoos. If we had not been involved, none of them would have done so. And for the Isiolo exercise, descendants of some of the rhino we moved to Solio are still alive.

Whether due to the nearness of "commercial extinction" — a chilling term to anyone concerned with conservation — or to increased surveillance and the placement of rhino in fenced or heavily guarded parks, as we head into the new century black rhino numbers seem to be creeping back up. One must be cautious about becoming over-optimistic.

In 1998, when we visited Kenya, three rhino were poached in the space of a few days, one within five miles of Nanyuki. By 2001, when a group of rhino specialists met in Lake Manyara, Tanzania, the numbers of all rhino in Africa were estimated to be about 2,700 black rhino and over 10,300 white rhino. A far cry from 19th-century numbers, and far fewer black rhino on the whole continent than had been present in Kenya alone when I first went back.

CHAPTER 25

LEMURS, PUPPIES, AND A PELICAN

Among my patients are a group of lemurs that have come to Nanyuki from their native Madagascar. A pelican becomes a patient and provides surprises, as well as a chance to test a new anesthetic. Jo has a brush with fame, and little Karen helps out at the clinic.

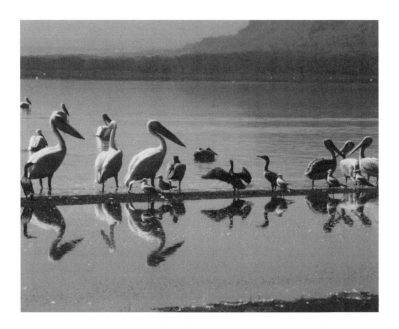

A wonderful bird is the pelican.

APART FROM THE ANIMAL orphanage, Don and Iris had some pens near their house in which they kept other creatures. Among these were a couple of cheetahs and a variety of lemurs. The latter had come from Madagascar, and were kept in quarantine in Kenya before being shipped on to the States. From time to time these beautiful little creatures would develop medical problems that needed attention, but it was impossible to get any information about them from my textbooks, and as they were not native there was no one else in the country to whom I could turn for advice or ideas. All I knew was where they came from, and that there were several types. The commonest were the striking ring-tailed species, but once or twice there were gorgeous black-and-white ruffed lemurs, looking for all the world as if they had been bestowed with Elizabethan collars, and also black lemurs, the males a deep black from head to foot, the females a brownish to russet colour, with black face and hands. All of these were no bigger than a domestic cat, but had the hands and feet of a primate and the pointed face, with its long nose, of a Chihuahua. They also had an impressive array of sharp teeth, as Iris found out one day, to her cost, when a male ring-tailed sank his fangs into the ball of her thumb and produced an ugly wound for Jo to look after.

It took me some time to find out that they were primitive primates, distant relatives of the apes and even us humans. Once again, my trusty *Guinness Book of World Records* came up with a little gem. It informed me that lemurs are not overbright, and in some tests appear less intelligent than pigeons. Now pigeons are fine birds, but intelligence is not one of their main attributes, and I wondered about these tests.

One morning, after a night of heavy thunderstorms, Iris found a ring-tailed lemur dead in its cage. Don sent it to me for a necropsy, which quickly showed the cause of death. The chest cavity was full of clotted blood, and there was a white cauliflower-like outgrowth just above the heart that had a small rent in it, to which were attached a few stringy clots. There was another similar, but smaller, lesion a couple of inches down the main artery. They were aneurysms of the aorta, the first of which was almost as big as the heart itself, and must have been present for quite some time. I placed the chest contents, minus the lungs, in a large jar of formalin and shipped the whole thing off to the pathology lab at Kabete. Within a couple of weeks the report came back. The aneurysm had had a double cause, the primary one being the presence of several worms in the aorta, on top of which a bacterial infection had become established. No doubt this had weakened the wall to the point where the sudden loud thunderclap had been too much for the system, and rupture had followed.

Over the next few months, I saw several more lemurs. Three had aneurysms similar to the first one I'd seen, and it seemed strange to me that this unusual lesion should be occurring so frequently. Far more, however, came in with war wounds. A typical entry in my medical records reads:

> Adult female black lemur. Attacked by male. Torn up.
> 0.05 cc Sernylan in 0.2 cc water for injection. 10 min-
> utes easily handled. Shaved, cleaned & stitched. Rt.
> shoulder, 6 stitches, Rt. wrist 5. Back 5. Rt. leg 5. 0.2 cc's
> Penbritin twice daily. One hour's work.

One day I was at the library at the vet college in Kabete, and quite by chance I saw a pile of pamphlets, looking slightly the worse for wear, lying in a cardboard box next to the rubbish basket. The top one caught my eye, as it had a picture of a lemur on the cover. Underneath were five more, and all of them were in French, which I could just about make out; one was titled "Mortalité, Natalaité et Pathologie." Browsing through, I found a list of causes of death among lemurs at the Tsimbazaza Zoo in Tananarive, Madagascar, and learned that our lemurs were, in fact, typical of their species. There had been 11 cases of aneurysm at the zoo in their native country, and 17 deaths caused by fighting.

A young female ring-tailed lemur presented me with an awkward surgical case. She had been bitten near the end of her tail, and the last two and a half inches of it were quite bald. When I examined it, it was immediately obvious that everything below the bite was dead tissue, cold and soggy. Worse yet, the necrosis was ascending up the tail, and I would have to amputate to save the little creature's life. If I didn't, there was every likelihood that gangrene would set in. My usual anesthesia with Sernylan ("angel dust" on the streets) worked well, and within 15 minutes I was able to instill some local anesthetic around the base of the tail, and shave and scrub the skin. The beautiful bushy brush, with its alternating rings of blue-grey and cream, is the crowning glory of the ring-tailed lemur, and to have it reduced to this skinny, bony stick, no more than about three-quarters of an inch in diameter near its base, was a trifle sad. Once I had taken it off the animal would no longer be able to curl it up over her head, or wrap herself in it like a blanket. However, there was no alternative, so I slipped a rubber band up the tail to make a simple tourniquet.

As Mutua prepared the patient and I started to scrub up for the surgery, two strangers walked into the clinic and introduced themselves. They were Marty Dinnes and Bill Boever, veterinarians visiting from the U.S.A., Bill from the St. Louis Zoo, Marty from the west coast. We chatted as I went through the relatively easy steps of the amputation, and Bill told me of a new anesthetic that had just become available in the U.S.A., which should work well on lemurs, and would also be useful for cats. It was basically a weaker version of Sernylan, with the marked advantages of having fewer side effects, and allowing a much quicker recovery.

This drug, called Ketamine, would become a staple in my own drug box, as well as those of many, many other vets, for a long time to come. It was useful for birds, llamas, big cats as well as domestic ones, and a variety of other beasts. I was soon able to use it on yet another lemur that needed stitches, and Marty and Bill's advice about the time it would work was very accurate. Within ten minutes of the first injection my new patient needed a top-up.

The pelican that Jo and I had watched as it gulped the fish thrown to him by a keeper became a patient. Brian Burroughs called, and I went up to the Safari Club to see what could be done. It was a surprise to see Jo's car near the front entrance, and, as luck would have it she came out as I entered.

She told me that she had been up to see the film star who had had a piece of flying glass in his eye, and who had visited her the previous day at the hospital. I had already heard how she had put him off work for three days, after removing the shard, and how the enraged producer had appeared in her office demanding that the star be put back to work because of the cost of the delay.

We caught up with the bird keeper, as he approached the wire-covered holding runs where some of his non-flying charges were penned at night, and he soon had the pelican in his hands, holding out the left wing and showing me the damage.

I could hardly believe my eyes. The front of the whole forearm of the bird was stripped of skin and feathers. About a foot of the bone was a dull white colour, and made a strange bridge between the elbow, which looked almost normal, and the feathers at the wing tip. Towards the elbow the skin had peeled back, exposing raw flesh, which was black and smelly, and a mass of maggots were burrowing and wriggling on the exposed tissue. On the other wing there was some minor damage on the top edge, and a few maggots were doing their thing.

"What happened?" I asked the keeper, trying not to make too much of it.

"He was attacked last week by a leopard. I told Mr. Burroughs, and he gave me some *dawa* to put in its drinking water," he said in a matter-of-fact tone.

"A leopard! Why isn't it dead? A pelican should be an easy meal for a leopard."

"Josphat told me he saw it attack, and that it ran away when he shouted."

I shook my head in wonder. To Jo, I said, "I suspect the word 'leopard' is being used incorrectly here. A real one would have made very short work of this bird. It was probably a smaller spotted cat, maybe a serval, and perhaps the keepers don't know any other Swahili word. Anyway, it doesn't much matter what happened, but it does look as if I'll have to amputate this left wing, so let's go and tell Jenny or Brian about the thing."

As we walked back to main club building Jo said — in a sort of half whisper, despite the fact that we were out of doors and there was not a soul in sight — "You'll never believe what I've just seen."

This was more or less rhetorical. "Go on," I rejoined, adopting the same unnecessary decibel level.

"Well, I was up to see some guest's new baby. They had brought her with them, as well as Scottish nanny. The babe just had a bit of sniffles, which I dealt with, and I had a good chat with the nanny, who is very sweet. She was trained in London, at a nanny school, and wears a smart blue uniform. Anyway, I noticed a pile of wooden crates of bottles in the suite. It was marked 'Scottish Spring Water.' I said to the nanny, 'I suppose that's for making up her formula. It must cost a fortune.' 'Oh no,' she replied with a secretive grin, 'It's no for the bairn. They have it delivered twice a week, by plane. It's just for bathing the babe.'" Jo gave me a special, skeptical look and shrugged her shoulders.

We arranged for the pelican to be brought to the clinic first thing in the morning, and sharp at eight o'clock the khaki Land Cruiser, shield and elephant's-head logo on its side, pulled up outside. My instruments were boiling away. This was my first bird surgery, and I had searched through a recent copy of *The Veterinary Record*, my only source of scientific advances, for a paper that I recalled seeing about bird anesthesia. It described how a friend and bird enthusiast from my Kabete days had tried an unnamed drug called CT1341 on chickens and birds of prey. That friend, John Cooper, had developed a reputation for veterinary interest and skill in non-traditional species while still a student at Bristol, and had also published his results for the benefit of the profession.

I had ordered some of the new drug, which was based on steroids related to cortisone, from Monks the chemist, in Nairobi, and a couple of boxes of it sat on my shelf, unused till now, and gathering dust, but waiting a chance to be tested.

The first challenge was a dose, and to estimate a dose I needed a weight.

The bird looked big. "What do you think it weighs, guys?" I asked

Mutua and Njeru. "Let's put ten cents each into a pool, and the closest one gets it all."

They thought for a moment and Mutua, looking at him, said "Maybe 20 pounds." I came in at 18. Njeru, who had the pelican under his arm, said, "Fifteen and a half." Then he put the bird on the office scale.

We were in for two surprises. The first one was the weight, which only a tad over 12 pounds. Njeru had won the pool.

The second surprise was for me personally, as I picked the patient off the scale to take him over to the operating table. I could feel a whole lot of air bubbles under the skin on his chest. It felt exactly like the bubbly plastic wrapping that some of our drugs were delivered in. It also set off alarm bells in my head, as this feeling, known as emphysema, would be a very bad sign under the skin of a mammal. It would indicate an active and fast-spreading infection which was badly in need of vigorous treatment. As it stood quietly, looking stately, but faintly ridiculous, on the table, I tried to think things through. I figured that it would be looking a whole lot sicker, if not dead, if the emphysema was really an infection, and that it was probably normal, explaining why pelicans float so high in the water, like a sailing ship. It was a built-in set of water-wings.

As for my 50% weight overestimate, the air under its skin, exaggerating its size, the bulk, but lightness of the feathers, and the lightweight bones probably explained everything. With time and practice I began to get better at judging the weight of large birds, but the scale remained an important part of the decision-making process.

Now that we knew the weight, I had to figure out an anesthetic dose. I knew that I was going to have to keep him sedated for quite some time, while I amputated the ruined wing at the elbow. So I drew up double the amount that John Cooper had used for large birds, and as Mutua applied pressure on the wing vein on the bird's "good" side, I injected the clear fluid.

The effect was almost instantaneous. As the drug reached the halfway level in the syringe, the patient suddenly relaxed. The head drooped, and all the tension went out of its muscles.

"You hold this syringe against his wing," I said to Mutua. "If it moves or shows any signs of pain while I'm working, give it some more." Almost in the same breath I said to Njeru, "Come and hold the wing away from its body. We'll try and clean the area as best we can, but we will have to work quickly, as this drug is supposed to only last for a short time."

Within a few moments we had applied some Savlon hospital solution to the skin, wrapped the feathery end of the wing in a sterilized green cloth, and I was working at the damage point. I cut as much good skin below his elbow as I could, flapped it back, and severed all the tendons and connections in his elbow, letting the cloth and its contents fall to the floor. The flaps that I had prepared then came into play, as I used them like a purse, sewing them together over the enlarged end of the humerus.

Twice during the procedure, which took about 20 minutes, Mutua gently pushed some extra CT1341 into the bird's vein. Seven minutes after I had straightened up, stretched, and laid down my forceps and needle, the bird woke up, moving from deep sleep to apparent full alertness almost instantaneously. We gave him an injection of antibiotics, dusted the wound on the "good" wing with some sulfa powder, and sent the driver home with the bird and a packet of more antibiotic to be added to his drinking water for ten days.

As I walked into the office one day after lunch, the telephone was ringing. Njeru, first out of the car, got it and passed it over to me. It was a local resident calling, in a strained voice, to tell me that she had just missed me at home, and would I please come quickly as her little terrier bitch Sally was having trouble delivering pups. I had met Sally on a few previous occasions. She came regularly for her vaccinations, and as her owner, Mrs. Emmerson, was none too adept at administering worm tablets, we had taken on that task as well. We took a few minutes to gather everything we might need, including the small delivery forceps, and I headed out the door.

As soon as I felt the little dog's abdomen I knew that there were probably several pups on the way. A further examination of her birth canal told me that I was not going to be able to deliver them by the normal route, not even with the forceps.

"Mrs. Emmerson," I said to the anxious owner, who had been hovering nearby, "I'm going to have to do a Caesarean to get these pups out and to save the bitch. If you'd like me to carry on, may I use your phone so as to call the office and get my staff to start sterilizing the instruments? If you've got her basket, I'd like to take that as well, so that when she's ready to come home she'll be in a familiar environment."

"Yes, please. Go ahead, I'll get the basket," was her prompt response.

Back at the office, knowing that I would need to draft some extra hands as neonatal nurses, I called Jo, who arrived 15 minutes later with Karen in tow. Ester was away on annual leave, visiting her mother near Kericho, so Jo was taking the afternoons off to be with Karen, who had started morning play school near the hospital. By the time they arrived from home, Mutua and I had prepared the surgery. The table had been scrubbed down, the instruments were ready, the angle lamp had been moved over the table, and a cardboard box had been layered with newspaper over the top of a hot water bottle.

As soon as Jo arrived I picked up the syringe of dissolved Themalon tablets that was to be our anesthetic. Themalon was a morphine-like drug developed for small animals that had the singular advantage of being reversible, somewhat like the much more potent things that I used for my wild animal work. This meant that we could wake the patient as soon as we were ready. If one was doing a Caesarean one had to remember to give each tiny new pup a small dose of antidote to counteract the narcotic that had crossed through the placenta into its bloodstream. Another essential job was to hold each pup and give it a vigorous rub, both to dry it off and to start it breathing. A veterinary equivalent of smacking a baby's bum to get it going.

While I carried out the surgery, with the help of Mutua, Jo handled the injections for the pups. Then she and Karen both dried off the pups and placed them in the warm cardboard box, Jo supervising the little girl all the while. This was the first time that three-year-old Karen had been involved in such a task, and of course the tiny live bundles were much more intriguing than mere dolls. At first she handled them too gently, but with encouragement from us she soon got the idea, and was delighted when her first little charge let out a squeak as she rubbed it with the towel.

"Is the next one ready yet, Mummy?"

Mrs. Emmerson was a senior member of Nanyuki society, a woman who was very much a pioneer. As a small girl, soon after the turn of the century, she had been part of a group who had walked up from the coast, a journey without roads under very tough conditions. She also had very definite ideas about what was proper. We were working in the back room, when I heard her strident tones booming through the building as she came through the front door. Njeru, acting as receptionist, suggested that we would soon be ready and that she could come back then.

She was obviously having none of this.

"*Hapana. Mimi kuenda ndani na nasema na bwana,*" (Oh no, I'll go in and speak to the *bwana*) she said in the up-country Kiswahili, known as Kisettla, that was typical of her generation. (A more literal translation would be "There is not. I to go inside and I say with *bwana*.")

Njeru, quite dominated by this *mzungu*, who also towered above his five feet six inches, could do nothing to stop her forward progress. He might as well have tried to stop a runaway bus. Carrying all before her, and also a great deal behind on her matronly frame, she swept past him into the surgery area.

For a moment she appeared to be nonplussed by the scene of activity in front of her, but only for a moment. Her first reaction had nothing to do with the pups or the sleeping bitch.

"Shouldn't that child be with her *ayah*? This is hardly a proper place for one so young."

"Oh, she has seen this sort of thing before, and anyway the pups need the help," I replied.

"Well done, Karen," said Jo, "keep rubbing, make sure he's dry. Here's another one for you."

The entire conversation appeared to go straight over Karen's head as she concentrated fiercely on her job, an enraptured look on her face. Soon all was finished, the pups and mum safely together, awake and warm. We took them from our cardboard box, transferred them to the basket that we had brought with us from the dog's home, and off they went in the *memsahib's* car.

Only much later, at home, did Karen ask why the pup's owner had seemed so concerned. Small pitchers have big ears. I don't think the lady was overly impressed with the modern approach to child rearing and sex education!

CHAPTER 26

THE MOMBASA QUARANTINE

I make the first of several trips to the animal quarantine station at Mombasa to run tests on a valuable cargo of African animals destined for zoos in the United States, a situation that presents several new challenges, including an acutely ill bongo.

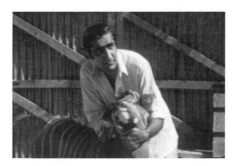

Haji Issak at Mombasa quarantine,
holding a partially drugged young bongo
ready for a blood sample collection.

CASUALLY, AS IF HE WERE asking me for the time of day, Don Hunt brought up a new subject. "Jerry, I'd like you to go down to the Mombasa quarantine station to check out the animals that we have there getting ready for a shipment state-side. Can you get away pretty soon?"

We were working together at the Animal Orphanage, trying see what was wrong with one of the rhino that we had recently brought down from Maralal.

"What's all involved?"

"Well, we have a bunch of stuff down there that needs to be screened before it can be allowed into the U.S. The Feds of U.S. Animal Health at Plum Island require two separate blood samples, drawn 30 days apart, to check for various diseases, including hoof-and-mouth disease and a bunch of others. Each animal will have to be bled twice, and the serum taken off and shipped. We need for you to go down there, link up with the owner of the quarantine — a guy named Haji — and do the job for us."

"Does he have any facilities for handling?"

"No, nothing like that."

"Hmm, so it'll be a case of drugging things. What species are involved?"

"There are some of the wildebeest, oryx, and impala that you've caught here, some bongo, and a bunch of West African animals like duikers. About 60 head in all."

"Bongo! They're worth a small fortune, aren't they? I'm not sure that I've ever read of anyone immobilizing one before."

"Yeah," he said casually, "about a 100,000 each to us."

Passing that by without worrying about it, at least for now, I added, "Phew, that'll take quite a bit of drug. I'll have to give Monks a call and see what they have in stock. I'll get back to you as soon as I can."

"Don't be too long. The shipment's due out on the 25th of next month, you need 30 days in advance of your second bleeding for the first one, and they want a few days at the other end to check the bloods before they agree to let us load."

We returned to the rhino, and I made a couple of suggestions for extra dietary items, but could not come up with anything concrete in the way of a diagnosis. Picking up some manure from his sleeping area, which was safely cut off for pen cleaning, I shoved it into a plastic bag, and hopped into my station wagon for the trip down the hill and back to town where I could check it for parasites.

As we prepared our gear, going carefully over a checklist, and making sure that we had more than enough of anything we might need, Njeru brought me up short with a question that seemed idiotic, until I remembered his lack of sophistication and level of education, as well as the absence of things such as television that we now take for granted. He had not been to high school, and I doubt that the textbooks at his primary school covered a huge range of subjects, or described them in any detail.

"What do the people breathe when they are on the ocean?" he asked.

Within a week, after a very early morning start, I was driving down to Mombasa, the luggage compartment loaded to the hilt with immobilizing drugs, darting equipment, antibiotics, and a small suitcase of clothes, as well as Mutua's overnight bag. I had phoned the Mombasa Club, who offered reciprocal visiting rights to members of the Nanyuki Sports Club, and I'd spoken at some length to Haji Issak at the quarantine. He told me that he could readily find accommodation for Mutua, and gave me explicit directions on how to find his facilities. It took most of a long day to get there, and as we crossed the causeway into the town, slowing down for the increasing traffic, and opening the windows against the heat that was building up in the car, we were assailed by the particular smell, among all others in Kenya, that identified the town. It was a mixture of the ocean, rotting vegetation and rubbish in the ditches, and a mass of people on the move.

We soon found the quarantine station, which was surrounded by a high stone wall, and knocked on the steel gate that kept the animals in and the curious out. It was opened by a slight, very dark, Swahili man who gestured for us to enter. We looked up, and there, standing in the centre of a group of four more men like the first was a slightly taller, smooth-haired man of Asian background, medium brown in complexion, about five foot seven inches tall, dressed in well-creased, pale khaki long trousers and a white, short-sleeved, open-necked shirt. He stepped forward at once, and greeted us with a proffered hand and a cheerful smile. "Good evening. Dr. Haigh, I presume," he said with a smile.

We went together round the pens, which were on the outside of a central concrete walk area. The animals I knew were easy to identify, each one in a small, shaded, concrete-floored pen, the largest of which was no more than about six feet by ten. Some pens, in which smaller animals were housed, had more than one animal in them. I did not comment, but wondered how we were going to be able to handle a pen with a group of animals in it, if some of them had not been treated, or were recovering after being given antidote.

Then we came to the bongos. What a spectacular sight. I had never before seen one close up, although I knew that they were supposed to be very beautiful. Each had dark, slowly spiraling horns, over a foot long, ending in a white, sharp, ivory-like tip. It was easy to distinguish the males, as their horns and body profiles were much more massive than those of the females, but there the differences ended. Both sexes were a glorious rich light orange-brown, with about half a dozen wide, creamy stripes on each side, running from their widest at the spine to a narrow point down near the belly. There were seven of them. With everything else inside the walls, the whole shipment was going to be worth over a million dollars! What a responsibility, especially as I would be working by the seat of my pants when it came to selecting doses.

There were more surprises in store. In a pen two down from the last bongo was a solidly built grey animal, about a third their size. "This is a Jentink's duiker," said Haji, rubbing his hands together. "They are very rare. I have never had one in here before."

Next to the Jentink's were two more duikers of almost the same massive form. They were mainly black in colour, or at least seemed black in the evening light and heavy shade. As Haji shone a torch on them I could see a broad dirty yellow stripe down the back of each one. "These are yellow-backed duikers. They come from West Africa, like the Jentink's. All three animals are coming in a shipment from Ivory Coast to be quarantined here. It's a long way, no?"

The final surprise were two tiny little duikers, no bigger than a medium-sized poodle, also smartly dressed with contrasting stripes down their sides. In this case the main coat was paler than that of the bongos, and had a reddish-yellow tinge. The stripes were black. As I admired them,

Haji said, "I thought you would enjoy these. They are zebra duikers."

Mutua took it all in, keeping his own counsel. This was his first trip to the coast, and he was no doubt undergoing quite a few cultural enlightenments.

We agreed to start work at first light, and I asked Haji to ensure that we had a couple of cooking pots on hand, as I would have to keep sterilizing my darts as we went along. Then it was off to the Mombasa Club for a cool beer, a swim, and a supper of fresh fish.

I also took the opportunity to try and clear up an old business debt of my father's. He had been posted to Mombasa to defend the port against a potential Japanese invasion after their army had taken Singapore. (Some chance! One bomber did visit when the officers were having a sundowner at the club. It flew in over the harbour and out again, and it was not until they saw the rising sun emblem on the wings that they realized what it was.) The Mombasa Club had needed funds to stay afloat, so my father took out a ten-pound debenture — about five days' pay for him at the time — and promptly forgot about it. Thirty years later, here I was, debenture certificate in hand, trying to see what his investment might be worth. The secretary was a trifle skeptical, but the shares — for that is what they were — were eventually redeemed after a lengthy correspondence. No interest was offered, so the ten pounds became the price of an adequate, but by no means superlative, dinner for two.

■

Luckily I had no trouble sleeping, although at first the humid heat threatened to prevent me getting off. The rhythmic swishing of the overhead fan acted as a soporific.

Before dawn I was up and away, and Mutua and I were soon filling darts and preparing syringes of antibiotic by the light of a couple of naked 60-watt bulbs hanging from the joists above us. I had prepared a record sheet that gave us the species, sex, estimated weight, drug dose, and time, and other similar information. There was also a column for notes and comments. My carbon-dioxide-charged pistol was going to get a work-out.

It seemed prudent to start with what I knew, so we got stuck in with the impalas, as they would be easy for Haji's staff to handle, and we would be able to sort out the issue of who did what before getting into unknown territory. I had done enough injections by now to be confident that I had made up the correct mixture of the morphine-like fentanyl and the additional sedative. Later I learned that fentanyl became *the* drug of choice for humans undergoing heart surgery. One of its main values is its wide margin of safety. The difference between a lethal dose and an effective dose is enormous, hundreds of times higher. I had been lucky in choosing it as a main ingredient in my immobilizing mixtures.

Mutua's extra duty was to clean the gunpowder from the inside of each dart as it was removed from the animal, take it apart, and put it into one of the two pots of boiling water. When half a dozen or so darts were in this state, he started up a new pot, so that we always had something ready to use. He also had to prepare all antibiotic injections — every animal would get one — and pass each tube of blood that I collected along to Haji. Haji, in turn, wrote the animal's tag number and species on each tube. By afternoon tea-time we had gone through everything except the West African visitors.

Haji called a halt. "Doctor," he said, "do you not think we should stop now? Everyone is tired, we have worked hard for many hours, and there are still a number of animals to be processing. Let us rest until tomorrow, and we can get going again at first light. At any rate, it will be cooler then." It took no effort for me to agree. I gave Mutua 20 shillings, telling him not to spend it all on riotous living. Smiling at the wide, pearly-white grin that he returned at once, with a chuckle, I headed once more for the club.

The next morning I had to tackle the most valuable, and worrying, animals at the quarantine. I felt more confident, now that my drug cock-tail had dealt smoothly and quickly with a variety of species.

I tried to decide which species, among the hoofed animals I'd worked with, most closely resembled a bongo. The answer seemed to be the eland. A cow eland is about the same size as a bull bongo. Both have spiral horns, and look somewhat similar, excepting, of course, the coat. At that time, the two species were placed in quite different genera in the taxonomic tree. The eland was *Taurotragus oryx*, the bongo, *Boocerus eurycus*. It was only much later that scientists determined that they were quite closely related. Close enough, in fact, for embryos of bongo to be successfully carried to term by eland. I mixed up a dose that would work on a cow eland, and was greatly relieved to see it work slickly on all seven bongo.

Basing the doses for the rare and beautiful West African duikers on the same mix, but in smaller quantities, we got through them without trouble as well, although we must have underestimated the weight of the Jentink's duiker. He took almost 15 minutes to go down, and we had to hold him while I struggled to collect his blood.

We were done in time for a late lunch. Not quite by the mid-day in which mad dogs and Englishmen go out in the sun, but enough to ensure that we could follow the normal tropical mode, and have a siesta. There was no point in rushing home, as we would not be able to make it in a day, so I headed for the club and a snooze.

I was just about to go out for an early curry when one of the club doormen came past bearing a board, and calling out my name. Haji, not being a member, and therefore not free to enter under any circumstances, was waiting in the car park, wringing his hands, and almost hopping up and down on one leg. "Oh Doctor, I am glad that I found you. We are having a problem with one of the bongos. He has yellow material com-ing out of his mouth, and is having trouble breathing. Please can you come quickly."

All my drugs were in the car, so I followed Haji back to the quarantine. One look at the bongo was enough to scare me. Since Haji had seen him, the "stuff" had trebled in amount. Moreover, it was not coming out of his mouth, but rather out of his nostrils. It was indeed yellow, and it was also frothy, hanging down from his face in a pear-shaped blob almost a foot long. I had never seen anything like it, and for a moment I could not even guess what was going on. Then my basic education kicked in. It could only be a frothy edema of his lungs, although what specifically was causing it I had no idea. No wonder he was having trouble breathing. If I didn't do something quickly the trouble would get worse, a lot worse, until he stopped breathing all together.

I realized that I needed two things, only one of which was in my drug kit. "Haji, it's not quite six o'clock. Can you get me to a big chemist's shop before they close?"

Without any hesitation he turned towards the gate, and we more or less dove into his Peugeot. Fifteen minutes later I had six human-sized doses of a rapid-acting cortisone in my hand, and we were heading back to the animal. I did not care whether or not the pharmacist believed my explanation. The main thing was that he had filled my prescription.

"Haji, we've got a problem. I can't go in to give these injections by hand, it's too risky, and the other animal there might attack me. I'm going to have to give it to him in three darts. Two with this cortisone that we bought at the chemist, and another one with this stuff, called Lasix, which should make him pee out the excess fluid in his lungs."

Despite the pain of the injections, which work when a minute powder charge empties the syringe in a fraction of a second, the bongo hardly moved. He was concentrating too hard on breathing to get upset at what must have seemed to be mere pin-pricks.

We waited anxiously for something to happen. I suggested to Haji that we find a hose and spray down the animals in the pen, to help cool them, and this took some time to organize. Just holding the nozzle and directing the jet seemed to provide some occupational therapy, at least for the humans. Within half an hour things had improved dramatically, and in another 15 minutes the bongo, and Haji, seemed to be well on the road to recovery.

I changed my supper plans, and told Haji that I would stay at the club all evening, so that he could call me if the need arose. Otherwise I would see him early in the morning, when I came by to pick up Mutua.

Later, browsing through the 1973 edition of the *Guinness Book of Records*, which turned up under the Christmas tree as an unexpected gift from Muffin, our miniature dachshund, who had cleverly managed to copy Jo's handwriting on the label, I came across the statement that the Jentink's duiker is probably the rarest antelope on earth, restricted to tropical West Africa.

There did not seem to be any previous account of immobilization of bongo, or of any of the West African duikers. Ignorance was indeed bliss.

CHAPTER 27

THE HORSE WHISPERER

*After a Christmas Eve treasure hunt, our night and Christmas
morning are unnecessarily disturbed. A few days later I witness
a horse whisperer in action. Her highly eccentric sister, visiting
from Ireland, tries to get me arrested.*

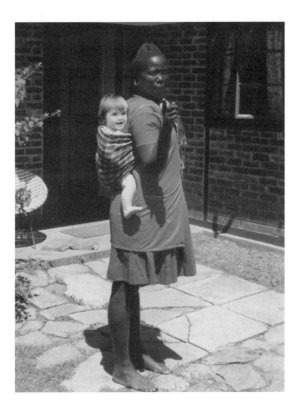

Traditional back carry. Ester and Karen return
from an afternoon walk.

BUNDY'S CHUTNEY

(This chutney was named for a Mr. Bundy who built the stone cottage at Wellow, Isle of Wight, England, in which Mrs. Mabel Haigh lived for many years after leaving Lee Farm (she was my grandmother, who trained as a *Cordon Bleu* cook before she married.)

INGREDIENTS
7 or 8 apples (3 lb.) or
2 lbs green tomatoes + 1 lb apples
    (also works with other fruits, e.g. bananas)
2 medium onions (¾ lb or 2 cups after
    chopping)
1 tsp chopped garlic
1 tsp ground ginger
¾ lb (1 cup) gooseberry, apricot or similar jam
½ lb (1.5 cups) sultanas
1 tsp mustard seed
¼ lb (1 cup) raisins (optional)
1 lb (2 cups) brown sugar
12 green chillies. (Use Thai dragon for hot,
    Serrano for milder)
1 pinch ground nutmeg
½ tsp curry powder (or to taste)
cayenne pepper to taste
1.5 pts (675 ml) white or apple cider vinegar

INSTRUCTIONS
• Mix all the ingredients except apples
(& tomatoes if used) and let them stand in vinegar overnight.
• Next day, chop the apples/tomatoes into ½"
pieces & boil in enough water to cover them, until soft.
• Crush the boiled fruit with a wooden spoon & drain the excess water.
• Mix in the reserved vinegar and all other ingredients.
• Boil for 20-30 minutes.
• Seal in sterile airtight jars.

Makes enough for about 4–5 pints. There's not much point in making less, as it will quickly disappear, and it will also make a welcome gift.

*Note, no two people make this recipe the same way, and even batches tend to differ, as the recipe is very flexible, and allows for different ingredients, depending upon what is available, e.g. zucchini can be used.

This recipe makes an ideal dish to accompany fish, cheese, salad and meat dishes of many types, including curries. It was a favourite in Karen's cooking co-op days at university.

JO AND I HAD BEEN TO A typical Sports Club social event on Christmas Eve. This one was a treasure hunt, and we had been challenged to find 20 items from a list of things that included men's coloured underwear, a bucket with a hole in it, and an unused roll of black-and-white film. The first person to arrive back at the club received a Christmas hamper that contained two bottles of champagne. For almost two hours we had driven around the town collecting bits and pieces, only to discover, when we pulled into the parking lot and grabbed our load to take into the club house, that we had been pipped at the post. It hardly mattered, and the rest of the evening was taken up with a marvelous spread of traditional Christmas goodies, such as mince pies, meringues, a rum-based punch that we both stayed away from, and various delicious but fattening chocolate concoctions. My favourite, sherry trifle, had also been on the table, and I had done my fair share of damage to that.

Shortly after midnight we made our way home down Lunatic Lane and fell into bed, exhausted and happy. Less than an hour later we were surfacing as the telephone rang and rang in the hall outside our little bedroom. At least we were no longer on a party line, as our line had been one of the very first to be converted when the system was upgraded. We were never sure, but we suspected that the other six people on the line had had enough of midnight calls, constant traffic all day long, and never being able to make a call out because one of us was always talking to someone.

This call came from a game lodge and was for Jo. The hoteliers there, whom I'll call Bill and Janet McDonald, had recently had their first baby, and she was not well. They were very worried about her; would Jo please come as soon as possible?

An hour and a half later a very disgruntled Jo arrived back and crept into the sheets next to me. "Bloody people," she said, with unusually vehement language. "The kid had been coughing for four days, but they decided to call me now, because they couldn't sleep themselves."

We wrote that one off to experience, and soon dropped off to sleep ourselves, knowing that Jo, who was two months pregnant and suffering from morning sickness, was going to need all the rest that she could get. Christmas morning at about eight o'clock, when we should have been having a lie-in, with no Abuyeka to bring us tea, the phone pealed again. It was Bill McDonald calling for me to go and see a dog who seemed to be suddenly very lame. After a quick snack, and wondering what I might be dealing with, I headed for the same hotel. The big black Labrador was lying outside, basking in the early morning sun, when I arrived. I could hardly believe my ears when, before I saw either of the McDonalds, the desk clerk told me that the dog had been lame for two weeks. Even the description of "very lame" was somewhat over the top. He was limping, and I tried to figure out what might be the cause, but very lame he was not.

I sent an invoice that had, clearly marked, "Out of hours emergency call" as an extra line item over and above the normal mileage and examination fee.

A week later, as we had long since booked our New Year's dinner at this same spot, we decided to take a lunch time spin up over the slopes above Timau, to see if we could see the mountain and to try and get a photo of the long-tailed Paradise Whydah birds — especially the spectacular males, which, with their two-foot-long black tails and bright yellow breasts, bounced up and down in the grass meadows beside the road.

We chatted about the future as we climbed up the slopes to the 8,000-foot-high crest of the road. With a new babe on the way, and Karen approaching the age when she would need more than play school, we began to wonder about leaving Kenya, much as it hurt to think about it. One thing that coloured our thinking was the Africanization program in which large-scale farms were being taken over and turned into small units of a few acres. It had already happened to several of my regular clients in the Mweiga, Naro Moru, and Nyeri areas, and there were rumours of more to come. These large farms provided my bread-and-butter, as I usually made once-a-month calls to them to carry out herd health visits. As they were bought out and divided, so my income dried up, because few, if any, of the new owners had any cattle at all, and those that did could not afford to pay me to come out to see an individual animal 30 or 40 miles from home.

We mulled over several possibilities, Australia and New Zealand being near the top of the list. It was not until Paul Sayer mentioned an advertisement in the British journal, *The Veterinary Record*, that Canada came into the picture. I wrote away, using a couple of local colleagues as references, as well as my former Dean, Sir William Weipers. In due course we received an acknowledgement, but thought no more about it for a few months.

All would have been well, and we would have made our dinner appointment, if my car had not been so easily recognized. As we sat by the roadside, a passing Peugeot van suddenly swerved, pulled to the side, and came to an abrupt halt. A man I did not recognize walked back from the van, waving at us. I wound down my window and he said, in Swahili, "*Jambo* Doctor. I was just going to come to Nanyuki to search for you. My cow is having trouble with the birth of her calf. Can you come and help?" Despite the complete lack of any equipment, I could hardly turn him down. If we were lucky, and the calf was not too difficult to remove, we could still make our dinner.

It was not to be. Three hours later, exhausted, hungry, and filthy, I drove Jo back to our home and collapsed into a bath. Jo dug out some leftover turkey from the fridge, and we had cheese and turkey sandwiches, with Bundy's chutney on the side. (This chutney, named for the cottage where my *Cordon Bleu*-trained grandmother lived for many years, was, and remains, a favourite accompaniment for many dishes.)

Ten days later we received two checks in the mail. One, for me, had an invoice clipped to it. The bill for the lame dog had been paid, but not in full. An itemized deduction, for exactly the same sum as my out-of-hours emergency call on Christmas Day, read: "For New Year's dinner, booked but not eaten."

Just after New Year an unexpected client walked shyly through the office door. I could never tell when she might appear, like a dumpy wraith, and ask for help. Mrs. Kenealy was tiny in stature, no more than five feet tall, but impossible to miss because she looked like a miniature Michelin man, and was always dressed in long, much-washed cavalry twill trousers and a once-white shirt, topped off, when she came into town, with a broad-brimmed khaki hat held onto her head by a wide cream-coloured ribbon tied under her chin.

After a quiet greeting, she asked when I might be able to come by and castrate three ponies that she had managed to sell to folks in Nyeri. Knowing that she must have hitched a ride to get into town from Naro Moru — 15 miles away — I told a little white lie and said I was planning to go that way later that morning, and would give her a ride back.

As Mutua loaded the station wagon for our pretend trip to go past Mrs. Kenealy's home, I checked that my fishing rod was in its rack on the ceiling of the car, my net in the luggage compartment, and my box of wet flies and nymphs in the glove compartment. I had long wanted to dip a line in the upper reaches of the Naro Moru river, above the forest edge, and Mrs. Kenealy happened to live nearby. As I swung the car round in front of her home to drop her off, I saw a couple of bearded visitors, their backpacks seemingly welded to their spines, emerging from the shady verandah that ran the full length of the old wooden house. It was a familiar sight. The old lady lived a tenuous hand-to-mouth existence, selling a few ponies each year for major cash injections (at least, major for her: 500 shillings each), and earning some petty cash by charging only five shillings for a night's room and board to young tourists who somehow learned of her existence. As she lived about three miles off the main road, and did no advertising, nor even hung out a welcoming board at her gate, the visitors must have heard of her through word of mouth. She always provided a large cooked breakfast, complete with eggs, bacon, bread, and marmalade, and how she made any profit from her guests — many of them Peace Corps, British vsos, and the like, all as poor as she was — I could never figure out.

As she got out of the car she said, "My sister is visiting from Ireland for a few weeks. I expect that you'll meet her when you come on

Thursday." I had heard rumours that she had a sister who had been committed and spent most of her time in a mental institution back where they had come from as young girls. "Barmy, she is," one Nanyuki resident had said. "Barmy, but harmless."

Two days later Mutua and I were back at Naro Moru, this time equipped to carry out the operations that we had been asked to do. Mrs. Kenealy greeted us as she emerged, hatless, from her house, halter in hand.

"Just a moment," she said, "I'll go and get one for you while you get your stuff ready."

With that she walked over to a small corral next to the house. We could see about 15 animals, of various shades and colour combinations, standing around in a paddock further back. Mrs. Kenealy returned with a smart-looking piebald, leading him by his mane, and talking quietly to him. As I drew up a syringe full of anesthetic she said, "He's never had a rope on him, but I think we'll be all right." With that she looped the halter over his neck and continued to blow down her nose at him and make comforting noises that I could hardly hear. He did not budge as I stuck the needle into his jugular vein. I connected the syringe and injected him with the yellow solution, a British product aptly named Immobilon that I had used in large elephants, as well as horses. Within about 30 seconds he pulled back and then subsided to the ground, out for the count.

I had never watched a horse whisperer in action before, and at first I didn't really appreciate what I was seeing. Only later, as we did another pony, did I realize what I had witnessed. Mrs. Kenealy had taken a young, unbroken, completely inexperienced horse from a mob of 15 or 20 animals, put him in a corral, and then caught him up again, brought him out on to her front lawn, where there was no fence at all, and made him stand, as a complete stranger came up and stuck a needle into his neck.

As I concentrated on tying up his legs, and preparing the site for my scalpel, I heard a voice say, "And what are you doing?"

I looked up, and there was another old lady, older even than Mrs.

Kenealy, but more or less the same shape, white haired, and dressed in a voluminous cotton skirt, and bright pink blouse.

Knowing to tread carefully, and quite unsure of myself, I said, "I'm doing what your sister asked me to do. I'm castrating him so that she can sell him for some children to ride. Training him will be easier then."

"You're hurting him," she responded, shaking a finger at me, and at the same time seeming to deliberately show off her knee-length, elastic-crimped bloomers, which matched her blouse, as she sat down next to his head and began to cradle him.

"No, no, he's under an anesthetic. Excuse me, I must get on with this." So saying, I dismissed her from my mind and finished what I had started.

I gave the Immobilon antidote, Revivon, also appropriately named, and watched him rise unsteadily to his feet. Mrs. Kenealy brought another candidate, and we went through the same scenario again, this time uninterrupted. Finally, she brought forward the last pony, a smart bay of somewhat stockier frame than the first two, again with only a rope around his neck. He too subsided without trouble, and I began to get things organized. As Mutua and I tied up his legs, a Land Rover drove into the yard and a smartly uniformed police inspector stepped out from the driver's side as the frazzled frame of Mrs. Kenealy's sister emerged from the passenger door.

She had walked all the way to the police post in Naro Moru village and laid a complaint of cruelty to animals, and the officer, no doubt acting in good faith, had brought her straight back to the farm. We soon cleared the matter up, but I never did hear how the two sisters resolved their differences over the affair.

CHAPTER 28

ELEPHANTS FOR NIGERIA

As Mutua and I prepare to head out for another trip to Maralal,
we receive a cable that vividly illustrates one of the hazards of
ranching in Kenya. We work on elephant capture, which has a
different set of dangers from rhino work. A young elephant is
rescued from a deep pit and becomes a challenging patient.

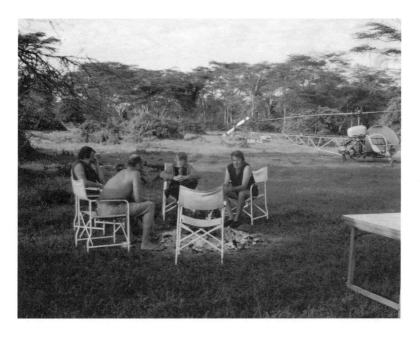

Tea-time at the Muramur dam.

I WAS UP AT THE ANIMAL ORPHANAGE, after trying yet again to catch some impala for Don, when Don himself put in an appearance, walking through the gap in the hedge with his partner William Holden.

"Hi Jerry," he said with his usual enthusiasm. "Glad we caught you. We've just been asked by President Kenyatta to catch some juvenile elephants for shipment to Nigeria. He has some sort of deal to help them restock a national park, and he wants them fairly soon. Will you be free the week after next?"

This would be my first venture into elephant capture, so I had a steep learning curve to climb. I had been able to get hold of a couple of articles from South Africa, where young elephants had been captured in the Kruger National Park, and so I had some background. I wrote to the director of the park, Dr. U. de V. Pienaar, who had been the author of one of the reports, and received a kindly and helpful reply. The elephant capture in the Kruger had been carried out in response to a concern about the young animals when the total numbers in the park had threatened to exceed the carrying capacity of the land. In the opinion of the park managers, disaster would follow if the population continued to increase unbridled. To prevent this they implemented a controversial program, under which elephants aged about nine years of age and up were killed. Those aged about two to eight were captured, held in *bomas* at park headquarters, and then moved to other parks in the country where all traces of elephant had long since disappeared under the twin challenges of excessive hunting in the 18th and 19th centuries and human population expansion since that time. The capture data collected by the scientists would prove vitally useful.

I paid another visit to Buster Cook and asked him to make up a set of needles, shorter than the rhino ones, but just as stout and barbed.

I planned to leave Nanyuki after lunch and stop overnight at Jasper Evans's ranch on the way to the Muramur camp. I'd met up with Jasper a few days earlier at the local annual tennis tournament, which was more of a fun event than a heavy-duty test of skills. I was competing, and he was in town strictly for the socializing. "I have a stallion that needs castrating," he had said, as we sat enjoying a drink at the Rumuruti Sports Club. "There's really no hurry, but if you can let me know a few days in advance, the next time you're coming up this way, I'll arrange to have him caught and you can do the job for me." So as soon as Don set the dates for the elephant work, I sent Jasper a cable, as this was the only really reliable way to communicate.

As Mutua and I were loading the station wagon with drug boxes, dart gun, camping gear, clothes, and other bits and pieces that we would need for the horse operation, a small man, dressed in the pale khaki uniform worn by most junior government employees, appeared at the clinic. He handed a cable to Njeru, who passed it on to me. I opened it up to read

a terse but precise message, which illustrated both a still-common problem of ranching in Kenya, and Jasper's famous dry wit:

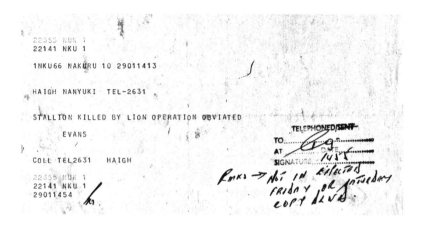

Naturally we delayed our departure, heading out early the next morning.
The camp site at Muramur was as beautiful as ever, and as we sat around
the table enjoying the evening sun as it set through the grove of yellow
fever trees, Don went over our instructions.

"If you see any rhino, we can catch them, but the main job will be
to catch ten juvenile elephants. Try not to get anything that is more than
52 inches at the shoulder, because we won't be able to get them into the
crates."

In the morning Punch and I took off and began to scour the wood-
lands to the west and north of the camp, searching for a herd of elephant,
or even a rhino. We headed south-west, over more open country, and soon
had a small herd of cows and calves in sight. Punch manoeuvered the chopper into position as the elephants took off at a run, and in less time than it
takes to tell I had a dart placed squarely in the backside of a young elephant.
Now came the tricky part, which was to separate mother and calf. Don had
given me a hand-held flash gun. I loaded a cartridge, which looked more
or less like a shot-gun shell, into the front of the thing, took aim and fired.
There was no recoil, but after a faint *shwoosh!* and with a small puff of

smoke, something headed off towards the low thorn scrub below. About 30 yards in front of us there was a sudden flash of bright light, just in front of the cow, who had turned to confront us as her calf began to slow down. She turned back at once, and took off to join the herd.

Punch came on the air again. "I'm going to put you down near the youngster, but I won't cut the revs. You keep an eye on junior, and I'll head straight off again to make sure that mama doesn't circle back."

So saying he circled quickly, descending towards a small clearing, and dropped me off with my drug box. By now the young elephant was walking very slowly, his trunk hanging loosely down. He came to a stop as I set up my new Super-8 camera, and obligingly leaned backwards and fell slowly on to his left-hand side.

I began to make the basic checks. He was breathing steadily, and his temperature seemed about normal, or at least normal for a horse, which seemed like a reasonable comparison. As I took out the dart I could hear the chopper returning, so my anxious over-the-shoulder looks for an enraged mother could stop. I moved over to the camera again and practised my amateur film skills by getting some material of the machine landing, and of Punch emerging and walking over towards the patient. Only when I reviewed the footage later did I realize that he walked with his right arm firmly tucked behind his back. He really was sensitive about that missing hand.

Don and the ground crew turned up within half an hour, and we soon had five gallon billy cans of water cascading over the elephant's head, ears, and back, in order to cool him down. After Mutua and I had injected him with antibiotics and a multivitamin shot, I gave him a partial dose of antagonist, which allowed him to stand rather wobbly. In this partially recovered state we were able to push and pull him into the crate, despite his bulk and 700-pound weight.

Punch and I were soon back in camp with Iris, drinking refreshing glasses of freshly-squeezed lemon and orange juice. Half an hour later, the trucks appeared through the trees, their engines grinding as they made the turn off the main road. We walked over, and saw that Don had a surprise for us. Held in the back of one of the two Land Cruisers by Ngatia and Nderitu, two of the orphanage crew, was another calf. It was much thinner than the butterball that we had captured earlier.

"The fellas found this little guy in the bottom of a huge pit," said Don. "We had the devil of a time getting him out. There were all sorts of marks where adults had scraped the sides with their tusks, but he was too far down for them. I've no idea how long he's been abandoned. We had to use all of our ropes to get to him. Nderitu went down to tie him on, and built a sort of harness."

The crew helped the unresisting little elephant down from the bed of the truck, then deferred to me; they weren't aware that this was only my second close-up look at an elephant. His temperature seemed low, but his breathing and pulse were OK, at least as far as I could tell. He seemed all shriveled up, and the skin on his head stood up like a tent when I took a small pinch between my finger and thumb, which indicated, not surprisingly, that he was badly dehydrated.

I looked round for Mutua, having some difficulty spotting him among the 30 or so people, as everyone in camp, including the kitchen staff, had heard the news and had come to see the new arrival.

"Please bring me some saline. There's about five litres in the wooden drug box. Don, can you get someone to cut me a forked stick, about six foot in length? I need something to hang the fluids bags on."

Very quickly we had everything ready to go. Now came the easy part, or at least it seemed easy. Looking behind the flapping ear I could see a maze of blood vessels, so it was surely just a question of choosing a large one, holding it off for a moment to check that it would swell, as a vein should when the flow is stopped, and inserting the intravenous needle. He was so dehydrated that I could run the first couple of litres of fluid into him almost as quickly as it would go.

I held off a vessel; it did not swell, but it was thin-walled and had no pulse, so I assumed it to be a vein. I slid the needle in, then turned back to my drug box to get some antibiotic, which this little fellow would surely need after his ordeal. The soluble penicillin would go directly into the intravenous line, where it could take immediate effect. At least, it should have been an intravenous line, but when I turned back to the patient, penicillin in hand, I got quite a shock. Instead of the bag collapsing as it emptied, it was rapidly filling, and the bottom half was bright red. I had inserted my needle into an artery, and his blood pressure was driving a red column up the plastic tube into the bag of saline. This was my first lesson in the distinctive anatomy of the elephant. His main method of cooling himself is to flap his ears, which act like a huge radiator. The arteries and veins that make for efficient cooling run all over the place, like a network of English country roads, lanes, and footpaths on a large-scale map. When the ears are flapped, cooling breezes remove the body heat from the blood. If the ear remains still, cooling is much less efficient, or non-existent.

Half an hour later, with three bottles of drip in his system, as well as an injection of cortisone to help him overcome the shock and bring up his blood sugar level, the elephant had perked up. While I had been working, Iris had started to "mother" him. She had fixed up a bottle of milk formula, and armed with a damp cloth, she was rubbing his lips and chin, trying to get him interested in something to drink. As I put away my bits and pieces I heard a sudden shout of pain from Iris. She was standing holding her right hand under her armpit and almost weeping.

"What happened?" asked Don and I, more or less in chorus.

"Ouch!" she responded, gingerly letting us look at her hand. "I was rubbing his gums, trying to stimulate him, when he suddenly began to move his mouth, and of course, wouldn't you know it, he chomped straight down on my finger."

He was very young, about three foot at the shoulder, and in his emaciated state no more than about 400 pounds in weight, but his teeth were huge. The last inch or so of Iris's index finger was a pulpy mass, bleeding like a stuck pig. Having banged myself on the thumb with a hammer more than once, I could only guess at how painful this much more serious injury must be.

"What should we do with it?" asked Don.

I went into my best doctor impression, using basic medical common sense and one of Jo's favourite remedies for anything from a sore throat to an infected nail bed. "Well, the first thing is to clean it up. Let's get you over to the mess tent and find a seat. Then we'll get some warm water and salt, and give it a good soak." I had often heard Jo say to patients with sore throats, over the phone, "Get her [or him] to do warm water and salt gargles several times a day."

As Don walked beside Iris I went over to my tent and tried to find something that would suit the job of clean-up. I had no idea what sorts of bugs might hang out in an elephant's mouth, but we certainly didn't want anything nasty to have a chance at infecting Iris. I grabbed the Betadine, and unable to find anything in the way of a good swab, I took my toothbrush out of my sponge bag, looked at it for a moment, and decided that it would have to do.

After the toothbrush had been steeped in boiling water, and then in a strong solution of the Betadine, I used it to try and clean up the debris at the end of Iris's finger. She bore it all stoically, and seemed much relieved when I gently lowered it into the bowl of salty water that was, by now, standing next to her on the table.

"Keep your finger in this for about 20 minutes, then we'll put some antibiotic cream on it, and make a dressing. I expect you've got some sort of painkiller in your first-aid kit. I'm afraid I don't have any other antibiotics for humans, only for animals, but I would think that you ought to get on to a course of something. Perhaps there's a medical clinic in Maralal to which you could go. And before I forget, what's your tetanus vaccination status? You'll need to get a booster if you're not up to date."

Next morning, instead of heading out to look for elephants, Don and Iris drove the 11 miles into Maralal for more expert medical attention. They returned at lunch time, with a smart new dressing on Iris's hand, her arm in a sling, and a brand new toothbrush, in its plastic wrap, for me.

While they were away I took on the duties of trying to get the newcomers to take to the bottle. The first one captured had already been fed the previous evening and had taken to it like a duck to water, polishing off an old wine bottle full of milk replacer in short order. The abandoned calf was much more of a challenge. He was rather too small to be sure of himself, and had not yet really found out what his trunk was for. At three feet tall he was probably not yet a year old, and would have been able to walk under his mother's belly. He was alert enough, as the injections seemed to have perked him up, but he did not seem to be able to grasp the principle of the artificial nipple that he was being offered. His trunk kept getting in the way, and nothing seemed to be getting into him. After about 45 minutes of futile effort I took a different tack. Nderitu and Mutua had been standing by, watching the proceedings with some amusement, so I asked for one of the metal bowls, shaped like a giant wok and known as a *karai*, and dumped the milk into it. The little elephant had already become used to human contact, and nudged me as he searched for comfort and possibly also for milk, although what I had to offer must have smelt very different from what he remembered. I waited until the right moment and then poured some of the milk directly from the bowl into his open mouth. He did not take more than a brief moment to assess the situation, swallowed quickly, and came back for more. By the time I had finished the process he had taken about 75% of the milk into his system. The other 25% was slopped down the front of my shorts, on the inside of my rubber boots, and over the water-proof coat that I had had the foresight to don before going in with him. However, we had found a method of meeting his needs, and he thrived for several months before coming to a sad end, dying of acute Salmonellosis back in Nanyuki.

Within five days we had a full complement of young elephants in camp. On the last evening, as we sat around enjoying a beer, Bill Woodley, the Aberdares National Park warden who had been flying reconnaissance for us in his small plane, said, "You don't know how close you were to buying it there back by the river this morning. As I watched you trying to manoeuver a group, an adult female stood on her hind legs and reached up towards the chopper. She missed the skids by no more than a couple of feet."

I shuddered at the near miss, imagining what a ghastly mess would have occurred if she had reached us. Dead humans, chopped elephant, and no doubt a ball of flame. It was not the only near miss we had had that week. Punch had said little about it, but I had felt a sharp bump as we had come in to land at lunch time on the second day. From about five feet above ground we had dropped like a stone, a marked change from the usual controlled descent. Punch had gone round the machine, as soon as he had turned off the engine, and inspected things. On the right-hand side, just behind where I normally sat on the floor, he leaned in further than usual and grunted. The throttle linkage had come loose, just above the carburetor. He had had no control over his engine speed, but luckily for us both he had not been up at 50 or more feet, trying to close in on a herd of frightened elephants.

Since my Kenya days, Clem Coetzee of Zimbabwe has pioneered the whole-family capture and translocation of elephants, as it is now understood that the capture and resettlement of young elephants is neither scientifically sound nor welfare friendly. There are many illustrations of this, including the story of the juvenile elephants — the four-to-eight-year-olds — which were removed from the Kruger Park. Some were moved to Pilansberg National Park, 250 miles west of the Kruger. Pilansberg, which is completely fenced, grew out of dry and almost useless ranch and farm land, and had no game in it when it was made into a park. As the young males went through puberty, they became virtual juvenile delinquents. Unfettered by parental discipline, or by any dominance from mature bulls, they began to run riot when their hormones started to kick into high gear. By the time they reached 18 or 20 years of age, they were larger than any females, and so were no longer under any sort of control. This led to the destruction of tourist vehicles, and at least one death: the killing of the father of an unfortunate family of tourists who were law-abidingly inside their car.

These delinquent elephants also took to attacking white rhinos, and in 1994 and 1996 there were 30 rhino deaths due to confirmed elephant attacks, with another 13 suspected. It's believed that the elephants, without big males to keep them in line, sought out the only large grey animals that they knew. When they first arrived at the park they were often seen grazing with the rhinos, appearing to "adopt" them as parental figures. Having been wrenched from their strong family groups, and orphaned, they seemed to be seeking companionship. When they went through puberty, a troublesome time for elephants as well as humans, they took up with — and, in at least one witnessed case, tried to mate with — the reluctant descendants of their "foster parents."

At a meeting held in Pilansberg in March 1998, a group of park staff, vets, and the elephant biologist Joyce Poole held a full day's workshop on this problem. On Joyce's advice, six adult bulls, aged between 35 and 45 years of age, were brought into the park to provide a more naturally balanced herd. Within a short space of time, these "super bulls" had "tuned in" the juvenile delinquents.

Even this elegant solution was not without its cost. The big males began to pay far too much attention to the mature trees in the park, and killed a good many of them.

CHAPTER 29

A PRESIDENT'S
DIFFICULT DECISION

*Mutua and I travel to Rwanda — his first trip outside Kenya —
and are engaged in an emotionally draining elephant capture and cull
in a country where elephants have been crowded into such limited
space that they have taken to destroying farms and houses.*

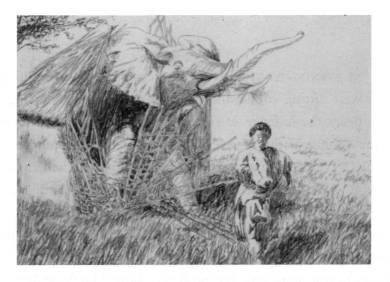

Artist's impression of real events. Terror for a Rwandan householder.

Artist Helmar Heimann

ONE EVENING AT THE Isiolo rhino camp, Tony Parkinson and I were sitting round the campfire contentedly nursing our beers, the cadence of conversation between the cooks mixing with the cooing of the doves as a vague background murmur. We reviewed the day's proceedings and then he abruptly switched channels.

"Can you work out a fee for an elephant project lasting a few weeks?"

"When did you have in mind?" I asked, wondering when I might hear about my job application in Canada.

"Well, we're not quite sure, but probably about March or April. If it comes off it will involve traveling to Rwanda. We may be working on elephants with Ian Parker on a joint cull and capture operation. We'd like you to supervise the capture side of things. Could you come up with some sort of daily fee, so that we can work out a budget?"

"Let me get back to you," I replied.

The first thing I did was to discuss the thing with Jo, who asked where Rwanda was. I got down the old atlas from the bookshelf and opened the blade of my Swiss Army knife to act as a pointer. "Here, it's over to the west of Lake Victoria, there's the Uganda border, and here's the Congo. That American woman, Dian Fossey, is working on gorillas here in the Virunga mountains."

"And what do you mean, cull and capture?" she asked.

"I'm not sure of the details, but basically it means that adults will be shot, and some of the young will be captured and translocated. I'll find out more when Tony gets back to me."

Within a couple of weeks Tony called with a firmer outline.

"The government has decided to cull all the elephants in the country, and they want help with the capture of some juveniles. We're probably going to start in late March or early April. I'd guess that the whole thing will take about six weeks, but we'll have to be flexible."

"Sounds fascinating," I said. "I think I should try to get down to Nairobi as soon as possible and meet you and Ian for more clarification."

Within a few days we were sitting in Ian's home in the Nairobi suburb of Langata, and I was learning something of the politics of elephant conservation. He was slim and very determined, no more than about five foot nine, but giving an impression of whipcord toughness.

"Elephants have become a serious problem animal in Rwanda," Ian told us. "The rapidly increasing human population has forced the animals into ever smaller and smaller areas, and they cannot get enough food without raiding *shambas*. Naturally the farmers object to the destruction of their crops, but this is nothing new. They have been struggling with it for years."

"Why was nothing done before?" I asked.

"Oh, it was," he replied. "The authorities tried to achieve a measure of control through individual culling, shooting individual problem elephants, just like we used to do in the Game Department here with so-called 'crop raiders.' But the situation has gone beyond their capabilities. The African

Wildlife Foundation, headed by the former U.S. ambassador to Kenya, Mr. Robinson McIlvaine, approached President Habyarimana of Rwanda for funding. The AWF wanted the money for Diane Fossey's gorilla conservation efforts, but the president said that the elephant problem was much more important to him, as people were being killed and crops destroyed. He could hardly support gorilla studies in the face of such a situation. McIlvaine suggested that the army be sent to shoot the elephants, but Habyarimana replied that that would be a disaster. They wouldn't be able to shoot straight, and there would be lots of wounded rogue elephants running about. So he ordered the Director of Wildlife of the Office of Tourism and National Parks [Office Rwandaise du Tourism et Parcs National, or ORTPN] to get things organized."

"How did you and John and Tony get involved then?"

"Well, my partner Tony Archer and I had done a fair bit of elephant culling in various places, and so they came to us. McIlvane also went to John Seago and then called a meeting at Seago's to which we were invited. He wanted to see some juveniles captured, instead of a total kill. Neither we, nor John and Tony P." — he gestured towards John's partner — "really wanted to get involved, so after some considerable pressure we set what we thought was an excessively high price. To our surprise, they accepted, so we were hoisted on our own petard.

"We've contracted to capture only animals between one and four years of age. Of course, we can't tell exact ages, but anything that can still walk under its mother is, for all practical purposes, less than one year old, and a four-year-old animal is about four feet high. The basic work plan is to capture as many young animals as possible and cull the large ones. We'll work out specific details onsite."

He explained the culling method to us: "The elephants will be driven by helicopter, in small groups, towards us as we wait on the ground. Tony Archer and I will do the shooting, you and Tony P. will work out the capture side of things."

"Will you be able to fire quickly enough to deal with a large herd? What sort of gun will you use?" I asked.

"Oh, don't worry, we'll each have an FN .762, with two magazines of 20 rounds each," said Ian.

"Hmm. I thought that only heavy rifles, a 375 magnum or bigger, were any good on elephants."

"That's generally true, but the basic issue is shooting accurately. Providing the bullets are in exactly the right place, even light calibres are effective. In any case, we'll have heavy rifles with us as back-up, and we'll probably use them on bulls because of the masses of spongy bone that they have in the front of their heads."

The notion of elephants being herded with helicopters seemed almost surreal, but Ian's matter-of-fact delivery made it all sound rather simple. We discussed the practical aspects of catching juvenile elephants, and the likely limitations of size.

"You and Tony, here, will carry dart guns and be responsible for selection of the young animals. I reckon we won't be able to handle anything bigger than about four feet at the shoulder," said Ian. "Also, very small calves will be impossible to keep. Anything under a year of age will be too small."

"Up at Maralal, working with Don Hunt, I've dealt with young elephants up to about 52 inches, and our main limitation was crate size and aircraft dimensions," I replied. "We might be able to go a little larger than four feet."

"Hmm . . . interesting!" was Ian's response. "Let's wait and see."

After more general discussion, the question of photography came up.

"Will I be able to bring my Super-8 camera?" I asked.

"Apart from the half dozen or so people with whom I've worked as shooters, and a couple of helicopter or fixed-wing pilots, there are less than five people" — Ian held up his right hand, fingers extended, for emphasis — "who have witnessed the actual killing, as we've never permitted filming. I'll bring along a young fellow to record it all, and we can use still cameras, but even then, no photos of the actual shooting. Anyway, you'll be far too busy to be able to take pictures."

The project sounded pretty complex, and I needed to work out many details and discuss the whole situation with Jo. Her main concern seemed to be with the time that I would be away, although I knew that she was not voicing her worries about my safety.

Another challenge would be obtaining a passport and entry permits for Mutua, who had never before been out of Kenya. He had become an integral part of the capture team, well able to supervise an immobilized animal while I looked after another, and I wanted to be sure he was part of the team.

Then there was the question of what clothes to pack. We would be in the bush for most of the time, and there would be no need for anything fancy. Or warm for that matter. I packed long trousers, and a long-sleeved shirt to keep the mosquitoes at bay in the evenings. Otherwise shorts, T-shirts, and a bush hat would just about cover my needs.

The work equipment was more of a problem. We might be completely out of touch with Nairobi. From previous experience I knew that I should over-budget drug supplies by about threefold. Missed darts, unexpected events, and Murphy's law would combine to make things thoroughly difficult if I did not. I had to have enough drugs to deal with possibly as many as 30 elephants, two dart guns (one as a spare), plenty of charges, and a large number of darts. Buster Cook had made sure that I had enough robust needles of the right size.

The negotiations about the project had gone on at top government levels, and Ian Parker had assured me that I need not worry about the little matter of taking large amounts of potent narcotics across international boundaries. I had enough narcotics in my kit to supply all the addicts of a large city for several months. Each vial contained enough drug to knock out about five baby elephants, or kill about 100 humans. The underworld term for one of the drugs that I had, which was in common use in many cities of the U.S.A., sums it up: "Elephant Tranquilizer."

So it was with some trepidation that I emerged from the Boeing 707 at Kigali airport carrying my lethal camera case, which contained no photographic equipment, just a mass of glass bottles encased in foam rubber. With me were the two Tonys, Miles Coverdale, a Thika coffee farmer who had come along to help, Ian, Giles Camplin, and Mutua. I envisioned the whole team being incarcerated. However, the papers that Ian produced, and the fact that the director of the ORTPN had personally met us at the airport, smoothed the way through. The customs inspector did not look at a single bag.

Mr. Falaise, a sallow-complexioned Belgian official with the Ministry, drove us to our hotel. It seemed strangely deserted, there being only two other guests in the large lounge. We sat around enjoying our Primus beer, the best beer that I've ever tried in Africa, which came in one litre bottles, large enough to make sharing no problem. From time to time, male guests would appear briefly and then leave quickly. The explanation for this odd behaviour surfaced only later, when I learned that the hotel was rated as the best of the local brothels. In order to make a good impression on our team, the police had, that afternoon, rounded up all the girls who used the hotel as a base and shipped them out of town in three five-ton trucks. They had been abandoned on the roadside and left to fend for themselves.

"The police chief proudly told me that they shipped out 15 tons of whores," said Ian. I could only imagine the contrast between the girls in their working outfits and the local peasants 30 miles out of town. High-heeled shoes were never designed to cope with rough country roads.

The next morning, Mr. Falaise led the convoy of two jeeps out to the site of the first part of the exercise at Karama, quite close to the southern border with Burundi, where we would be based for at least a couple of weeks. Mr. Falaise spoke almost no English; in a mixture of schoolboy

French, tortured English, and a little Swahili we were able to make way, although his Flemish accent and colloquial usage made the whole thing rather difficult for everyone.

The fact that the Swahili used in Rwanda is substantially different from that spoken in Kenya made it even harder. While Swahili is the "lingua franca" of all of east and some parts of central Africa, local dialects had developed over the centuries, reflecting influences of the mixing of tribes, as well as Arab, Indian, British, French, Belgian, German, Portuguese, and other European traders and rulers in the various regions. Beautiful poetry has been written in the purest *safi* form of Swahili, which is nearly 2,000 years old. Julius Nyrere, the first president of Tanganyika (later Tanzania), translated some of Shakespeare's works into Swahili.

"*Ici votre maison,*" said Mr. Falaise. The abandoned wooden house looked particularly unprepossessing.

"How will we cook our food?" I tried in my schoolboy French. No response other than a blank stare. I tried again in Swahili. A light went on in his hawk-like face.

"*Nalete le chop avec l'auto kilasiku.*" The first and last words were Swahili and we understood them easily. *Avec l'auto* I knew to be French for "with the vehicle." "We will bring . . . with the vehicle every day." *Le chop* had us foxed.

"*Qu'est que c'est le chop?*" I ventured.

"*Chakula. Á manger,*" he replied in both languages, and mimed filling his mouth with a spoon.

"*A bon, mzuri.*" (Good, good.) I unconsciously mimicked in both languages.

To illustrate his point he took us to the back of the jeep and showed us a trolley of the type used on airplanes for passenger meals. Each tray held two plates of pre-cooked food that was to be our lunch and supper for the day.

With that apparently sorted out, Tony Parkinson and Miles went off to look at the elephant *bomas* as I started to check out and sight the guns. Tony was back in no time flat. "Jerry, come and take a look. We have our hands full, the *bomas* are hopeless. These people haven't followed my instructions at all."

We walked over to the site where six square pens had been constructed by vertically standing heavy logs in a ditch. Cross members had been loosely tied onto the logs with the occasional strand of wire, but we could easily push our way through the walls, moving the vertical pieces aside with ease. Even a tiny elephant would make short work of them and be gone in no time.

Luckily, Tony had made sure that there was a generous supply of number nine wire on site. Using only the simplest of tools — a pair of pliers, a tire iron, and a large screwdriver — we spent the next two days reinforcing the entire system. The local staff were detailed off to cut new lengths for use as horizontal members. Miles and Mutua trimmed the new poles and cut lengths of wire and bent them double. Tony and I used the tire iron and the screwdriver to twist the wire around the lumber at 12-inch intervals. By the time we had finished, we had built a virtual fortress.

The *bomas* were not our only problem. Despite Mr. Falaise's assurances, we didn't see another soul from Kigali for two more days. For sustenance on day two, after waiting in vain for a food run, we ended up buying fish and yams from the locals and cooking them over an open fire.

The house was about a stone's throw from one of the many lakes in the area, so obtaining fish was not a problem. However, water was a challenge, as it resembled strained hippo dung in both colour and smell, and the ceramic core of the drinking water filter quickly clogged. As our need for body fluids exceeded the capacity of the filter to produce potable water, we had to find a solution. While boiling the water no doubt sterilized it, the addition of tea bags made no difference to the colour, and not much to the taste. As for washing, we opted to stay dirty until we could rectify the situation; we were also in need of a supply of disinfectant. On the third day we rebelled and made a trip into town in our own jeep for supplies.

Ian and Tony Archer, meanwhile, had stayed in Kigali dealing with a series of political and other issues. The worst of these had been the sudden death of the youngest child of the director of wildlife. When the director left home to put the final signature on the contract — in effect, to sign the elephants' death warrant — the little boy had had some mild flu-like symptoms. When the man returned home, his son was dead. The coincidence was taken as a sign of extreme ill omen by many officials and Rwandans in the know.

Five days after our arrival, it looked as if the project was finally a go. Another jeep rolled into camp and Ian and Tony Archer emerged carrying guns. Several cases of ammunition were unloaded.

As the distant and distinctive sound of the helicopter turbo increased to a racket that made conversation impossible, the team gathered on a large patch of open ground. Heavy trucks had already arrived from town, and a substantial crew of Belgian expatriates had gathered. Among them were a strongly built young blond man, Daniel Gallez, and his father, whose shape had probably been the same as his son's in youth, but whose hairy stomach now served as a substantial preamble to a large paunch. Also there were Charles Mahouden, who had been a mercenary fighting for Tshombe, the brothers Siko and Hubert Verhulst, and Alain and Nicole Monfort, a married couple, both biologists.

Ian Parker went up with the Belgian pilot for a reconnaissance and found a family group of elephants about three miles away. The time had come. Nervous chatter, mostly mine, gave way to concerned silence and we boarded the Alouette 3, which had been provided by the Rwandan Air Force. Looking down as the chopper ascended and turned away from the lake, I got a better idea of the layout of the land. Thickets of bush were dotted on numerous termite mounds. The rest was rolling grassland.

That first day, especially, sticks in my mind.

We overflew the mob and Ian and the Belgian pilot discussed the lay of the land. Those of us in the back seats had little idea of what was going on. I simply sat, letting my mind go blank, and hoping that I had not forgotten any of the critical elements that we would need in the next few hours.

The helicopter banked and moved away from the herd. About half a mile away it set us down and took off again without reducing engine revs. Ian and the two Tonys knew what to expect. I was the complete greenhorn. We lined up in a small semi-circle, about five yards from each other in front of a large bush, the FN riflemen on the outside, Tony P. and me in the middle, our dart guns about as useful as pea shooters if things went wrong.

I had decided upon the use of a single-sized drug dose. I knew we might be dealing with elephants of several different sizes, ranging in weight from 650 to 1,800 pounds; we could fire extra darts into larger animals. Worrying about this, and fiddling with the holsters that I had designed to hold up to ten darts each, was really only a displacement behaviour as the sound of the helicopter grew louder.

Before I knew it the herd was almost on us, led by a matriarch who was showing her displeasure, head up, trunk waving. At the same moment that she saw us, her knees buckled and she fell dead. I hardly heard the shots as two more adults fell near the back of the group, and I selected a youngster for a dart. A single juvenile broke from the side of the mob and took off through the bushes, one dart in his backside.

It was all over in about 90 seconds. Seventeen adult and teenage elephants lay dead in front of us, and five juveniles were milling about in shock. The cracks of the rifle shots cutting through the roar and throb of the helicopter were replaced by almost complete silence, allowing Tony and I to discuss the need to give top-up doses to a couple of animals that had had less than the required number of darts. We could hear the distant buzz of the machine as it went off in search of the escapee.

It was surreal. Despite Ian's clinical descriptions, both in Langata, and again here in Rwanda, I could hardly believe what I had seen. During the actual darting I'd had to suppress my feelings about the destruction, as I had a serious job to do, but the pile of carcasses was an amazing and moving sight.

I did not have long for reflection, for now my task really began. I had to decide when it would be safe to approach the youngsters, keep an eye on each one to ensure that it did not become too deeply anesthetized, and ensure that all of them received their protective doses of antibiotics.

There was a further problem. What to do about the single youngster that had escaped?

"I can go up and shoot him, unless you can dart him, Jerry," said Ian.

"If he's not moving far, and you can give me five minutes, I'm sure we can do something," I replied.

The ground crew, who had been waiting about half a mile away, appeared. Giles had the responsibility of recording everything on both Super-8 and print film. Miles and the Belgians waited for instructions. Now Mutua came into his own, as his rhino and elephant work over the preceding four years paid off in spades. Tony Parkinson and I made estimates of the weight of the five calves, and based on these, Mutua could work out the doses of antibiotic and multivitamins for each.

I left him and Tony to get on with it, and boarded the helicopter after filling up a couple of extra darts. It took only a couple of minutes to find the elephant. It was wandering about in a daze about 300 yards away, as the drugs had done most of their work and it had been just one dart short of its requirement. This was soon remedied, and I hopped out of the machine, which had put me down in a convenient clearing, and was left to my own devices.

I quickly dispensed the antibiotics and vitamins, after which I had only to find some shade and wait. And wait, and wait. I learned later that the heavy machinery had been used to pull some of the carcasses aside so that the youngsters could be led out of the centre of the destruction and loaded on to the trucks. Waiting elephants had been tied with stout ropes to stakes driven into the ground, to nearby dead adults, or to the sides of the trucks themselves. Three hours passed before all the live animals had been loaded and the crew could turn their attention to me and my patient.

Within an hour, the effects of the darts had begun to wear off the young bull that I was tending and a top-up dose was needed. Soon afterwards, one of the Belgians came over to see how I was doing.

"Je veux des . . ." I had forgotten the French for rope. *"Nataka kamba ine kubwa."* I need four big ropes. The lingua franca of East Africa, unadorned with plurals or syntax in order to be comprehensible in Rwanda, came to the rescue. While Swahili is a hard language to learn perfectly, it is an easy one to learn badly.

Before the patient began to come around for a second time, I tied each leg to a different tree, and hobbled its hind legs. I did not need 1,500 pounds of groggy pachyderm loose and distressed.

Eventually the entire crew turned up, but not before I had had to administer two more top-up doses. I was contemplating yet another, as the elephant had stood up and was swaying groggily, its legs apart like a Saturday night drunk.

Now Tony's brief career as a stunt man in the movies came in handy. He had worked on a Hollywood film called *Cowboy in Africa*, where the real cowboys had taught him to use a lariat, and he quickly constructed a makeshift one out of one-inch manila rope. I would wager that this is the only time that a lariat of such a size has been successfully thrown over the head of an elephant at a range of five yards. Just twirling the thing around his head and opening the loop was a major achievement.

Before we left the scene of the carnage, I watched in amazement the events unfolding there. Ian and Tony Archer were using blackboard chalk to map lines for cutting on each elephant's body. Men with sharpened *pangas*, the machetes of East Africa, were slicing through the skin and peeling it back. Others were hacking off the heads, and a crane was picking them up and loading them onto a truck. At the demand of the Rwandans, they would be buried, tusks protruding from the ground, to speed up the loosening of the ivory from its sockets while reducing the accompanying stench.

Ian explained, "Nothing will be going to waste. Every marketable item will be sold to defray the huge costs of the operation, the money going back to the Rwandans. Hide, especially ear skin for boots, feet for umbrella stands or waste paper baskets, and of course the ivory."

The meat, too, was not being wasted. Large crowds of men had honed in on the killing site and were hacking huge steaks off the carcasses. These they skewered onto poles about eight feet in length. Men in tandem, each end of the pole on a shoulder, disappeared into the surrounding bush bearing their giant kebabs. Within two days every edible scrap of meat had disappeared.

When we measured it later, we found that the matriarch had dropped a mere 20 feet from the guns, and that the other side of the circle of carcasses was only 60 feet further. Pacing these distances out some 24 years later, they seem hardly credible. I asked Ian how he had managed to keep everything in such a tight circle.

"Well, of course, the first animal shot has to be the matriarch, as she makes all the decisions for the group. After that, we have to take out a couple of adult females near the back of the mob, to stop anything from breaking back. The rest, now leaderless, will just bunch; and as the shooting takes only a few seconds, they never have time to get their act together."

"But how can you be so certain of a kill, with animals facing every which way?" I asked, thinking of the consequences to both the people and the animals if these men missed.

"We simply shut out the bulk of the animal and visualize the brain stem. In that way, we shoot at a small area, ignoring the rest. You saw the results."

"About the only animal you can't kill is one facing directly away from you," I said.

"Precisely."

Not a nice subject or activity; but, as it had to be done, this was the best way, the most efficient and effective, and least painful for the animals.

■

Within a very few days the new residents of the *bomas* had settled nicely. We were even able to let the smallest one out for some exercise, and he followed the food bowl like the best-trained Labrador. Siko named him Minus (Titch) and he became a real pet, chasing anyone who showed fear of him (which included most of the local peasants in our work force) and getting his trunk into places and things where it did not belong.

In one day we had exceeded all expectations. The *bomas* were full, and we needed to build more. Moreover, we had far exceeded the size limitation of four feet, or four years old. The largest animal was a female of six feet four inches, probably about ten or 11 years old, and weighing over 3,300 pounds. The work that we had done on the *bomas* was thoroughly tested.

Next morning, after ensuring that all my charges were in good order I grabbed a ride to Kigali and called Jo to ask how she was doing, and how her pregnancy was progressing.

"Oh, I'm fine," she said over the cracking line. "Karen has been staying with Julie for the weekend, and I've had no calls at all. There is some big news. A man called Dr. Nielsen called from Canada — " The line went dead.

It took another very anxious ten minutes to re-establish the connection. Jo continued where she had left off: "They have offered you the job in Saskatoon. I told them you were away and would get back to them."

Luckily, I was able to get to a telegraph office and make myself understood to the clerk. The cable I sent apparently caused some amusement at the other end.

> "UNDERSTAND JOB OFFER SASKATOON STOP ON SAFARI IN RWANDA TRANSLOCATING ELEPHANTS STOP WILL MAKE CONTACT ASAP ON RETURN TO KENYA STOP HAIGH."

Within ten days we had captured another eight youngsters, and apart from a few solitary old bulls there were no plains elephants left in the southern part of the country. Adult bulls had been shot with the heavy rifles. We had a couple of casualties in the *bomas*. A stray bullet had gone into one female's right flank, and another had a puncture wound in her foot that looked as if it had been caused by a tusk. We immobilized them both and cleaned things up as best we could. After that, there was no point in my staying in Rwanda until the next phase of the project was ready to go.

Leaving Mutua to act as headman and look after the animals, the two Tonys, Ian, Miles, and I took the opportunity to return to Kenya. I wanted to get back, not only to see Jo and Karen, but to get down to the Mombasa quarantine station where another group of animals belonging to Don Hunt was ready to be tested for shipment to the U.S.A. I also had to sort out my possible Canadian future.

Nanyuki first. Jo, fit and well, but getting decidedly large, was amazed at the accounts of the Rwandan work. She was still working at the Cottage Hospital, and the first night I was home she had to go out at some ungodly hour and deliver a baby. Not, however, until she had woken me and given me the phone numbers of two of her corps of potential blood donors scattered around both the town and the compound at the new military airfield. Happily, I did not need to make the calls.

Next afternoon, trying to match local office hours in Canada, I struggled to place a call to Saskatoon through the operator. We ended up leaving a message.

"This is Dr. Haigh calling for Dr. Nielsen. I am at Nanyuki, Kenya. The number is Nanyuki 2271. I'll wait for his call."

Within a couple of hours, over a remarkably clear line, the dean of the Western College of Veterinary Medicine repeated the offer that had come through to Jo two weeks before.

"Ole Nielsen here. We'd like to offer you the job. Sir William Weipers came through about a month ago and thinks that the job would suit your abilities. How do you feel about it?"

"Well, I'm delighted, but I don't know the first thing about Canada. Could I come and see you about it?"

"That sounds like a good idea. When could you get here?"

"Well, I have to go back to Rwanda to finish up that project in about two weeks time, but I should be able to get to you after the end of April. How does that sound?"

"That's all right. We'll be happy to see you. If you decide you like it here, when can you start?"

"Well, my wife is due to have a baby on the fourth of July, so we obviously won't be able to come before that, or even right away afterwards. Let's discuss it when I see you. I'll call you as soon as I know my flight details."

As Mutua was still in Rwanda, I closed up the Nanyuki office and took Njeru with me to Mombasa. We completed the task of bleeding yet another group of antelopes from various regions of Africa in order to test them for infectious diseases. Among them were four of the most beautiful little zebra duiker, which stood no more than about 20 inches at the shoulder. One of them appeared to be heavily pregnant. How heavily I would find out in a month's time, after another session in Rwanda and a quick trip to Canada.

CHAPTER 30

RWANDA REVISITED

*More work in Rwanda. The horrifying consequences of a mistake
made by an American camerawoman. A look back and
an attempt to explain the ABC of wildlife/human interactions
to a city-raised journalist.*

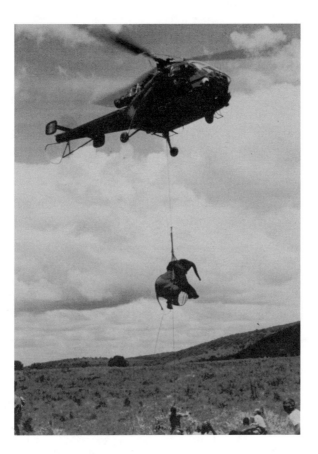

Unusual cargo. Rwanda 1975.

THE RETURN TRIP TO RWANDA in Ian's Cessna 185 was slower and somewhat hairier than the first one. As we crossed Lake Victoria I noticed what I took to be small whirlwinds moving along above the surface of the water. However, they were not quite right, as they kept changing shape — sometimes resembling a column, then quickly becoming an irregular mass. I tapped Miles, who was sitting next to me, on the elbow, pointed, and half-shouted above the noise of the engine, "What are those funny things over there, that look like low clouds or water spouts?"

He leant over and said loudly, about three inches from my ear, "They're clouds of lake flies. They appear from the surface of the water almost daily, but I don't know much about their life cycle. They can be very dangerous in large numbers and it has even been reported that people can choke to death if they sail into a cloud of them."

I wondered what "large numbers" of them could mean. A crude guess put the total in any one of the clouds we could see in the millions, or perhaps even the billions. We flew over and between some tall thunder-heads on the western shores of the lake and slipped between rain showers down to Kigali airport. The place was bristling with armed militia men who seemed to eye us with considerable suspicion.

There was no big welcoming committee this time, and we went straight to lunch at the hotel-cum-brothel where the professional ladies had been so disrupted on our previous visit. At this time of day there was no sign of them.

■

There was an unwelcome surprise. We had all agreed that there was to be no filming of this exercise. It was an unpleasant, if necessary task, and there was no need to broadcast such a potentially emotional scene. However, somehow one segment of the press had got wind of things, and a camerawoman who had been filming gorillas was also at the hotel.

She was a gorgeous dark-haired Californian named Lee Lyon, who had been employed by the British nature series *Survival Anglia* to film gorillas in Zaire. Bernard Grzimek, who had initially not wanted to get involved in the project, had had a change of heart, and John Seago, who had not been averse to the publicity, had some personal contacts in England. Through one or another of these channels, *Survival* had arranged to send Lee to Rwanda. Speaking to Ian, she referred to the elephants as "beautiful people," showing an unrealistic bias that seems to have spread throughout western society, but that has no credibility amongst people who have to live with elephants as neighbours. Her good-looking com-panion was introduced as Adrien Deschriever.

"Aren't you from Zaire?" I queried him. "You work with gorillas over there on the other side of the Virungas, don't you?"

"Oh yes," he replied in excellent English. "I am with Lee, and I wanted to see how things are done." It soon became clear that when he said "with," he meant something more than a professional relationship.

Lee told us that Adrien's wife, a native Zairean and mother of their children, no doubt incensed at the situation, had consulted a witch doctor to arrange a curse to be put on her.

As far as we were concerned this was an unwelcome intrusion, and we were on the brink of closing down the entire project. Only some furious politicking by the Rwandans and the director of the ORTPN changed the course of things, with, as it would turn out, terrible consequences for Lee.

Over a brief lunch we discussed the new situation. The only stipulation made by Ian was that Lee would not film the actual moments of the culling itself, as the scenes were going to be horrifying enough without that. We also met the new helicopter pilot, a local Rwandan captain, who was replacing the Belgian with whom we had been working. It was most disconcerting to see him down a whole litre of Primus just a couple of hours before he was to fly to the site of the second leg of the operation. I was happy to let Ian and Tony Archer travel by air while we went overland in the jeep.

The new camp, located on a hill above the banks of the Nyaborongo River at a place called Rwinzoka, looked out over a large swamp. The river itself, no more than 20 yards wide at this point, fed into Lake Victoria and thence the Nile.

New elephant *bomas* had been constructed, this time according to instructions, and we were ready to get going right away. Diminutive Siko Verhulst, with his balding head carrying a wisp of pale blond hair in the middle, led us down a rough track to the water's edge, and I got a closer look at the tall stands of papyrus that were the predominant vegetation.

"How on earth are we going to get elephants out of that lot?" I asked the group, no doubt voicing a concern of all of the Kenya crew. "No trucks can get in, and the helicopter can't lift more than about 2,500 pounds. I guess we'll have to stick to little guys."

Despite his lack of English, Siko got the drift of the question, and as we

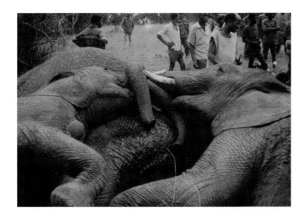

Day 1. Ninety seconds later. Seventeen dead elephants.

Tony Archer surveys the scene, in the swamp at Rwinzoka.

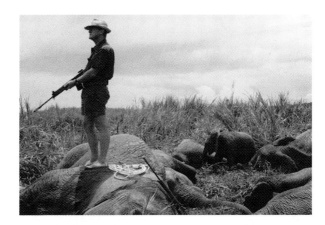

The consequences of snaring: this young adult has lost virtually all of its trunk and had to enter the lakes and rivers to drink. It could also not hope to reach for grass or pull down branches from above. The two tiny youngsters beside it were too small to have any chance of being successfully raised in the conditions we were working under.

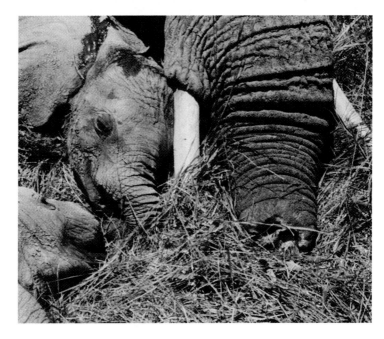

Tony Parkinson puts his lassoing skills to good use on a partially drugged elephant.

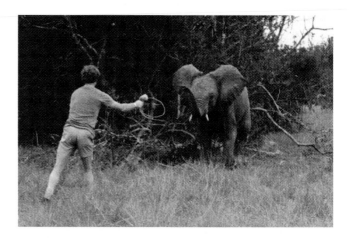

Tony Parkinson and the author load darts into specially prepared holsters that held up to ten syringes.

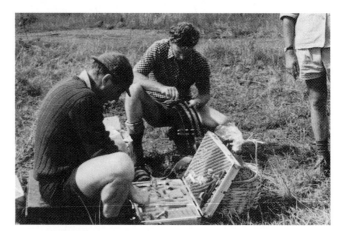

Tony Parkinson restrains Minus, who soon after capture became the camp pet, but tended to be a trifle boisterous.

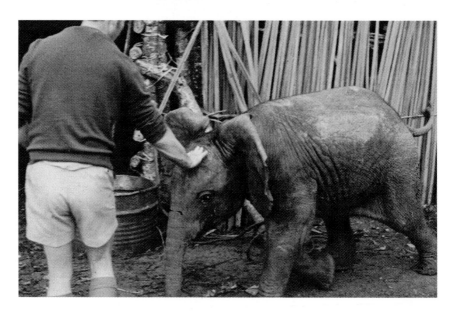

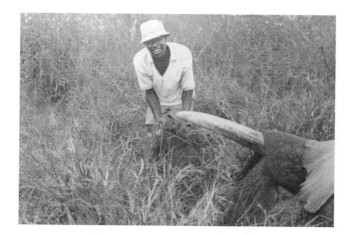

Mutua checks out a large elephant's damaged trunk. Thirty-six of 106 elephants had some degree of trunk missing or severely damaged.

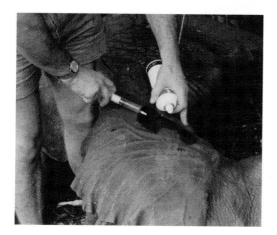

Like roads and lanes on a large scale map, the veins and arteries on the back of an elephant's ear are vital to its ability to keep cool. An intravenous injection of vitamins helps to overcome some of the stresses associated with capture.

Once the injections are finished, the author demonstrates to a hired man how water is to be used for cooling the patient. The ear will be flapped back and forth until the animal is given the drug antidote, is able to stand, and can regain its normal functions.

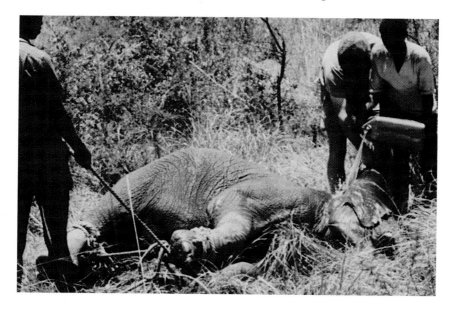

The catamaran "Queen Mary" descends the Nyaborongo River.

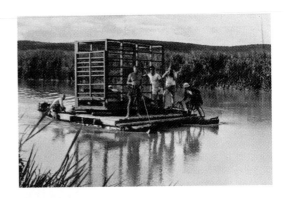

In the Papyrus swamp at Rwinzoka a partially drugged large juvenile is pulled towards a cage by a band of willing helpers. Stay ropes were tied to every corner and the operation was supervised by Ian Parker (left), Giles Camplin (nearest cage), and the author in a "deerstalker" hat.

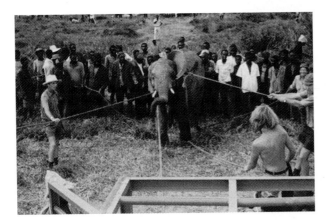

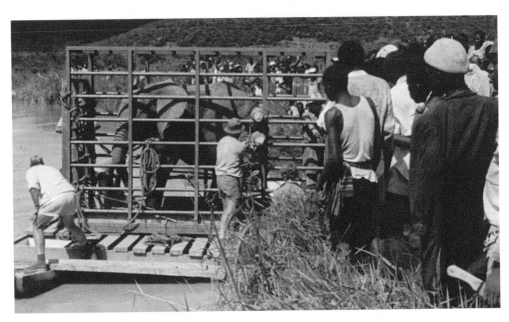

With the elephant loaded, the freeboard will decline to zero. Siko Verhulst checks the knots behind while Mr. Gallez prepares to cast off. The crowd looks on.

rounded the corner he said, in Swahili, "Don't worry, we shall get them out with the boat." The boat turned out to be a rusted old catamaran, about 15 feet long, the two hulls having no more than about nine inches of freeboard. An antediluvian five-horsepower engine, its brand name long since covered in grime and rust, seemed to be the only means of propulsion.

A team of Belgian workmen, aided by a substantial number of locals, dragged one of the heavy steel cages down to the water's edge by main force, and thence up on to the catamaran, which had promptly been christened the *Queen Mary* by the skeptical Kenyan group. The freeboard decreased to about four inches.

In the morning, hoping that the effects of the pilot's beer had worn off, Ian, Tony P., and I decided to go up and have a look at the scene. It took no time at all to see that we would be dealing with a very different set of problems. There were numerous tracks leading from the swamp up onto the riparian farmland, and several fields of green maize lay waste where elephants had been feeding at night. In one spot an abandoned set of family dwellings appeared to have been randomly demolished. Ian pointed down, and over the noise of the helicopter shouted, "Elephant damage." I nodded, as conversation was not really possible.

We returned to camp, and as I prepared the syringes, Ian and the pilots left to try to find an elephant group. It took longer than expected, as the animals were dispersed in the swamp up and down the river over several miles.

Our driving, culling, and capture techniques changed hardly at all, the main difference being that we had to tie the immobilized youngsters to the legs of their dead relatives, as stakes could not possibly hold in the swamps. Beneath our feet was a shifting substrata of many years' worth of packed, rotting vegetation; it felt like walking on a water bed. One just hoped the thing would not rupture.

We had planned to airlift the smallest of our new charges out of the swamp in a small metal cage. The pilot returned to camp to fetch it, and at this point the effects of the Primus made themselves known. The rope attached to the cage was easily fixed to the helicopter hook and the pilot took off, gingerly lifting the new weight. But then he forgot the principles of loads and pendulums. As he pulled away, the cage trailed 50 feet behind him. Instead of flying slowly he accelerated, and the angle of the rope grew even more acute. He then banked left to head for the swamp. The cage carried straight on at 30 knots, and the pilot suddenly had an extra problem to contend with as he found himself being pulled in the wrong direction. Having reached the end of its arc, the cage swung back, and suddenly it appeared on the other side of the helicopter, which began to yaw in concert with the load. The pilot did the only possible thing. He pressed the emergency release button. From 200 feet up the cage, which weighed about 1,100 pounds, instantly followed the same trajectory as Newton's apple and plummeted earthwards. On contact with the sloping ground it crumpled like chicken wire, leaving a swath of destruction in the banana plants beside the river as it rolled down the hill. By the time it came to rest it looked like a badly made pretzel.

There was only one thing for it if we were to get the animals out in any sort of sensible time. We rigged a harness with stout ropes and airlifted the smallest of our new charges direct to the *bomas*. A baby elephant swaying under a military helicopter was the picture that appeared in the world's media a few days later. I went with it to administer antidotes and ensure a safe transfer to the pen.

We soon saw gruesome evidence of one of the problems faced by the elephants. Three of the six adults in our first group had trunks that had been damaged by snares some time ago. Two were grim, the third less severe. One had only about a foot of trunk left, and another's trunk had been severed about three-quarters of the way through, so that a useless five-foot-long lump of meat hung down from her face, impeding her ability to feed. The only way that either animal could possibly drink was to go right into the river and dunk their heads. The least seriously damaged animal had lost only about six inches off the end of its trunk. The Swahili word for an elephant's trunk is *mkono*, which means hand. The two pointed tips with which the most delicate of tasks are performed are naturally known as *vidole* (fingers). Both names are appropriate, and anyone who has watched the incredible sensitivity with which an elephant uses the hundreds of muscles in this vital organ, and seen the multitude of uses to which it is put, could not fail to be appalled by the mutilations they had suffered.

The villagers used snares indiscriminately to try to trap antelope and other game, no doubt hoping to enhance their meagre diets, so deficient in protein other than fish. The elephants, finding the strange objects in the grass as they searched for food themselves, would pick them up and examine them. Some would spring shut or pull up tight, and terrible damage would ensue.

On the second day, we ran into trouble. We had set up in a handy spot and were waiting for the helicopter to herd the elephants to us. As they got within about a hundred yards a group of about 20 buffalos broke out of the greenery in front of us. The pilot had not seen them, as they were less than half as tall as the papyrus stalks. Self-defense was the only recourse, as they were only about 30 yards away, and thoroughly frightened. We stood up. Ian politely raised his hat and we waved, keeping silent, hoping to turn the mob aside without alarming the elephants. The buffalo scattered, some of them turning right round and charging off through the elephant mob, which themselves scattered. Consternation. I turned to Ian, and between us we reached a quick decision.

"If you can shoot the adults from the air, I can dart the youngsters, unless you think we can get them again tomorrow," I said.

"Right. Let's get on with it. Tony, you stay here with the crew and we'll try to keep everything fairly close."

A lot of contorted flying followed in short order. Eventually we had darts in five animals scattered over an area the size of two football fields. We could not see any one of them from any other, and so we had to change strategy for loading. I had to stay on the move, checking the depth of anesthesia of each catch, while Tony P., Ian, Miles, and Mutua monitored and did the antibiotic treatments. Tony A. supervised the loading of the two smallest animals, that would go out by airlift direct to the *bomas*. By now we had all become comfortable working together, and he had no trouble administering the antidote once the animals were safely inside their new pens.

We had to use second darts on four occasions as the day wore on. The experience gained on that first day proved valuable. At one point Mutua was badly shaken when, moving between two downed animals, he almost bumped into a patient that had partially recovered from its immobilizing mixture. It was staggering slowly down a path that had by now been created in the papyrus, so Mutua dived into the greenery and did not emerge for a few minutes, a greyish pallor to his normally dark skin.

When I got to the third animal, I saw that we had a problem — another example of the conflict between the villagers and the animals. Low down on his foreleg, a piece of half-inch wire cable was sticking out of the skin. Part of the end of his trunk was missing. I called over to Ian and the two Tonys.

"Fellows, come and look at this. I don't think that there is much point in continuing." As they stood there I showed them the extent of the mess. "This is the end of a snare. Look, the skin has grown back over, but it's paper thin, and if I put my finger down this track you can see that it goes right around the leg and cuts into the deep tissues. It has even damaged the bone over here on the inside."

"Can you fix it?" asked Ian.

"Given a pair of bolt cutters, time, daily hosing with cold water, about a month's course of antibiotics and some luck, and assuming that the blood supply to the leg below the snare is still functioning, probably," I replied. "But remember that he will be very stressed once we get him in the *bomas*, and that may alter the outcome."

The solution, although unpalatable, seemed obvious. However, it was not ours to make. The animals belonged to the Rwandan government, and we had already shown that we could capture and keep much larger animals than had originally been thought possible. As luck would have it, Mr. Falaise had abandoned his desk job for the day and taken a cruise on the *Queen Mary* in order to see how we were doing. As the government representative, he had to be consulted.

Ian's French was better than mine. "Look at this wound, caused by this heavy cable snare. Dr. Haigh tells me that it will be very difficult to treat, and will take a long time to heal, if it heals at all. We have caught many animals already, and this one will be a real problem. What should we do?"

"You say it is possible to fix?" said Mr. Falaise, turning to me.

I marshaled my thoughts and worked out a response in French, using what was left of my schoolboy memories and the refresher course that I'd had over the last few weeks in Rwanda. *"Possible, mais seulement avec beaucoup de bonne chance, beaucoup de temps, et beaucoup d'argent. Ici, dans les bomas, il faut tres difficile."* (Possibly, but only with luck, and a lot of time and expense. Here in the *bomas* it will be very hard.) I used the Swahili *boma*, which I knew he'd understand, as I could not recall, or had never known, the correct French word for "pen."

Ian added weight by pointing to the trunk. "Even if his leg gets better in time, he will always have trouble feeding."

Mr. Falaise bit the bullet, so to speak, and a single loud crack from the FN told all within earshot that Ian had done the necessary.

Loading 1,800 or 2,200 pounds of elephant on to the *Queen Mary* presented its own special challenge. On dry land, during the first part of the exercise, we had been able to place heavy ropes around the forelegs and heads of the beasts and use trucks to more or less drag them into the cages. My task had been to gauge the antidote dosages so that each animal would be able to stand, but not much more. The crates had then been lifted by a huge crane onto the back of a flat-bed truck. Now, in the swamp, there was no question of trucks. It was manpower or nothing. The same doses of antidote seemed to work, and we placed heavy ropes on all four legs of each animal, as well as its head. Dozens of willing hands joined in on each rope, as the locals had by now gathered in droves to get their slice of the vast quantities of meat that would soon be available, and we dragged, pushed, and prodded the dopey animals on board into the cage.

With a ton of elephant on board, the freeboard diminished to a theoretical zero. Even at minimum speed the brown waters of the river constantly lapped over the hulls. They must have been entirely waterproof, or else we would have become a second *African Queen* and a disaster would have overtaken the animal in its cage. Crocodiles would no doubt have feasted on the humans, but might have been foxed by the bars when trying to get at the larger meals.

Meanwhile, back in the field, Miles had a surprise encounter with President Habyarimana. As he recounted at dinner that evening, "I was looking after the elephant that Jerry had delegated to me, and just getting ready give it its intravenous vitamin injection when the president came up, walking unaccompanied, and introduced himself. As I was holding off a vein and trying to stick the needle in I just leaned across, put out my right hand which held the syringe, and he bent over and shook my wrist. I said 'Excuse me' and carried on. He didn't seem the least bit put out."

Checking the *bomas* the morning after the next group of three youngsters had been brought in, I noticed a problem. At breakfast I said to Tony P, "That single female we caught the day before yesterday is very lame. Can you come and look at her when we've finished eating?"

"Mind if we come too?" asked Ian.

"Sure."

To the group of us standing beside the pen it was not at once apparent that the animal was doing anything more than resting one hind leg, a stance that elephants often take.

"Miles, please can you go round to the other side of the *boma* and try to move her?" I asked.

Normally a newly caught animal would turn and confront such a challenge. Not this one.

"Wave something at her," I suggested. Miles took off his hat and tried that. Still nothing more than a concerned turn of the head. Without further ado, Miles picked up a handy stick and waved it over the wall of the *boma*, tapping the calf on her backside.

It was immediately obvious to all that this elephant was not just resting. As she turned her left-hind-end half collapsed, and she let out a squeal of pain.

"She may have been hurt when an adult fell on her. I should like to examine her more closely," I said.

Half an hour later she was on the ground, sleeping soundly under the effects of a narcotic mixture. Luckily, she had gone down on her right side, so the damaged limb was uppermost. Now the challenge began. One can examine a lame dog singlehandedly; a lame cow needs one, or sometimes two people; three of us had to work on this one.

"Pull the leg forward and then swing it back as far as you can," I said. Tony P. and Mutua lifted the foot and obliged.

"Again, two or three times, slowly." I could not feel much in the heavy muscles under my hand. The knee seemed fine. There was no abnormal movement lower down the leg, where the bones are close to the surface and no apparent damage in the foot.

"Now lift it up as high as you can." A slight crackle, like an exaggerated rustling of silver paper on a chocolate bar, more felt than heard, emanated from deep inside the thigh muscles. I put one hand underneath what seemed to be the spot, and one on top.

"Again, slowly." There was no doubt now.

"I think she's got a broken femur."

"Then she's had it," said Ian.

"Not necessarily," I replied. "Of course, I can't do anything fancy like operating out here, but even in a fully equipped hospital I probably wouldn't. If we can keep her confined for a longish period, and make sure she rests the leg, it should heal."

"Doesn't she need a cast?" asked Tony.

"You'd never get one to hold, and those heavy thigh muscles act as a natural cast. No, we're far better to leave her. We call this treatment 'masterly inactivity.' It sounds good, but it just means benign neglect. The key is at least six weeks of rest, with minimal movement. You must make sure she gets plenty of good food, and as she's so young, the bones should heal quickly."

We wrapped up this part of the project in another ten days. Other than the 27 youngsters in captivity, there were now virtually no plains elephant left in Rwanda. Some smaller forest elephant no doubt existed on the western border, and a few solitary bulls probably roamed at large. It was time for Mutua and me to head back to Kenya.

Four weeks later, I was in a plane from Canada back to Nairobi, having been over to look at the possibilities for a new job. Jo, now even larger and more uncomfortable, met me at the airport. As ever, our friends Paul and Elma offered unstinting hospitality and we stayed with them for a couple of nights.

"What was Canada like?" asked Elma. "I've got a cousin in L.A. and I've been to see her a couple of times, but I've never been to Canada. What's the place called?"

"Saskatoon. The University of Saskatchewan. The Western College of Veterinary Medicine. The worst thing was the change of weather. I arrived late in the evening of May the first. When we stepped out of the airport it was snowing! And I don't even own a coat. Luckily, my host lent me one, and the weather smartened up a bit during the week."

"Do you think you'll take the job?" asked Paul.

"I'm not sure. Jo and I'll have to discuss it."

In the morning, we drove down to Tony Parkinson's house on Lower Kabete Road, about two miles from Paul and Elma, to try to get the news of the second half of the Rwandan exercise. Over tea, I enquired how everything had gone.

"Oh, we had a disaster," he replied. "As you know, we planned to release all the young elephants onto a peninsula in Lake Hago in the Akagera National Park. We were to hold them there for a while behind a palisade, and then let them find their own way out into the park once they had become acclimatized and formed a group. We hoped that that large female would act as a sort of matriarch."

He took a mouthful of tea and paused.

"What went wrong?" I asked.

"Well, everything went smoothly, and we were down to the last elephant in the *bomas*. It was just a little one, not much more than 50 inches. The one with the broken leg had already gone, and seemed fine. The weekend was coming up, and I wanted to wait until the Monday. As you know, I never work on Sundays. It's not a religious thing, I just believe that one must rest."

"Mm-hmm. We've never worked on a Sunday in the last four years together. No reason to."

Tony continued, almost as if reciting a nightmare.

"Unfortunately, I caved in to pressure from the Rwandans. They insisted that we move the last animal on a Sunday, as they wanted to make a big production of it. Invite out some of the politicians, have a bit of a celebration. Lee Lyon was to film the successful culmination of the whole exercise.

"Things started to go wrong almost at once. We loaded the animal OK, but then I found out that there was no water *en route* for cooling him. We had arranged for it with all the other animals, but somehow it did not happen this time. We got to the release site and Lee got her camera ready. The guests were all on the backs of lorries, and we opened the crate. Several of us were standing by the big Dodge that had been provided.

"The elephant came out part way, but backed in again. The staff pounded on the roof, and shoved sticks through the slats. Eventually he came out, almost at a dead run, straight towards the Dodge. I shouted at everyone to get in and close the doors. We all moved back, and Lee, who had the furthest to move, suddenly found herself at the end of a cable attached to the camera. Her battery packs were on her belt, the cable plugged in for filming."

He paused and licked his lips, took another sip of tea, and continued.

"Then I don't know quite know what went through her mind. Instead of unplugging the cable at her belt, she moved back to the camera, which was in front of the bonnet. She seemed to even try to take some more film, as she put her eye up to the viewfinder. I shouted at her, and she tried to get back. It was too late. The elephant came around the side of the truck, knocked the tripod and camera for six, disconnecting the cable, and kept on coming, slamming the doors as it chased her. She backed up, her hands on its forehead. Then she tripped. As she fell on her hands and knees, the elephant began to thump her with its head. Why she didn't simply dive under the Dodge I can't understand. Then she fell right down. The elephant immediately knelt astride her and began to pound her belly and chest with its forehead. We jumped out of the vehicle and tried to wrestle it off, but it was too much for us."

"Ghastly. A 50-inch elephant already weighs as much as a Jersey bull — at least 1,100 pounds," I said.

"The thing must have hit her 20 times or more, and as we struggled to push it away and pull her out she rolled over, which was the worst thing that could have happened. Then the calf began pounding her back. Anyway, by the time it quit, she was dead."

The flow of words dried up as Tony relived that horrible moment. I, too, was dumbstruck.

"I don't know what the elephant would have done after that. Alain Monfort, the Belgian biologist who worked with us, shot it almost at once."

Did that witch doctor's curse play a role in that terrible scene?

■

Twenty-four years on, in the face of the twin horrors of AIDs and massive genocide, the entire Rwandan elephant exercise palls into complete insignificance. Nonetheless, we did achieve some interesting results. The tallest of the captured females did not turn out to be the matriarch of the herd; instead, it was the third largest. Perhaps she was the calf of a matriarch. There has been considerable breeding activity in the group, indicating that the males must have become fertile at a much younger age than had previously been recognized. The oldest male we moved was no more than about eight years of age. The herd now numbers 60 animals and there is a third generation of calves. Sadly, almost two-thirds of the Akagera Park has been de-gazetted and turned over to cattle grazers. Only the southern section remains, and it is here that the elephants live, again crowded into a shrunken environment.

When we published the account of our experiences in the scientific journal *Environmental Conservation*, we concluded with the following paragraphs, little knowing how sadly prophetic they would be:

"Rwandans live at subsistence or near subsistence levels. It is difficult to see how they will maintain current standards, let alone raise them, in the face of their projected population increase. In these circumstances we do not see how the 484,200 ha that are currently set aside as national parks and game and forest reserves can be kept free of settlement.

"The 25 elephants in Akagera will be barely halfway through their potential lifespan of 63 years by the time Rwanda will, according to projections, have eight million people. At that time the 'new' elephant population will be under much the same pressures as those which led to the elimination of its immediate forbears."

Twenty-five years after the event, I was interviewed by a well-known Canadian journalist to whom I had sent an early draft of this account. I was amazed when he asked me, "Why didn't you move all the people away from the places where the elephants were? Then you wouldn't have had to kill any of them. That's what people in Toronto would think was correct."

As the interview progressed it turned out that he had never lived outside a large city, nor even in a detached house. He had lived in apartments all his life. His understanding of the real workings of nature were tenuous. Perhaps it was entirely based upon the sanitized version presented on most of the "nature" television shows. I'm not sure he believed my assertion that his idea was totally impractical, and that there had been no choice. It would have involved moving hundreds of thousands of people into urban settings where they would have had no imaginable means of support, no food, no homes, nothing. In any conflict between wildlife and humans, the wildlife almost always lose out. When the wildlife are destroying homes, terrorizing the community, and killing people, there is only one solution.

Modern approaches to elephant management, such as have been developed in Zimbabwe and other southern African countries, have a chance of working. They are designed to involve the villagers in the management of, and decision-making about, their own resources, which include elephants.

CHAPTER 31

THE SECOND SURGEON

*A breech presentation leads to an unusual demand
on a very involved vet.*

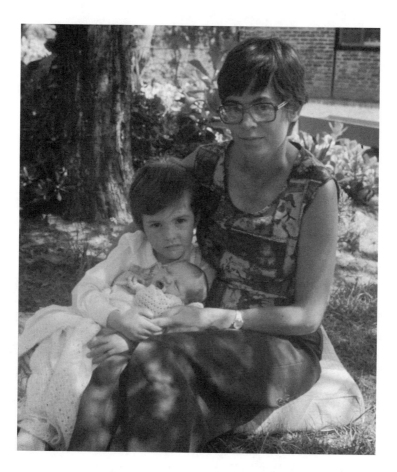

In front of the cottage on Lunatic Lane.
Jo, Karen, and one-week-old Charles.

WHEN SUPERVISING MIDWIVES in Meru, and looking after expectant mothers in Nanyuki, Jo had ensured that regular ante-natal examinations be carried out. Of course, when pregnant herself, she had let this sound practice slide by her. Some doctors can indeed be their own worst patients.

Donald Gebbie had been Jo's obstetrician during her first pregnancy and the birth of Karen, and we visited him in Nairobi at about the six-month stage of this one. However, he had recently accepted an overseas post and would not be there at the critical moment. He referred us to his colleague, Dr. Khehar, who did his best to keep an eye on things. But Jo was not as frequent a visitor as perhaps she should have been. Her own busy practice took priority over visits to Nairobi via rough roads.

She finally realized that her practice must take second place when, late in her eighth month, a Peace Corps volunteer appeared at the cottage hospital with a broken leg. I had already persuaded her that she should not use the ancient X-ray machine during the pregnancy, as we had no idea how safe it really was, so I was drafted to help out. Once the X-rays had been developed and examined, it was time to apply several layers of plaster of Paris. Jo found the task almost beyond her. After applying the first few layers, she could hardly stand up. Luckily I was on hand to finish off under her watchful eye.

"Okay," she said to the patient. "For your next visit, you go to Nairobi. My back hurts and I will be otherwise occupied."

At the end of June, a week later, we traveled to Nairobi to see Dr. Khehar. Like most expectant fathers, I sat in the waiting room, only half-reading an ancient magazine. She came out of the examining room wearing a severe frown.

"What's up?"

"Well," she said, "if he's right, and I'm right, we are due for twins!"

"What do you mean?"

"Well, this here — " she patted her upper mid-section " — feels too hard to be a bum, I say this is a head. He says it's head down, so I'm for an X-ray."

After piling into the hot car, which had no air conditioning, and driving up the hill to Nairobi Hospital, we were lucky to find no line-up in the radiology clinic. An hour later we knew that Jo was not pregnant with twins, but was almost certainly in for a breech delivery. Dr. Khehar tried to turn it, but it was too large and near term for him to have any luck.

Five days later Jo's contractions began, and soon her waters broke. Off we went to Nairobi Hospital, where Dr. Khehar soon arrived.

The struggle seemed to go on for ever, and I lost all track of time. Jo made no noise, but her fierce grip on my hand, and the strain in her face, told me a great deal. Dr. Khehar popped in. With skill developed from long practice, he calmly encouraged her and, in so doing, helped to settle me down.

After what seemed an eternity he returned, and made another examination.

"Well," he said, "there are his testicles, purple and swollen, and if I can't deliver his bum there is no way that I will be able to deliver his head. It's a Caesarean section for you, young lady."

Jo's recollection is that the young lady just looked at him and wished he'd get on with it. It seemed to take ages, ages, ages. "More pain . . . hurry up. . . ." drifted through her mind. "In my hospital it would have been done by now, hurry up, hurry up, hurry up."

Of course in a large hospital there was a good deal of protocol to go through, but mercifully, and far sooner than Jo, in her pain cloud, realized, she was going under the anesthetic. The nurses were all geared to go, and the resident on duty had been paged.

I had asked, and been granted, permission to attend as an observer, and planned to remain as a fly on the wall throughout the procedure. This was not to be. As Dr. Khehar went into his final scrub it became increasingly clear that the resident had somehow vanished and an assistant surgeon was needed.

Dr. Khehar turned to me with a piercing look. I felt like a child caught in some mischievous act; the look on my face said, "Who, me?"

"Jerry, we need some help. You know how to do this. Can you scrub in?"

As I look back on that strange event, it's obvious that for a time my mind went into a sort of blank-out mode. A draped white abdomen became a draped orange abdomen as the iodine soaked sponges were applied by the nurse. Once the patient had been draped she became just that, a patient. Her head was concealed from my view by a drape, as the anesthesiologist sat and monitored her. I had to concentrate on my role as an assistant.

Then the big moment. I took my beautiful blue-gray son, sore scrotum and all, from his living bed and moved him to a crib where an efficient nurse took over. He quickly voiced his objection to being removed from his familiar environment. His yells, and the air that he breathed in as he yelled, turned him from that strange colour to the more familiar and healthy pink. Now back to finish the job. Forceps! sponge! swab! forceps! suture! cut! So the terse instructions were made. So I complied.

It was an astonishing experience. There are all sorts of anecdotal accounts of the importance of early bonding between parents and young. It would be hard to imagine an earlier bonding event between father and son. Unusual challenges call for unusual solutions. As the great Canadian physician Sir William Osler said, "you must put your emotions on ice."

CHAPTER 32

SACH-SASSA-SASKATCHEWAN

The move to Canada is on, but first there is some tidying up to be done, and some last cases to be attended to. A dog is poisoned, but its alert owner smells a rat. Tick-borne disease ravages a beautiful dairy herd. On one last trip to see a sick rhino, I meet a Canadian couple who are on leave from the very city we're moving to.

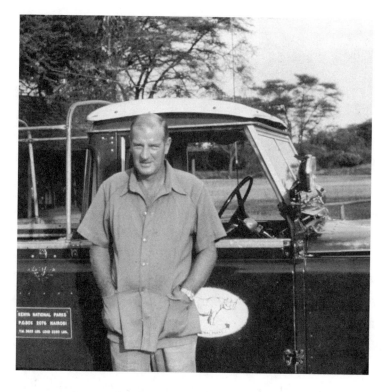

Peter Jenkins, warden of Meru National Park.

WE DECIDED THAT I WOULD accept the job in Canada, as it was too good an opportunity to pass up. After the birth of Charles, we stayed a few days extra in Nairobi at the home of Paul and Elma Sayer. Jo gradually recovered from her difficult Caesarean, enjoying the unstinting hospitality of Elma and the Sayers' motherly, gossipy *ayah*, Selena. Meanwhile, Paul and I made a trip to the Mombasa quarantine, where I showed him and our colleague Dieter Rottcher how to immobilize and handle the various species. I gave Paul a complete list of the immobilizing doses that I had developed over the last few years, and after I left, he worked for Don Hunt until exports were banned.

I picked up Jo, Karen, and baby Charles at Kabete, and we headed home. When we got back to Nanyuki, we had an unpleasant surprise. Ester had disappeared. Her room was completely empty. Abuyeka then let on that she had been gradually moving her stuff out of the house over the last three or four weeks, and had taken the opportunity to move her bed and other furniture while we were in Nairobi. We never did find out exactly what became of her, which was really sad, as she had played such an important role in our lives, especially Karen's life. With Jo not fully recovered, Ester's absence made life a little difficult.

We began the paperwork and interview process with the Canadian High Commission in Nairobi. The interview was easy and relaxing, despite our trepidation. The Canadians had obviously done their homework, as our interviewer made reference to my parents and their Kenyan history with the British military.

We were told that even though he was only a few weeks old, Charles would need his own passport. So we half-sat him in a wicker-work chair, wrapped in a warm blanket, and snapped a photo of his little baby face. How any immigration officer was going to identify him from that was beyond us.

We organized for a moving company to come and pick up the bits and pieces that we felt we could not part with. The double bed, custom-made of beautiful pale Meru oak, went into a crate. The crate itself was also made of Meru oak, and in due course became a full suite of sitting-room furniture in our new home in Canada.

As the move loomed, and time seemed to accelerate, I carried on with my veterinary practice. The usual run of small animal cases turned up in the office: vaccinations, sales of de-worming pills, a couple of cat spays.

One afternoon, just as we were going to call it quits, the Burguret estate's Peugeot pick-up arrived at the door. The farm headman, arap Ruto, and a couple of others emerged from the vehicle, with Mike Littlewood's handsome yellow Labrador, Bimbo, at the end of a length of twine. A year-old adolescent, Bimbo was usually all go–go–go. Today he seemed quieter, though still fairly bright-eyed and alert.

After our brief Kipsigis greeting, I said, *"Shauri gani?"* (What's the problem? or, What's up?)

The author Errol Trzebinski has called *shauri* "a wonderful all-embracing Swahili word meaning troubles or any complication of an adverse nature, which, in a word, saves the victim of all necessity of recounting the tedious and harassing details to the listener." It can also mean "business."

There are a few standard responses to *"Shauri gani?"* They include:

"Shauri la serikali" (The government's business)

"Shauri la Mungu" (God's business)

"Shauri lako" (Your problem)

In this case none quite fitted. Arap Ruto handed me a note and said, simply, *"Sumu"* (poison).

Mike's note was brief and to the point. "I'm sure Bimbo's been poisoned, in his feed. Can you *fanya?"* *Fanya* (*ku-fanya*) is another all-embracing Swahili word that means different things in different contexts. Here it meant "do" or more expansively, "sort it out."

I asked arap Ruto for more details and learned that, following a quarrel, Mike had overheard a discussion between his kitchen staff that made him suspicious. He had gone into the kitchen and seen Bimbo devouring the last of a bowl of maize meal and meat scraps. The timing was off, and the staff ought not to have been doing the feeding. This was enough to convince Mike to ship the dog off with all haste.

For about eight years, I had had in my drug-safe a small bottle of a morphine derivative called apomorphine that had only one reported use: it was supposed to make dogs vomit. I had never used it, and it had sat in the dark all that time, the stopper unbreached. Luckily I had not yet cleared it out from my stock, and so I went to the back of the office and got it out.

Within five minutes of his arrival at the clinic, and no more than 40 seconds after the injection, Bimbo had deposited a large bolus of virtually undigested food on the floor. I scooped some up with a plastic cup, and then asked Njeru to get rid of the rest. Bimbo went home, none the worse for wear, and never having shown any of the pronounced signs of being poisoned.

Ten days later I was able to show Mike the lab report that had come back from Kabete. Someone had had it in for Bimbo, or indirectly for Mike. The maize meal had been spiked with two poisons. One was the same toxaphene that had so nearly done for the little boy in Meru six years ago, and the other was an organophosphate. Either would have been fatal if left untreated. Both were used as cattle dips for tick control, and had been in the store at Burguret.

■

About three weeks before we left, a slim man, whom I recognized as a former colleague from my Meru days, entered the office.

"*Jambo* Doctor Haigh! Do you remember me? Mwangi is the name. I was a livestock officer when you first came to Meru, but I was soon posted to Nyeri district."

He explained that he was now a farm manager for a group of farmers who had formed a co-operative, and who had received government funding. "There is a problem at the farm we have purchased. Several of the cattle are very sick, and I was hoping that you come and help me. It does not look good."

"How so?"

"Well, the government only funded the farm purchase. I was given no float for day-to-day management. When I went to the KFA store [the Kenya Farmers Association, a private business that sold all kinds of farm supplies], they refused to let me have any cattle dip on credit, so we have not been able to dip or spray the animals for almost a month."

This did indeed sound serious. I promised to come round the next day, mindful of the fact that if Mr. Mwangi had no cash float, it would probably be a charity visit.

My worst fears were confirmed. A dozen milk cows were standing in line in a cattle chute, several of them looking thoroughly dejected. The first two told the story. They both had elevated temperature, over 104 degrees, or 40 centigrade on my new thermometer, as well as several hemorrhages inside their mouths and on the membranes inside their mouths, around the eyes, and inside the vulva. To add confirmation to these were the very swollen lymph nodes just in front of their shoulders. The nodes in the first one were quite a bit bigger than my closed fist; a normal one would probably have been no bigger around than a breakfast sausage. It was easy to pop a needle into the node and squeeze out a drop of fluid on to a glass slide. Every cow in the line had similar signs of disease.

Mr. Mwangi knew very well what he was seeing, and had a worried look on his face. Although I could not be completely certain until I had seen what the slides might reveal under the microscope, we both knew this was probably East Coast Fever, something we had seen before, but not in what amounted to an outbreak form. It was frustrating and distressing, because there was absolutely nothing I could do in the way of treatment. These beautiful cattle were almost certain to die. As their condition deteriorated they would develop pneumonia-like symptoms, go downhill rapidly, and proceed to the inevitable end. All the money that had been spent on the farm purchase, would have to be repaid, and no doubt Mr. Mwangi would be blamed, which was grossly unfair. Funding for cattle dip would have entirely prevented this catastrophe.

I take my hat off to Mr. Mwangi. He somehow managed to get his Nairobi head-office staff to process my invoice with much more than usual speed, and a cheque arrived in good time for me to bank it.

■

There was one more trip to Meru park. Warden Peter Jenkins called me in to look at a rhino with a large wound on its side. This was the last time I would ever see this herd of white rhino, with which I had had professional dealings at least a dozen times over the years. They would all be killed by poachers before we got back to Kenya.

"What was that place you said you were going to in Canada?" Peter asked as we drove away from the rhino *boma*. "Sach — Sassa — "

"Saskatoon, Saskatchewan."

"Really? What a coincidence. We have a couple from there studying in the park."

We headed back to the park headquarters and to the thatched house next to his own, the same house that Jo and I had stayed in when I had given the giant enema to the lovelorn rhino. Here Peter introduced me to a slim, fit-looking couple, Dick and Jenny Neal, whose English accents, like my own, indicated origins outside of Canada. We chatted over cool drinks, as their two young children played on the verandah, and I learned that Dick and Jenny had obtained their biology degrees at Southampton, right next to the spot from which my mother's flight had left for Kenya in 1939.

It turned out that Dick, who was on faculty at the Department of Biology at the same university where I had accepted my post, was on sabbatical leave. He was in the park to study the elephant shrew — a little animal on the other end of the mammalian scale from what I was used to!

We talked about Canada and Saskatoon, and they extolled the virtues of the small prairie city. I'm sure they mentioned the winters, but I'm not sure I believed them. Perhaps I didn't want to?

This entirely fortuitous meeting was to play a vital role in helping us settle in Canada. Dick and Jenny offered us hospitality and unstinting help as soon as we arrived, and also came up with an absent colleague's house for us to live in, rent free, as we tried to find our feet.

Finally, the day of our departure arrived. We went first to Scotland for a few days, then on to Holland, where Jo continued her recovery, relaxing among her family. After three days in Holland I moved on to Munich, to attend my first international conference, a Wildlife Disease Association meeting.

One of the people I met there said something that gave me a bit of a turn: "Ah! I've always wanted to meet someone going to Saskatoon. I know plenty who have left, but never before met anyone going there."

As we flew across the Atlantic, I pondered the changes in my life over the past ten years. I had grown as a professional, which was no surprise. The superb education at Glasgow had equipped me as well as it could, but as any new vet realizes, graduation is just the beginning of the process of learning your profession. Perhaps the most important thing I had learned was the importance of observation and reasoning. My senses of sight, sound, smell, and touch had all been put to use on my first wildlife patient — that towering giraffe.

But more important, by a country mile, were the personal changes. I had left Glasgow as an unattached bachelor, and now I was part of a new and much larger family: Jo, Karen, and baby Charles, as well as lots of Dutch relatives.

Our first days in Saskatoon were packed with new cultural experiences. For a start, we found ourselves living in a city environment — something we changed as soon as we could. Of course there was no Abuyeka to clean the house, bring in the early morning tea, and prepare delicious meals at short notice.

Work at the local zoo kept me busy, and within a few short weeks my luck held and I was involved in a big moose research project with the provincial government. For Jo there was, at first, no work outside the house. She became a full-time mum. As we found our financial feet, and Jo felt an ever-increasing need to get back into medicine, we found a nanny through an agency, and Jo started up at the Department of Paediatrics at the university.

Winter was indeed a revelation, but if everyone else could manage it, why not us? The house was well-designed, draft-free, and warm. We took some lessons in cross-country skiing, and tried to integrate ourselves into the new culture. In our first summer we bought a canoe, and discovered a recreational activity that is second to none. Charles went canoeing before he could walk. All of us find the remote regions of Saskatchewan, and its 97,000 and something lakes, to be absolute magic. We have become Canadians, but our roots lie in the tropics.

The Haigh family motto is "Tyde what may," and for me that has been an ideal dictum. Who could have imagined that my youthful boyhood wish to be a zookeeper would have led to a career in veterinary medicine, lots of wildlife cases, a job in Canada where I would spend over half my time looking after animals in a zoo setting, and a deep involvement in the world of zoo and wildlife medicine? Certainly not my worried parents, and certainly none of my classmates or professors at Glasgow.

RETURN TO THE HONEYPOT

On a return visit to the country, we see many things that make us sad, but also many that give hope. The population has exploded, wildlife is dwindling, AIDS is wreaking havoc, the roads are a shambles; but the society has matured, and we are royally entertained by a theatrical group who show that one can laugh at misfortune.

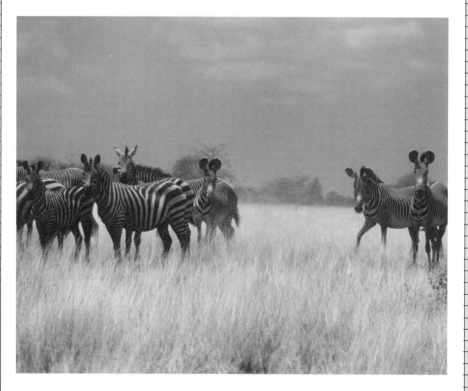

A mixed herd of Grevy's and Burchell's zebra in the Isiolo Triangle.

SINCE MOVING TO CANADA, we've made several trips back to Kenya to see old friends and favourite places. During the most recent, in 1998, we saw that the land we knew had undergone many changes.

Many of our Meru friends had prospered. Even by 1970, a strong middle class had grown up, and would continue to do so. These people owned land and healthy cattle. Kipsiele and Mutua were two examples. By 1998, Lily Mwenda and several others who had worked with Jo in the Meru hospital had also become independent business people, running their own clinics. Their children had good jobs, or were overseas at university.

There were also many friends left in the Nanyuki area. Some who had been parents were now grandparents, but otherwise they had changed little. Nanyuki itself had more than doubled in size, but its roads were a nightmare. On the other hand, the road to Chuka, once famous for its many hairpin bends, had been straightened and tarred — a huge job which had started near the end of our time in Meru.

By 1998 Paul Sayer's sandy hair had turned to an elegant white, but his slim frame showed not the slightest trace of middle-aged spread. He had dealt with the loss of his wife, our dear friend Elma, to the scourge of cancer. He had not so much "got over" her loss but, as all who lose a loved one must, in order to continue, he had come to terms with it, overcome his despair, and soldiered on.

Shortly after we moved to Canada, Paul had found Mutua a post at the small animal clinic at Kabete. Mutua also helped out at the Mombasa quarantine. Paul and I later funded him for a year at a technical school in England, where he did extraordinarily well as the only foreigner among a group of local young men. He also developed special skills in dog handling. Back in Kenya, however, the collapse of the infrastructure, and the well-publicized government corruption, hurt him and his family. When we saw him in 1998, he was frustrated by the fact that he had not been paid a cent for the last few coffee crops he and his wife had produced. With half a dozen children, including two in high school, the missing income was making life awkward, but he was battling on, just like so many of his countrymen.

Lunatic Lane has undergone a name change, which comes as no surprise. It is now Simba Lane, which may reflect the presence of lions many years ago, but hardly fits the current situation. Estimates vary, but we were told that about 10,000 squatters occupy a shanty town between the rutted murram road and the Liki river a hundred yards to its north. When we were last there, all water for the settlement was hauled from the river, which also acted as the local drainage for all waste material. Even if there were any trout a mile downstream by the back gate of what was our home for almost five years, I doubt that they'd be fit to eat.

Many government programs appear to have collapsed. The Kenya Meat Commission is long gone. And the cattle artificial insemination scheme in Meru, which I had a role in developing, has folded. Kipsiele's prediction of this failure, made in 1969, had come true. Cattle numbers were way down; the beautiful Guernsey cattle, once the mainstay of so many small farms, had become scarce as dipping programs had fallen apart. We looked up David Mbuko, who had been one of the dozen or so members of the *piki-piki*-riding AI team. David was doing AI on a free-lance basis, and told me that he was one of only three people so engaged. There simply wasn't enough work for more, and he did not get called every day.

■

Some very serious problems now plague Kenya. There are masses of dispossessed people in its cities; population growth rates peaked in the eighties. AIDS has done more than rear its ugly head, it has eaten at the heart and soul of the country, much as it has in many parts of Africa. At the entrance to every town there are now huge billboards warning people about the disease and urging safe sex.

The media have made a meal of other problems, such as lawlessness and corruption.

Wildlife numbers continued to decline, which is nothing new. Wildlife numbers had begun to dwindle long before African governments took over, and the great pandemics of the late 19th century decimated animal populations and the people that herded or hunted them. Rinderpest took out a huge proportion of the hoofstock, and distemper is reported to have killed masses of carnivores. (Very recently this deadly disease of the dog family extended its target, and killed as many as one-third of the lions in the Serengeti.) Smallpox and measles devastated the human population.

With vast areas of grazing, the wildlife numbers rebounded somewhat. Teeming millions of wildebeest, zebra, and other antelopes roamed the plains. Elspeth Huxley, in her book *Out in the Midday Sun*, described a scene she saw when traveling up from Mombasa by train, before the First World War. At dawn, she writes, "the white dome of Kilimanjaro seemed to hover in the western sky. But it was the animals that brought life and wonder to the scene. Thousands, tens of thousands of them could be seen from the carriage window. . . ."

But what the wildlife could not deal with was human competition.

By the time Huxley returned to Kenya in 1933, she saw changes. Outside the game reserves, "[the game] were already being harried in places and 'shot out,' not by sportsmen, whose bags were strictly limited by licence, but by farmers, black and white."

These animals lived in areas where humans wanted to settle and farm, so their fate was sealed. The wildebeest of the Mara and Serengeti were probably saved by the tsetse flies, which made ranching an unprofitable business well before the wildlife parks there were gazetted.

In the years since my stint in Kenya, the rhino has been the most highly publicized victim of the various effects of poaching and human population growth in Africa, but others have taken a similar hit.

One small microcosm illustrates this decline. The Isiolo Triangle, a tiny patch of waving grass, no more than about six kilometres along any of its sides, used to hold a wide variety of species when I first traveled along the gravel road that formed one of its borders in 1965. One could be absolutely certain of seeing herds of wildlife there: eland, impala, Grant's gazelle, reticulated giraffe, and even lions. On one occasion I saw the unusual sight of a mixed herd of Grevy's and Burchell's zebra with their contrasting narrow and broad stripes, and the large mule-like ears of the Grevy's. By 1970 most were gone, and by 1975 none remained. Instead the grassland was dotted with small houses, some with corrugated iron roofs. A wide tarmac road had been cut along the edge of the area in 1971, and in a few spots landowners had tried to plough the land and even cultivate some ground, with absolutely no success. The climate was simply too dry. In 1998, when we visited the area, many of these houses were unoccupied.

On a more upbeat note, there are now at least five private game parks in the Mount Kenya area. They are home to a variety of wild animals which include rhinos and elephants, and several species of hoofed stock behind high fences. They have been developed on land that once carried cattle, was owned by former clients, and from which game species were actively discouraged. Three of them are open to tourists and one, which borders the old Triangle, is run in close collaboration with a neighbouring operation owned by Samburu people.

Meanwhile, the current state of the so-called "human-elephant conflict" is not much different from what it was in Rwanda in 1975, but it has become more widespread. All over Africa, elephants are reported to be creating problems for people (or should that be the other way round?). A set of 13 articles published in *The East African Standard* in the first week of October 2001 highlight the situation; emotional headlines shout "Jumbos killed my husband, says distraught mother of ten" and "Elephants send farmers on leave in Laikipia."

According to *The Standard*, "From January 1989 to June 1994, wild animals in Kenya killed 230 people and injured 218, which is an average of 42 deaths and 40 injuries per year. Elephants perpetrated 173 of these attacks." The accuracy of numbers like these is difficult to determine, but even one person's death is a disaster for that family.

Richard Hoare, a member of the International Union for the Conservation of Nature's African Elephant Specialist Group, has written, "The realities of survival faced by rural Africans mean that little attention will be paid to the debate on conservation philosophy in the developed world."

While a farmer in Canada or the U.S.A. may see damage to a hay crop from marauding elk, or the loss of a few sheep to wolves, as a major nuisance, the loss of an entire year's crop of maize, intended to feed that family of ten and perhaps bring in some cash, is more than a nuisance. Not many ranchers or farmers in North America or Western Europe are killed by wild animals. For the African small holder facing nightly raids, the elephant may rightly be thought of as a predator. It is not just in Africa that such raids occur. In Indonesia, exactly the same challenges face elephant conservationists and villagers.

Another item in *The Standard* quotes the Kenya Wildlife Service's list of "Causes of human-wildlife conflict." The first four in the list of 29 are:

1. Loss and damage of agricultural crops.
2. Damage of forest plantation trees and seedlings.
3. Human beings killed or injured by wild animals.
4. Loss of livestock killed by wild animals.

The problem of human-wildlife conflict is massive and widespread; elephants are simply the largest and most obvious examples. People take notice of elephants, and become emotional about them, because they are truly "charismatic megafauna." But ever-increasing human populations are having an equally serious impact on much smaller and less visible species.

But these problems are hardly unique to Kenya, or even to Africa. In the words of David Quammen, "All over the planet humans are at war with wildlife." Birds, plants, insects, even the tiny microorganisms that make up the soil matrix are being affected by what we do. After over a hundred years of cultivation the prairies, where I now live, is one of the most radically altered environments on earth. Cultivation, the introduction of exotic crops (exotic to North America), chemical fertilizers, and lately the development of genetically modified plants, have wrought irretrievable changes.

In Europe, the giant Irish elk, with an antler spread of up to four metres, was hunted to extinction centuries ago. Then during the middle ages, carnivores were actively extirpated from the British Isles; bounties were places on some species because they killed livestock. Later, in North America, the passenger pigeon disappeared due to rapacious market hunting, and because the trees in which they nested in huge colonies were logged out. The superimposition of some deadly pandemic on an already stressed population may have been a factor as well. The North American bison, variously estimated to have numbered from 30 to 60 million in the early 1800s, had long been hunted by many indigenous peoples for food, shelter, and clothing. Then European settlers arrived, and wanted the bisons' grazing land for their own cattle and sheep. It has been well documented that some United States government officials actively encouraged the slaughter of millions of bison in order to deprive the Plains Indians of their traditional and fundamental means of support. Bounties were paid for tongues, and carcasses were left to rot. Bison bones, shipped by the ton, ended up in fine china in England. The animal was soon virtually extinct.

Despite all its troubles, the Kenya we visited in 1998 was far from bleak. One of the most memorable events of that visit was our trip to the Christmas pantomime with Paul and his delightful new partner Olwen.

In a traditional British pantomime, fairytales like *Cinderella, Jack and the Beanstalk,* or *Puss in Boots* are set to music, and interwoven with lame jokes, topical satire, and plenty of slapstick. The principal boy is usually a pretty girl with the minimum of clothing allowable for a family show, and there is always a villain, and a "mother-in-law" figure played by a man, preferably an ugly man.

The Nairobi panto that year was titled "Aladdin and His Magic Lamp." Every single player was a dark-skinned native Kenyan. The cast were obviously drawn from several different tribal groups. It was easy to recognize the aquiline features of a girl with a Somali background, and the part of the obligatory granddam — in this case the "Widow Twanky" — was played by the brilliant Kikuyu Ian Mbugua. He's a good six feet, and skinny. The director had cleverly costumed him in a dress that only came down to mid-shin, which showed off his spider-thin legs to great advantage and much laughter.

During the show, which was very loosely derived from the children's classic, the actors sang songs from many sources. Somehow there was a troupe of policemen, and every time that they appeared on stage (naturally singing pieces from *The Pirates of Penzance*) they promptly hit someone over the head with a convincing-looking stage truncheon or stole a wallet or two from a back pocket. It did not take a genius to deduce that there might be some level of dissatisfaction with the national police force. The appalling, car-swallowing state of Nairobi's roads and their potholes and the lack of attention to the pervasive heaps of rotting garbage in every suburb were mercilessly lambasted. The school system was targeted with a version of Tom Lehrer's satirical song, "New Math": "In the new approach the important thing is to understand what you're doing rather than to get the right answer." Just about anything and everything that was deemed wrong with the state of the country seemed to be fair game. There were, however, no overtly obvious jokes about the president.

The audience joined in as prompted. Every time the wicked landlord appeared on stage there were boos and hisses, and when Aladdin (played non-traditionally by a very funny comedic actor, Charles Kiari) appeared with his girl, the audience sighed with mock love. The jokes and skits flew so fast and furious that the very mixed audience (European, local Asian, African, and even an East Asian couple) hardly had time to get over their laughter from one before they were on to the next.

We left with our sides aching, and have often since reflected that only a mature society would be able to poke such fun at itself and its institutions and icons. There are other parts of the world in which such irreverence would most likely lead to severe consequences for all involved.

We will surely visit Kenya again, having already fulfilled the old Swahili proverb with which Elspeth Huxley concluded the second volume of her autobiography:

"He who has tasted honey will return to the honeypot."

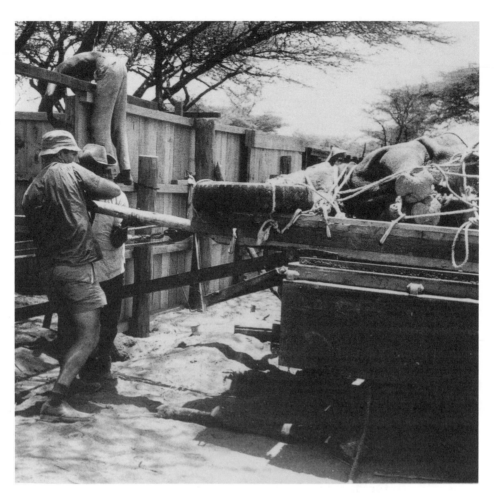

It is not real work unless you would rather be doing something else.
— Sir James Barrie.
Rectorial address, May 3, 1922, St. Andrew's University, Scotland

SWAHILI PRIMER

Technically, I should have used the term Kiswahili, which refers to language, rather than merely Swahili, which refers to an ethnic group, throughout, but the shorter term is in common use for the language, and both books that I used as sources use the latter term.

I have used two small books as the source for most of the terms listed below. The first is my mother's 1964 edition of Le Breton's 1936 *Up-Country Swahili*, the second is Steere's 1938 *Swahili Exercises*, which my father used as his source for exams he had to pass in order to attain promotion. This is the Swahili that I learned and used between 1965 and 1975. It does not entirely reflect the Swahili spoken today (what language has not evolved in 25 years?) Furthermore the widespread improvement in Swahili around the countryside today can probably be ascribed to its use on the radio, where virtually everyone can now hear it.

The Steere has a revealing first page titled "Pronunciation," which is worth quoting:

"Swahili is an easy language because there is no new alphabet to learn, and because the rules are fairly simple and exceptions hardly exist.

The **consonants** are pronounced as in English, but *q* and *x* are not wanted, *c* only occurs in *ch*, *g* is always hard as in *go*, and *y* is always a consonant as in the English word *yet*.

The **vowels** must *on no account* be pronounced as in English; it is usual to say that the vowels are Italian, but this does not help you much unless you know an Italian vowel when you hear one! When in doubt make the vowel as full and rich as you like, and remember that there are no diphthongs. Bad pronunciation comes most often from speaking with short clipped vowels, and this is both ugly and unintelligible. The following five English words give pretty nearly the sounds of the five Swahili vowels **a e i o u**.

far   fail   feel   foal   fool

When the vowels are short they are pronounced much as in

pat   pet   pit   pot   put

Bata, a *duck*, does not rhyme with either *hater*, *hatter* or *water*, but it does sound very much like *barter*.

Like most languages there are degrees of regional difference. The purest forms are spoken by the coastal peoples of Kenya and Tanzania, and these varieties have specific terms that are not used elsewhere. In general, as one goes east into central Africa the language becomes simpler, often losing prefixes, suffixes, and tense. The counting cadence in Rwanda bears only faint resemblance to the Arabic of 20, 30, 40, and so on as used throughout Kenya. The word for "butter" used in Kenya is *siagi*, which according to Colin Clarkson of Cambridge University derives from one of two possible Arabic words. Either "siyagh" in the sense of "to soak bread, & c, in fat, & c" or "siraj" meaning "melted butter" or sesame oil.

In Rwanda butter is *manteka*, which is a direct transcript from Portuguese. I can only speculate the source of this change. There was a long-time Portuguese colonial presence in Angola, 2,000 odd kilometres to the south-west. There was also a strong Portuguese presence on the Kenya coast, where Fort Jesus in Mombasa was named. Did *manteka* come from travelers heading north-east in the form of slave traders, ivory gatherers or missionaries, or maybe all three rolled into one, or did it move west? Mombasa is only 1,000 kilometres away, even if you have to go around Lake Victoria. My bet would go here.

Kiswahili

Asante	thank you
Askari	guard, policeman, soldier
Banda	large shed, thatched house
Barazza	meeting, an official assembly
Boma	fenced enclosure, corral (also an adminstrative centre, although this meaning had largely been dropped by 1965)
Bui-bui	black covering worn by Muslim women. Equivalent to the chadoor
Chai	tea
Chakula	food, a meal
Choma (ku)	to burn, scorch, scald
Daktari	doctor, veterinary officer (the latter usually qualified by the addition of "ya ngombe" = of cow)
Dawa	medicine

Enda (ku)	to go
Fanya (ku)	to do
Gani?	what (as in habari gani, what news?), which?
Habari	news, information
Hamjambo	Hello, plural, said to more than one person
Hapana	there is not. Often used to mean "no" "none" "not," especially in "up-country Swahili"
Heshima	prestige, pride, face, dignity
Hodi	May I come in?
Ine	four
Jambo	universally understood greeting. Equivalent to hello.
Kali	multi-use, depending upon context. UCS lists fierce, sharp, cross, acid, strict, savage. Others include, spicy and angry.
Kamba	rope, also cord, rawhide thong.
Karai	metal bowl (wok-shaped, about 18"–2' in diameter)
Kidole	finger, toe (plural is vidole)
Kikoi	cotton garment worn around the waist by males. Used at any time of day, especially at the coast. Similar to a sarong. Originally (1940, UCS) a white cloth with coloured border.
Ku-	used as the infinitive in front of verbs: i.e. to go
Kuenda	to go
Kufanya	to do
Kusema	to say
Kumbe	Wow!
Lugga*	water-course, usually dry, often in desert regions
Mabati	corrugated iron sheeting, often refers to a roof
Manyatta	group of family dwellings, often enclosed by a thorn barricade. Originally used for Masai homesteads only.
Maridadi	smart, pretty

Matatu★	taxi
Mawingu★	cloud
Memsahib or	
Memsaab	Hindi term for a European woman
Mia	a hundred
Mimi	I, as in "Mimi nafanya," I am doing
Mira'a★	tree growing in parts of Meru that produced twigs chewed by many people in East Africa. Also known as Quatt, or Khatt. Contains an amphetamine-like substance.
Mkono	hand, arm
Mkubwa	large, great, important, the eldest, big
Moja	one
Moto	hot, fire
Munanda★	cattle crush
Mungo	God
Mzungu	European (plural is wazungu). Also any white person; for instance, an American or Canadian.
Na	and, also, by, with
Nasema	I say — often used with the word "mimi" (I) in front of it. Personal form of verb Ku-sema.
Ndio	yes, it is so
Ndume	bull, a male animal
Nguo	clothes
Nyama	animals, meat, flesh
Panga	sword, large chopping knife (machete)
Piki-Piki	motorized bike, ranging from a 50-cc motorized peddle bike to a powerful machine like a BSA 650 or a Harley
Pole-Pole	slow, gentle
Pombe	beer (UCS gives only "native beer")

Rondavel★	single room building with (normally) a circular footprint
Safi	clean, pure (smart, polished, high quality)
Sana	very, much (it intensifies any word)
Sema (ku)	to say
Serikali	the government, the law
Shamba	farm, cultivated land, garden
Shauri	a matter, business, negotiation, affair, dispute
Shenzi	barbarous, uncivilized, unrefined, make-shift (also of poor quality). Often used in a very derogatory sense, even as a noun.
Shifta★	bandits, usually of Somali extraction, operating in the NFD
Sumu	poison
Syce★	groom
Tano	five
Tinka–Tinka	power driven machinery. By 1965 had become more specific to a diesel engine (sound it out by repeating the words several times)
Tyari★	ready
Ugali	porridge, mush meal made from maize. A staple diet item.
Ulaya	England, Europe
Nguo	clothes
Vidole	fingers (singular is kidole)
Wazungu	plural form of mzungu — European
Weka (Ku)	place, put away, put down
Ya	of
Yako, lako	your (depends upon context of pronoun)

★do not appear in either of the source books but are in common usage

Kimeru terms in common use

Ale	(or Are, the "L" and "r" are pronounced interchangably. This one sounds like an r to English speakers. It means "no."
Katheroko	native beer
Muga	Hello
Muno	very (when used with muga, it implies superlative, as in "very many hellos.") Like the Swahili *sana* it emphasizes any word.
Muthee	Old man — equivalent to Swahili mzee
Mwekuru	Old woman — similar term of respect to Muthee

My very limited Kipsigis

Ajamage	Hello
Mising	very. Used with ajamge or sai seri, to indicate extra emphasis. Emphasizes any word.
Sai seri	Goodbye
Weri	chum, friend

FURTHER READING

The Peoples of Kenya. Joy Adamson. 1967. Collins and Harvill Press. London.

Facing Mount Kenya: The tribal life of the Gikuyu. Jomo Kenyatta. Vintage Books. Random House. 1962.

The Great Safari: The Lives of George and Joy Adamson. Adrian House. William Morrow and Company Inc. New York. 1993.

White Man's Country. Lord Delamere and the Making of Kenya. Elspeth Huxley. Chatto and Windus. London. 1935.

Out in the Midday Sun: My Kenya. Elspeth Huxley. Chatto and Windus. 1985. Penguin Books. 1987

The Flame Trees of Thika. Elspeth Huxley. Chatto and Windus. 1959. Penguin Books. 1962.

The Mottled Lizard. Elspeth Huxley. Chatto and Windus 1962. Penguin Books 1981.

Nine Faces of Kenya: An Anthology. Elspeth Huxley. Collins Harvill. 1990. Harvill. 1991.

The Man Eaters of Tsavo and Other Adventures. J. H. Patterson. The Macmillan Company. 1927.

The Iron Snake. Ronald Hardy. Collins. London. 1965.

The Lunatic Express: An Entertainment in Imperialism. Charles Miller. The Macmillan Company. 1971.

Battle for the Bundu; The First World War in East Africa. Charles Miller. Macmillan Publishing Co. Ltd. 1974.

West with the Night. Beryl Markham. Houghton Mifflin Co. 1942, and North Point Press. San Francisco 1983.

No Man's Land: The Last of White Africa. John Heminway. E.P. Dutton Inc. 1983.

No Picnic on Mount Kenya. Felice Benuzzi. Dutton. 1953. Peregrine Smith Book. Layton, Utah. 1989.

Bwana Game: The Life Story of George Adamson. Collins and Harvill Press. London. 1968.

My Pride and Joy: An Autobiography. George Adamson. Collins Harvill, London. 1986.

The Spotted Sphinx. Joy Adamson. A Helen and Kurt Wolf Book. Harcourt Brace & World Inc. New York. 1969.

A Love Affair with the Sun. Michael Blundell. Kenway Publications Ltd. Nairobi. 1994.

Karen Blixen: Out of Africa. (First published 1937, Putnam, London.) My copy. Penguin Books. 1954.

Mau Mau: An African Crucible. Robert Edgerton. The Free Press. A Division of Macmillan Inc. New York. 1989.

Africa: Despatches from a Fragile Continent. Blaine Harden. HarperCollins. 1990.

White Mischief: The Murder of Lord Errol. James Fox. Random House. New York. 1982.

Silence Will Speak. Errol Trzebinski. William Heinemann. 1977. Grafton Books. 1985.

The Desert's Dusty Face. Charles Chevenix Trench. William Blackwood & Sons Ltd. London. 1964.

Ivory Crisis. Ian Parker & Mohamed Amin. Chatto & Windus Ltd. London. 1983.

The Song of the Dodo: Island Biogeography in an Age of Extinctions. David Quammen. Touchstone Books, Simon & Schuster. 1996.

Run Rhino Run. Esmond and Chryssee Bradley Martin. Chatto and Windus. London. 1982.

Up-Country Swahili Exercises: for the soldier, settler, miner, merchant and their wives. And for all who deal with up-country natives without interpreters. F. H. Le Breton. Printed by R. W. Simpson & Co Ltd. (1st edition October, 1936, enlarged March 1940. 15th edition, July 1964.)

Swahili Exercises. Edward Steere. The Sheldon Press. London. 1938.